FERTILIZATION AND EMBRYONIC DEVELOPMENT
IN VITRO

FERTILIZATION AND EMBRYONIC DEVELOPMENT
IN VITRO

Edited by

Luigi Mastroianni, Jr.
University of Pennsylvania
Philadelphia, Pennsylvania

and

John D. Biggers
Harvard Medical School
Boston, Massachusetts

PLENUM PRESS • NEW YORK AND LONDON

Library of Congress Cataloging in Publication Data

Main entry under title:

Fertilization and embryonic development in vitro.

  Bibliography: p.
  Includes index.
  1. Fertilization in vitro. 2. Embryology, Experimental. I. Mastroianni, Luigi. II.
Biggers, John D., 1923-   . [DNLM: I. Fertilization in vitro. 2. Embryo transfer.
3. Embryo. 4. Embryo, Non-mammalian. WQ 205 F411]
QP273.F47   599.03'3   81-13829
ISBN 0-306-40783-3   AACR2

CONTRIBUTORS

D. H. BARRON Department of Obstetrics and Gynecology, University of Florida, Gainesville, Florida 32611

BARRY D. BAVISTER Wisconsin Regional Primate Research Center, Madison, Wisconsin 53706

FULLER W. BAZER Department of Animal Science, University of Florida, Gainesville, Florida 32611

DALE JOHN BENOS Department of Physiology and Biophysics, Laboratory of Human Reproduction and Reproductive Biology, Harvard Medical School, Boston, Massachusetts 02115

JOHN D. BIGGERS Department of Physiology and Biophysics, Laboratory of Human Reproduction and Reproductive Biology, Harvard Medical School, Boston, Massachusetts 02115

BENJAMIN G. BRACKETT Department of Clinical Studies–New Bolton Center, University of Pennsylvania School of Veterinary Medicine, Kennett Square, Pennsylvania 19348, and Department of Obstetrics and Gynecology, University of Pennsylvania School of Medicine, Philadelphia, Pennsylvania 19104

LUDEMAN A. ENG Department of Anatomy, University of Virginia School of Medicine, Charlottesville, Virginia 22908

CHARLES J. EPSTEIN Departments of Pediatrics and of Biochemistry and Biophysics, University of California, San Francisco, California 94143

v

MITCHELL S. GOLBUS   Departments of Obstetrics, Gynecology, and Reproductive Sciences and of Pediatrics, University of California Medical Center, San Francisco, California 94143

M. H. GOLDSTEIN   Department of Physiology, University of Florida, Gainesville, Florida 32611

GARY D. HODGEN   Pregnancy Research Branch, National Institute of Child Health and Human Development, National Institutes of Health, Bethesda, Maryland 20205

OLIVIER KREITMANN   Pregnancy Research Branch, National Institute of Child Health and Human Development, National Institutes of Health, Bethesda, Maryland 20205

ALINA C. LOPO   Department of Anatomy, University of California Medical Center, San Francisco, California 94143

LUIGI MASTROIANNI, Jr.   Department of Obstetrics and Gynecology, University of Pennsylvania School of Medicine, Philadelphia, Pennsylvania 19104

WILBERT E. NIXON   Pregnancy Research Branch, National Institute of Child Health and Human Development, National Institutes of Health, Bethesda, Maryland 20205

GENE OLIPHANT   Department of Anatomy, University of Virginia School of Medicine, Charlottesville, Virginia 22908

G. E. SEIDEL, Jr.   Animal Reproduction Laboratory, Colorado State University, Fort Collins, Colorado 80523

BENNETT M. SHAPIRO   Department of Biochemistry, University of Washington, Seattle, Washington 98195

VICTOR D. VACQUIER   Marine Biology Research Division, Scripps Institution of Oceanography, University of California, San Diego, La Jolla, California 92093

DON P. WOLF   Division of Reproductive Biology, Departments of Obstetrics and Gynecology, and Biochemistry and Biophysics, University of Pennsylvania School of Medicine, Philadelphia, Pennsylvania 19104

R. YANAGIMACHI   Department of Anatomy and Reproductive Biology, University of Hawaii School of Medicine, Honolulu, Hawaii 96822

CONTENTS

Chapter 7

GAMETE INTERACTION IN THE SEA URCHIN
A Model for Understanding the Molecular Details of Animal Fertilization
Alina C. Lopo and Victor D. Vacquier

Chapter 8

AWAKENING OF THE INVERTEBRATE EGG AT FERTILIZATION
Bennett M. Shapiro

Chapter 9

CHROMOSOME ABERRATIONS AND MAMMALIAN REPRODUCTION
Mitchell S. Golbus

Chapter 10

THE EFFECTS OF CHROMOSOMAL ANEUPLOIDY ON EARLY DEVELOPMENT
Experimental Approaches
Charles J. Epstein

Chapter 11

BLASTOCYST FLUID FORMATION
Dale John Benos and John D. Biggers

Chapter 12

WATER AND ELECTROLYTE TRANSPORT BY PIG CHORIOALLANTOIS
Fuller W. Bazer, M. H. Goldstein, and D. H. Barron

Chapter 13
CRITICAL REVIEW OF EMBRYO TRANSFER PROCEDURES WITH CATTLE
G. E. Seidel, Jr.

EPILOGUE
Luigi Mastroianni, Jr.

INDEX

PROLOGUE

JOHN D. BIGGERS

By 1882 enough was known about the preimplantation developmental stages of mammals that a laboratory course was offered to students at the University of Cambridge in which they recovered and examined these stages from rabbits. The course was part of a larger embryology class given by the brilliant young biologist Francis Maitland Balfour. Balfour's research concerned the embryology of the chick, elasmobranchs, and the invertebrate *Peripatus*. In 1879 Walter Heape, at the age of 25, abandoned a business vocation and joined Balfour's laboratory. A distinguished career followed, for Heape was destined to discover the estrous cycle, perform the first transfer of a mammalian embryo from one female to another, describe the uterine changes in primates during the menstrual cycle, and discover nonspontaneous ovulation.

Balfour set Heape to work on the developmental changes in the 5- to 7-day-old rabbit blastocyst (Balfour, 1880). The work was stimulated by different interpretations of development during this period by Van Beneden on the one hand and Kölliker, Rauber, and Lieberkühn independently on the other. Although they did not resolve the problem, Heape became experienced in handling preimplantation mammalian embryos. Tragedy was soon to strike the laboratory, however, for in 1882 Balfour, at the age of 32, lost his life while climbing in the Swiss Alps. At the time of his death Balfour was writing the second edition of his book with Michael Foster, *The Elements of Embryology*. The work was only half done but it was completed by Balfour's main associate and successor Adam Sedgwick, and Walter Heape. The book finally appeared

JOHN D. BIGGERS • Department of Physiology and Biophysics, Laboratory of Human Reproduction and Reproductive Biology, Harvard Medical School, Boston, Massachusetts 02115.

1

in 1883 (Foster and Balfour, 1883). At the end of the book (p. 460) is a section—which I suspect was written by Heape, for Sedgwick never worked on mammals—that describes the laboratory course. The section dealing with preimplantation development reads:

PRACTICAL DIRECTIONS FOR OBTAINING AND STUDYING
MAMMALIAN EMBRYOS.

XI. Animals and breeding.

For class work the Rabbit is the most convenient animal from which to obtain embryos, it will breed freely in the early spring months of the year and will give ample opportunity for the student to observe the exact time when the female is covered. A number of does should be kept together in a large pen, and two or three bucks in separate small cages also placed within the pen; at the period of heat, the doe should be temporarily placed with the buck and the exact time of copulation noted, the age of the embryo being calculated from that hour.

XII. Examination of segmenting ova.

It will be well to mention here that although a doe may have been satisfactorily covered, embryos are not always obtained from her. A superficial examination of the ovaries will determine whether or no fertilized ova are present. If ova have been recently dehisced from the ovary, the Graafian follicles from which they were discharged will be found to be of a distinctly red colour. In case no such "corpora lutea" as they are called are present further search is useless.

A. *To obtain ova from 1 to 60 hours old.*

Cut open the abdomen from pubis to sternum, and from the pubis round the thigh of each side, and turn back the flaps of the body wall so formed. Remove the viscera and observe below (dorsal) the single median vagina, from the anterior end of which the uterine horns diverge.

Observe at the anterior end of each uterine horn a small much coiled tube, the oviduct (Fallopian tube) near the anterior end of which a little below the kidney lies the ovary. Cut out the uterus and oviduct together and lay them in a small dissecting dish. Carefully stretch out the oviduct by cutting the tissue which binds it, and separating it from the uterus, taking care to obtain its whole length, lay it upon a glass slide.

With the aid of a lens it is frequently possible to distinguish the ovum or ova, through the wall of the oviduct. In this case cut a transverse slit into the lumen of the duct with a fine pair of scissors a little to one side of an ovum; press with a needle upon the oviduct or the other side of the ovum, which will glide out through the slit, and can be with ease transported upon the point of a small scalpel, or what is better spear-headed needle. In case the ovum cannot be distinguished in the oviduct by superficial observation, the latter must be slit up with a fine pair of scissors, when it will easily be seen with the aid of an ordinary dissecting lens.

B. *Treatment of the ovum.*

The ovum may be examined fresh in salt solution, it is however more instructive when preserved and stained in the following manner.

a. Immerse it in a 1/5 p.c. solution of osmic acid for 5 or even 10 minutes, transfer it thence to the picro-carmine solution described above (I). After staining the ovum should then be washed in distilled water and placed in a weak solution of glycerine in a watchglass—half glycerine, half water. It should be allowed to remain thus under a bell jar for several days (7 to 14 or longer) in a warm room until the water has evaporated. By this means shrinkage and distortion are avoided, the glycerine becoming very gradually more and more dense. It should be mounted in glycerine in which 1 p.c. formic acid has been mixed to prevent fungoid growths. Care must be taken that there is no pressure upon the ovum this being insured by the insertion of a couple of slips of paper one on each side of the ovum under the cover glass.

b. Another method of preservation is used, but does not appear to us so successful as the one already described. It consists of an immersion of the ovum for 5 minutes in 1/5 to 1/2 p.c. osmic acid, subsequent treatment with Müller's fluid for two or three days, and finally mounting in glycerine.

C. *Examination of the ovum.*

The most instructive stages to observe are ova of

a. 18 hours old, when four segmentation spheres will be observed.
b. 36 hours old, when segmentation is more advanced and the spheres numerous.

The chief points to be noted are:—

1. The number and size of the segmentation spheres; in each of which, when treated as described in B.*a.*, a large deeply stained nucleus will be visible. The spheres themselves are also stained slightly.
2. The presence of one of two polar bodies on the outer side of the segments in ova of not more than 48 hours old: these also are slightly stained.
3. The zona radiata immediately surrounding the segments, and
4. The thick albuminous coat, marked with concentric rings.

D. *The fully segmented ovum. 70 hours old.*

The fully segmented ovum is found in the uterus at its anterior end close to the place where the oviduct opens into the uterus.

To obtain this stage the uterus must be slit open and examined carefully with a dissecting lens: the ovum will be seen as a somewhat opaque spot on the glistening moist mucous epithelium of the uterus.

It may be treated in the manner described under B.*a*., but the segments being closely pressed together their outlines are not rendered distinct by this method. A more advantageous mode of treatment is the following: wash the ovum rapidly in distilled water, and place it in a 1 p.c. solution of silver nitrate for about 3 minutes: then expose it to the light in a dish of distilled water until it be tinged a brown colour.

The brown colour is due to the reduction of the silver, which takes place chiefly in the cement substance between the cells and thus defines very exactly their size and shape. The ovum may now be treated with glycerine and mounted as described in B.

The points to be observed are:—

1. The division of the segmentation spheres into the layers—an outer layer of cubical hyaline cells, and an inner of rounded granular cells.
2. The blastopore of van Beneden.
3. The presence of a thin layer of mucous outside the concentrically ringed albuminous coat of the ovum.

XIII. Examination of the blastodermic vesicle, 72–90 hours.
    A. *To obtain the embryo see* XII.D.
    B. *Prepare the ovum either as in* XII.B. or D.
        or in picric acid see I.B.1.
    C. *Surface view, or in section see* I.B.3.

Observe:—

1. The great increase in size of the ovum and the reduction in the thickness of the membranes.
2. The flattened layer of outer cells enclosing a cavity.
3. The rounded cells of the inner mass attached as a lens-shaped mass to one side of the vesicle.

Walter Heape resigned his Demonstratorship at Cambridge in 1885 and became Superintendent of the Laboratory at Plymouth that was being constructed by the Marine Biological Association. In 1890 he was awarded a Balfour Studentship—a program founded in honor of his mentor—and, with a grant from the Royal Society of London, traveled to India to work in the Zoological Gardens in Calcutta with the expressed purpose of studying the early development of primates. His mission was doomed, however, for he soon found that it was very difficult to recover preimplantation embryos from monkeys, and after four months he contracted a disease that forced him to return to England. Nevertheless, he collected sufficient material from two species of monkey, *Macacus rhesus* and *Semnopithecus entellus*, to enable him to describe the uterine changes in the menstrual cycle (Heape, 1894, 1897a). Later he extended this work to women (Heape, 1898).

Early in 1890 Heape, with the assistance of a surgeon, Mr. Samuel Buckley, performed the first transfer of embryos between mothers. He states his reason for the experiment as follows (Heape, 1890):

> The experiment . . . was undertaken to determine in the first place what effect, if any, a uterine foster-mother would have upon her foster children, and whether or not the presence and development of foreign ova in the uterus of a mother would affect the offspring of that mother born at the same time.

To test these ideas the following experiment was done:

> On the 27th April, 1890, two ova were obtained from an Angora doe rabbit which had been fertilized by an Angora buck thirty-two hours previously; the ova were undergoing segmentation, being divided into four segments. The ova were immediately transferred into the upper end of the fallopian tube of a Belgian hare doe rabbit which had been fertilized three hours before by a buck of the same breed as herself . . . .
>
> In due course this Belgian hare doe gave birth to six young—four of these resembled herself and her mate, while two of them were undoubted Angoras. The Angora young were characterized by the possession of long silky hair peculiar to the breed, and were total albinoes, like their Angora parents.

The experiment is of further interest since it anticipated the use of genetic markers used in more recent work.

Heape, however, was not entirely successful with this technique, for in subsequent years he had several failures and only repeated it once (Heape, 1897b). Unfortunately Heape gives no details of how the embryos were collected and transferred. If physiological saline was used it is very unlikely it would have the appropriate osmolality since the work was done before the first physiological saline for mammalian tissues was introduced (Locke, 1901).

Between 1933 and 1951 successful embryo transfers were done in other species (Table I). The reasons for the work varied. The studies of Nicholas (1933) on the rat were done for basic embryological research. The transfer of mouse embryos was done in studies of breast cancer in mice. Little transferred fertilized ova from *dba* mice, which suffer from a high incidence of breast cancer into the oviducts of CS7 mice, which have a low incidence of the disease. The *dba* offspring lived many months and none developed tumors. By

Table I
First Reported Transfers of Preimplantation
Embryos between Females in
Different Species

Species	Reference
Rabbit	Heape (1890)
Rat	Nicholas (1933)
Sheep	Warwick et al. (1934)[a]
Goat	Warwick et al. (1934)[a]
Mouse	Little (1935)[b]
Cow	Willett et al. (1951)
Pig	Kvasnickii (1951)[a]

[a]Quoted by Austin (1961).
[b]Quoted by Bittner and Little (1937).

this time the value of embryo transfer in the livestock industry was recognized for the study of infertility (Willett et al., 1951), for the shortening of the generation interval to accelerate the improvement of livestock by selective breeding (Adams, 1954), and, in the words of McLaren and Michie (1956), "to multiply the genetic contribution to the breed made by outstanding females, just as artificial insemination can be used to propagate the good qualities of outstanding males."

The fundamental understanding that fertilization involves the union of the nuclei of one sperm and one ovum was discovered by the efforts of several investigators using sea urchins, starfish, rabbits, and bats between the years 1875 and 1880 (see Austin, 1961, for a review). Attempts to fertilize rabbit and guinea pig ova *in vitro* were made during this period by Schenk (1878). He incubated follicular oocytes with undiluted epididymal spermatozoa in the presence of a fragment of uterine mucosa. His experiments, unfortunately, were not successful. Many investigators tried to fertilize mammalian eggs *in vitro* over the next 80 years and several claims of success were made. The field became very controversial because of the difficulty of proving that the sperm had entered the ovum. A detailed critical review of the work is given by Austin (1961). Final unequivocal proof of successful *in vitro* fertilization was obtained by Chang (1959) using rabbits and the technique of genetic markers.

Brachet (1912) appears to be the first investigator to have cultured mammalian embryos. This work was done only five years after the introduction of tissue culture techniques by Ross Harrison at Yale. Brachet incubated 5½- and 6½-day-old rabbit blastocysts for 48 hr on a plasma clot. The blastocysts continued development and doubled their size. Major contributions were next made by Lewis and Gregory (1929), also using rabbit embryos. They cultured one- or two-cell embryos on plasma and obtained some blastocysts. They also incubated late morula embryos for 7–8 days and obtained normal blastocysts. During the study they made the first time-lapse movies of early mammalian development. Lewis and Gregory were impressed with a change in the appearance of the embryo that occurs at about the 16-cell stage and coined the word *compaction* to describe it. Only recently has compaction been associated with the development of tight junctions between the outer trophoblast cells to form the trophectoderm. The development of this epithelial structure allows the embryo to control the composition of its extracellular fluid.

Following these pioneer studies several attempts to culture mammalian preimplantation embryos were made (for reviews, see Pincus, 1936; Austin, 1961; Chang, 1981). An important contribution was made by Hammond (1949), who devised a complex biological medium that supported the development of eight-cell mouse embryos to blastocysts. Subsequently Whitten (1956) showed that eight-cell mouse embryos would develop into blastocysts in a simple defined medium based on Krebs–Ringer bicarbonate solution. McLaren and Biggers (1958) then demonstrated that mouse blastocysts produced by Whitten's technique could develop into normal adult mice, capable of reproduction, after transfer into uterine foster mothers.

In 1947 Chang obtained normal rabbit young following the transfer of fertilized ova that had been stored at 5 or 10° C (Chang, 1947). Later Chang and Marden (1954) collected two-cell embryos from a white California breed of rabbit in Worcester, Massachusetts, and placed them in serum in small glass containers. The temperature was lowered to 10° C and then the vials were placed in a vacuum flask and sent by a commercial airline to London and thence to the School of Agriculture in Cambridge. There the embryos were transferred to black recipient foster-mothers. About 30 hr elapsed between collection of the embryos and transfer into the recipients. In due course rabbits of the California type were born.

The first attempt to freeze preimplantation embryos was reported by Smith (1953). She summarized her results as follows:

> . . . these results are sufficient to prove that exposure to very low temperatures is not incompatible with the further development of mammalian eggs . . . there is little doubt that with appropriate modifications in technique a high survival rate will be obtainable.

The breakthrough occurred independently in two laboratories 19 years later (Whittingham *et al.*, 1972; Wilmut, 1972).

The techniques whose historical origins I have described are now widely used all over the world. They have applications in many areas, which will be described in this volume. These areas include:

1. The study of development and differentiation at cellular and molecular levels.

2. The study and treatment of infertility in women and domestic animals.
3. The analysis of disease conditions (for example, the use of mouse chimeras to study the etiology of neuromuscular diseases with a genetic background).
4. The improvement of animal production by the storage of embryos to save the cost of maintaining expensive animal colonies and to save endangered species, thus preserving the genetic pool.
5. The improvement of animal stocks to shorten the generation time and speed up genetic selection.
6. In disease control by the introduction of new samples of the gene pool into countries with strict quarantine regulations.

This diversity of applications justifies widespread interest in the field of *in vitro* fertilization, embryo culture, and embryo transfer.

References

Adams, C. E., 1954, The experimental shortening of the generation interval. *Proc. Br. Soc. Anim. Prod.* pp. 97–108.
Austin, C. R., 1961, *The Mammalian Egg*, Charles C Thomas, Springfield, Illinois.
Balfour, F. M., 1880, *A Treatise on Comparative Embryology*, Vol. 2, Macmillan, London, pp. 218–223.
Bittner, J. J., and Little, C. C., 1937, Transmission of breast and lung cancer in mice, *J. Hered.* **28:**117–121.
Brachet, A., 1912, Développement *in vitro* de blastomeres et jeunes embryons de mammifères, *C. R. Acad. Sci.* **155:**1191–1193.
Chang, M. C., 1947, Normal development of fertilized rabbit ova stored at low temperature for several days, *Nature (London)* **159:**602–603.
Chang, M. C., 1959, Fertilization of rabbit ova *in vitro*, *Nature (London)* **184:**466–467.
Chang, M. C., 1981, My life with mammalian eggs, in: *Cellular and Molecular Aspects of Implantation* (S. R. Glasser and D. W. Bullock, eds.), Plenum, New York, pp. 27–36.
Chang, M. C., and Marden, W. G. R., 1954, Transport of fertilized mammalian ova, *J. Hered.* **45:**75–78.
Foster, M., and Balfour, F. M., 1883, *The Elements of Embryology*, 2nd ed. (A. Sedgwick and W. Heape, eds.), Macmillan, London, pp. 460–470.
Hammond, J., Jr., 1949, Recovery and culture of tubal mouse ova, *Nature (London)* **163:**28–29.
Heape, W., 1890, Preliminary note on the transplantation and growth of mammalian ova within a uterine foster-mother, *Proc. R. Soc. London* **48:**457–458.
Heape, W., 1894, The menstruation of *Semnopithecus entellus*, *Philos. Trans. R. Soc. London Ser. B* **185:**411–471.
Heape, W., 1897a, The menstruation and ovulation of *Macacus rhesus*, with observations on the changes undergone by the discharged follicle, *Philos. Trans. R. Soc. London Ser. B.* **188:**135–166.
Heape, W., 1897b, Further note on the transplantation and growth of mammalian ova within a uterine foster-mother, *Proc. R. Soc. London* **62:**178–185.
Heape, W., 1898, On menstruation of monkeys and human female, *Trans. Obstet. Soc.* **40:**161–174.

Lewis, W. H., and Gregory, P. W., 1929, Cinematographs of living developing rabbit eggs, *Science* **69**:226–229.

Locke, F. S., 1901, Die Wirkung der Metalle des Blutplasmas und verschiedener Zucker auf das isolierte Säugetierherz, *Zentralbl. Physiol.* **14**:670–672.

McLaren, A., and Biggers, J. D., 1958, Successful development and birth of mice cultivated *in vitro* as early embryos, *Nature (London)* **182**:877–878.

McLaren, A., and Michie, D., 1956, Studies on the transfer of fertilized mouse eggs to uterine foster-mothers, *J. Exp. Biol.* **33**:394–416.

Nicholas, J. S., 1933, Development of transplanted rat eggs, *Proc. Soc. Exp. Biol. N. Y.* **30**:1111–1113.

Pincus, G., 1936, *The Eggs of Mammals*, Macmillan, New York.

Schenk, S. L., 1878, Das Säugetierei: Künstlich befruchtet ausserhalb des Muttertieres, *Mitt. Embr. Inst. K. K. Univ. Wien.* **1**:107.

Smith, A. U., 1953, *In vitro* experiments with rabbit eggs, in: *Mammalian Germ Cells* (Ciba Foundation Symposium), Churchill, London, pp. 217–232.

Whitten, W. K., 1956, Culture of tubal mouse ova, *Nature (London)* **177**:96.

Whittingham, D. G., Leibo, S. P., and Mazur, P., 1972, Survival of mouse embryos frozen to −196°C and −269°C, *Science* **178**:411–414.

Willett, E. L., Black, W. G., Casida, L. E., Stone, W. H., and Buckner, P. J., 1951, Successful transplantation of a fertilized bovine ovum, *Science* **113**:247.

Wilmut, I., 1972, Effect of cooling rate, warming rate, cryoprotective agent and stage of development on survival of mouse embryos during cooling and thawing, *Life Sci.* **11** (pt. 2): 1071–1079.

1

COLLECTION OF GAMETES IN LABORATORY ANIMALS AND PREPARATION OF SPERM FOR *IN VITRO* FERTILIZATION

GENE OLIPHANT and LUDEMAN A. ENG

Collection of Ova for *in Vitro* Fertilization

Ova to be used for *in vitro* fertilization are routinely collected after superovulation. In small animals and depending on the species, 5–150 IU of pregnant mare serum gonadotropin (PMSG) is administered 2–4 days prior to an ovulating dose (5–125 IU) of human chorionic gonadotropin (hCG) (Yanagimachi, 1969; Iwamatsu and Chang, 1969; Barros *et al.*, 1973; Brackett and Oliphant, 1975). Superovulation procedures, for example in rabbit, can produce as many as 60 ova per rabbit but will more commonly result in 20 ± 3.0 ova recovered from the oviduct. There is some evidence that superovulation may cause chromosomal abnormalities (Fugimoto *et al.*, 1974; Maudlin and Fraser, 1977).

Given that many investigators utilize hormonal stimulation to increase the recovery of ova, there are three commonly used techniques to harvest ova. Ova can be collected: (1) from follicles before ovulation, (2) from the surface of the ovary after ovulation, or (3) from the oviduct after ovulation. Collection of ova from follicles usually involves excising the ovary and rupturing the follicle with a needle, after which the ova are recovered by pipet. These manipulations often are carried out with the ovary immersed in medium that is covered with oil and at a temperature of 37°C (Barros and

GENE OLIPHANT and LUDEMAN A. ENG • Department of Anatomy, University of Virginia School of Medicine, Charlottesville, Virginia 22908.

Table I

Effect of the Ovum Source on *in Vitro* Fertilization

Source	Ova fertilized/inseminated	Percent fertilized	Reference
Rabbit follicular	171/345	50	Mills *et al.* (1973)
Rabbit ovarian surface	241/328	74	Mills *et al.* (1973)
Rabbit oviductal	35/54	65	Brackett (1968)
Hamster follicular	123/262	47	Barros and Austin (1967)
Hamster oviductal	94/160	59	Barros and Austin (1967)

Austin, 1967; Pickworth and Chang, 1969; Edwards *et al.*, 1970; Gould *et al.*, 1973; Mills *et al.*, 1973; Rogers and Yanagimachi, 1975).

Ova collected from the surface of the ovary have been limited to rabbits (Brackett and Server, 1970; Mills *et al.*, 1973; Brackett and Oliphant, 1975); the advantage here is that the ova are fully mature but have not been exposed to the oviductal environment. In these experiments, ovaries are excised exactly 12 hr after the ovulating dose of hCG and placed in medium. Ova adhering to the surface of the ovary by their cumulus mass are then pulled off the surface with forceps, collected, and transferred to fresh medium for fertilization.

Tubal ova are the most common source of ova used for *in vitro* fertilization in small animals. These ova are collected after excising the oviduct and either retrograde flushing, as in rabbit (Brackett and Williams, 1965), or in the case of smaller animals, a small cut in the oviduct is made and the cumulus mass containing the ova is teased out (Yanagimachi and Chang, 1963; Yanagimachi, 1969, 1972; Iwamatsu and Chang, 1969; Pavlok and McLaren, 1972; Toyoda and Chang, 1974).

Comparison of the fertilizability of ova from these sources is difficult because experiments have usually been designed to accomplish *in vitro* fertilization and not necessarily to compare different sources of ova. Table I compares the results from two studies along with the data of rabbit tubal ova fertilized in the same laboratory but in a different set of experiments. These results would suggest that rabbit ovarian surface ova have some advantage over ova recovered from follicles or from the oviduct. Both studies suggest a slight advantage of oviductal ova over follicular ova. In any case it is apparent that successful *in vitro* fertilization can be accomplished with ova from any of these three sources, and they can thus be used to fit into the desired experimental design of the investigator.

Methods Presently Used for Sperm Collection

Epididymal sperm are routinely used for *in vitro* fertilization of hamster, mouse, guinea pig, and other small mammals (Yanagimachi and Chang, 1963;

Yanagimachi, 1969, 1972; Iwamatsu and Chang, 1969; Oliphant and Brackett, 1973b; Rogers and Yanagimachi, 1975; Noske, 1972). In the technique generally used, the cauda epididymis is excised, placed in a drop of medium under oil, and either minced or several cuts made through it. At this point, sperm are either squeezed out of the epididymis by light pressure or they are allowed to swim out over a standard period of time. This technique produces sperm of good motility and fertilizability. An alternate procedure for collection of cauda epididymal sperm, usually used in the rabbit or larger mammals, is to place a clamp between the distal corpus and the cauda epididymis after excision of the epididymis. Medium is flushed out retrograde via the vas deferens and the cauda epididymis is distended. Progressive distension is observed and when 75% of the tubule is distended a small cut is made with scissors at the site of distension closest to the corpus. An additional 1–2 ml of medium is then flushed through the epididymis and the very clean cauda epididymal sperm recovered in a sterile petri dish (Brackett *et al.*, 1978).

Ejaculated sperm have rarely been collected from small mammals and to date little has been published on the use of ejaculated sperm from these animals for *in vitro* fertilization. However, techniques have been established for the collection of electroejaculated sperm. The technique used for rats, mice, and guinea pigs has been described by Scott and Dziuk (1959). They used unipolar rectal electrodes in conjunction with electrodes placed around the base of the penis and 60-cycle AC current at low voltage given intermittently to stimulate erection and ejaculation. Of the female rats inseminated with electroejaculated sperm, only 18% became pregnant. With regard to the mouse, sperm were entrapped in the coagulum and fertilization thus could not be achieved. Recently, Oswald and Zaneveld (1980) have reundertaken the evaluation of mouse sperm collected by electroejaculation and are attempting to utilize the sperm for *in vitro* fertilization (Zaneveld, personal communication). A problem associated with this method of collection is that the coagulation plug prevents further manipulation of the sperm, and under some conditions after collection the copulation plug has blocked the urethra and resulted in uremia and death of the animal (Scott and Dziuk, 1959). This complication can be overcome by removing the seminal vesicles. However, the ejaculate without seminal vesicle components could not be considered normal and thus comparison of fertilizing capacity, *in vivo* or *in vitro*, with other sperm sources would have to be carefully considered. Such blockage of the urethra by copulation plugs does not seem to be the case when semen is collected by electroejaculation from monkeys as reported by Mastroianni and Mason (1963) and Fussell *et al.* (1967). Sperm collected by electroejaculation have been utilized successfully for *in vitro* fertilization of the squirrel monkey (Gould *et al.*, 1973; Kuehl and Dukelow, 1975).

Ejaculated sperm have been utilized for *in vitro* fertilization of ova from cats, dogs, rabbits, cows, and humans (Hamner *et al.*, 1970; Mahi and

Yanagimachi, 1978; Brackett and Oliphant, 1975; Brackett et al., 1980; Edwards et al., 1970). These ejaculated sperm were collected either by use of an artificial vagina or by digital manipulation in the case of the dog and human. Collection of semen by means of an artificial vagina has been carried out in many species (reviewed by First, 1971). The general construction of the artificial vagina can be described as a water-jacketed soft rubber tube. Into one end a test tube is placed to collect the ejaculate and the other end is open for intromission of the penis. As the warmth of the artificial vagina is important in inducing ejaculation, the water temperature employed is approximately 50° C. Commonly, the male is induced to mount a "teaser" female. At this point the penis is directed into the artificial vagina and ejaculation allowed to occur. Using rabbits this laboratory has found it optimal to use as a teaser an ovariectomized doe given bimonthly injections of 200 μg ECP.

Differences in Sperm as a Function of Collection Method

The amount of sperm available varies considerably according to the technique used for collection. Table II reports the amount of sperm available after collection from one pair of epididymides or from one ejaculation. Certainly the amount of material varies with the collection method used. This seems especially true for electroejaculation.

As indicated above, much of the success and advances in methodology for *in vitro* fertilization have been accomplished with epididymal sperm. It is well established that the swimming patterns of sperm and their ability to fertilize develop during epididymal transit (reviewed by Turner, 1979). Less

Table II

Total Number of Sperm Available for *in Vitro* Fertilization[a]

Animal	Epididymal ($\times 10^6$)	Ejaculated ($\times 10^6$)
Cat	—	28–45[b]
Bull	—	1200–8000[b]
Dog	—	260–1300[b]
Gerbil	7.5–10[b]	—
Guinea pig	2.5–10[b]	4–8 (5–235)[c]
Hamster	480–810[b]	—
Mouse	2–8[b]	—
Rabbit	300–1200[b]	100–300[b]
Rat	2.5–7.5[b]	— (0.4–342)[c]

[a] Based on one pair of epididymides or on ejaculate.
[b] Source used for *in vitro* fertilization.
[c] Electroejaculation.

emphasis has been placed on the possible effects of ejaculation on sperm, partly because of the lack of experimental models where both ease and/or expense of semen collection and *in vitro* fertilization exist together. Weil and Rodenburg (1962) demonstrated that an antigen from the seminal vesicle coated both rabbit and human sperm during ejaculation. Recently, after iodination of surface components of ejaculated and epididymal rabbit sperm, Oliphant and Singhas (1979) demonstrated the loss or masking of a 63,000 (molecular weight) component present in epididymal sperm and the appearance of a new, 20,000 (molecular weight) component after ejaculation. Likewise, a 34,000 (molecular weight) component from vas deferens has been shown to bind to mouse sperm (Herr and Eddy, 1980). Other changes in rabbit sperm have been demonstrated. Exposure of epididymal sperm to seminal plasma resulted in decreased wheat germ agglutin-induced agglutination (Nicolson and Yanagimachi, 1972). There is also decreased binding of ferritin-labeled plant lectins. *Ricinus communis* and wheat germ agglutin, to sperm after ejaculation (Nicolson *et al.*, 1977). Gordon *et al.* (1974) also suggested decreased concanavalin A binding to rabbit sperm after ejaculation, but the conditions used by Nicolson *et al.* (1977) did not allow confirmation of this observation. It is of great significance that when rabbit epididymal sperm were compared to ejaculated sperm under *in vitro* fertilization conditions, 79% of the ova inseminated with epididymal sperm were fertilized compared to only 36% for ejaculated sperm. This strongly suggests that the changes (sperm coating or other surface modifications) occurring during the process of ejaculation likely affect the fertilizability (Brackett *et al.*, 1978). When rabbit sperm were incubated with high concentrations (40%) of follicular fluid, these differences were overcome, as ejaculated sperm and epididymal sperm from the same buck showed virtually identical percentages of acrosome-reacted sperm when incubated for 2 hr (Oliphant, 1976). Such studies strongly warrant that the differences between epididymal and ejaculated sperm be more closely scrutinized and that attempts be made to compare these sources of sperm in other animals utilized for *in vitro* fertilization models.

Preparation of Ejaculated Sperm for Use in *In Vitro* Fertilization

Conditions for the preparation of sperm for *in vitro* fertilization are, in essence, those required for sperm capacitation. A requirement for capacitation has been demonstrated in mouse, rat, hamster, guinea pig, cat, dog, rabbit, pig, bull, and human (Greep and Koblinsky, 1977). However, the time and conditions required to capacitate these sperm vary from 1–2 hr for mouse to 6–12 hr for rabbit. Capacitation initially was defined as all the changes that the sperm underwent in the female reproductive tract to acquire the capacity to fertilize the ova (Austin, 1952). However, many of these changes have now become classified as separate events in the process of fertilization; therefore, for the purposes of this discussion, capacitation will be considered as sperm surface and metabolic events prior to the acrosome reaction. Indeed, some investigators have classified these metabolic changes as a separate entity (activation) and this may be justified, as will be discussed later.

Before reviewing the actual preparation of ejaculated sperm for *in vitro* fertilization, a brief background of metabolic and membrane changes and the factors associated with capacitation will be presented.

Metabolism

Increased sperm metabolism as a result of capacitation was first indicated by Hamner and Williams (1963), who demonstrated an increased utilization of oxygen by rabbit sperm after a sojourn in the female reproductive tract of the rabbit. This has been repeated by several investigators (Mounib and Chang, 1964; Murdoch and White, 1967; Brackett, 1968) and also shown to occur when sperm are incubated *in vitro* in reproductive tract fluids (Iritani *et al.*, 1969). This increased oxygen utilization may be reflected in hamster and guinea pig (Yanagimachi, 1975) spermatozoa when after 2–4 hr of incubation in defined medium they begin to swim extremely vigorously with a whiplash movement of the tail. A similar tail movement does not appear in rabbit spermatozoa, at least not to the extent observed in these two species.

Membrane Alterations during Capacitation

It could have been inferred from Chang's recapacitation experiment in 1957 that the process of capacitation involved surface changes of the spermatozoa. He demonstrated that rabbit sperm could be capacitated after a period of time in the female reproductive tract, after which reincubation of these capacitated sperm in seminal plasma concentrations as low as 5% resulted in their "decapacitation." A further sojourn of these "decapacitated" sperm in the female reproductive tract resulted in a "recapacitation" with subsequent ability to fertilize ova.

Evaluation of sperm surface characteristics associated with capacitation was expanded by Vaidya *et al.* (1971), who showed that capacitated sperm had a lower electrophoretic mobility than freshly ejaculated sperm or sperm incubated shortly thereafter. The phospholipid content of rabbit spermatozoa has been probed by Snider and Clegg (1972), who found that phosphatidylinositol (PI) is barely detectable in uncapacitated sperm. However, PI was found to increase to a peak of 2.2% of the total phospholipids after a 90-min incubation in the estrous uterus and up to 2.3% after only 30 min in the oviduct. PI percentages declined after these times, however, and the relationship of PI content to the capacitation process remains speculative.

An immunological approach to assessing the surface change in capacitated sperm was advanced by Johnson and Hunter (1972) by the use of immunofluorescence with antisera to antigens on washed rabbit sperm (ARS) and to antigens in the seminal plasma (ARSP). Ejaculated sperm showed bright fluorescence with ARSP and dull fluorescence with ARS. After a 10-hr incubation in an estrous uterus, however, spermatozoa were observed to show a dull fluorescence with ARSP and a bright fluorescence with ARS. These results were interpreted as being due to the removal of sperm-coating antigens from the surface of the sperm, thereby unmasking sperm-specific antigenic sites. Sperm would therefore appear bright with ARSP before capacitation and with ARS after capacitation.

Oliphant and Brackett (1973a) showed that antiserum to rabbit seminal plasma caused rabbit sperm to agglutinate. This agglutination reaction was undiminished even when the sperm had been extensively washed for up to 18 hr. When sperm were incubated in an estrous uterus, however, the agglutinability decreased as incubation time and fertilizing ability increased. The diminution of agglutination with increasing incubation *in utero* was regarded as a reflection of the removal of seminal plasma components from the sperm membrane during capacitation. This interpretation was confirmed and quantitated by ^{14}C-labeled antiserum, i.e., the uptake of ^{14}C-labeled antiserum by sperm cells was constant during incubation for 24 hr in a defined medium but decreased significantly during incubation in uterine fluid.

Aonuma *et al.* (1973) showed that guinea pig antigens could be released from sperm into the medium during incubation in calcium-free Krebs Ringer phosphate buffer. These antigens showed reversible decapacitation activity, and an antiserum was raised against them and labeled with ^{131}I. Binding of the ^{131}I-labeled antiserum was greatest in uncapacitated sperm and decreased by 30% when sperm were recovered after a 6-hr incubation in an estrous uterus, thus confirming the results obtained in the rabbit by Oliphant and Brackett (1973a).

Plant lectins have been observed to bind and readily agglutinate rabbit and hamster sperm (Nicolson and Yanagimachi, 1972). Concanavalin A (Con A) binds uniformly over the head of ejaculated sperm but after capacitation is found to bind only to the postacrosomal region. The loss of Con A binding to the periacrosomal plasmalemma in capacitated spermatozoa is interpreted as providing visible evidence for the removal of seminal plasma glycoproteins during the capacitation process (Gordon *et al.*, 1974). This removal has been found to be a prerequisite for the induction of the acrosome reaction (Oliphant, 1976).

This hypothesis is supported by the work of Koehler (1976), who prepared antiglobulin against rabbit sperm and labeled it with hemocyanin. Transmission electron micrographs revealed that ejaculated or epididymal sperm showed a uniform distribution of labeled antibody over the sperm head. In capacitated sperm, however, antibody binding was patchy or completely abolished by freeze-etching, which demonstrated that the distribution of a surface coat layer over the sperm head in capacitated and uncapacitated sperm was correlated with that of the labeled antibody.

A change in membrane fluidity with capacitation was demonstrated immunofluorescently by O'Rand (1977) with antibodies specific for a single glycoprotein on the membrane surface of rabbit sperm. Epididymal and ejaculated sperm that had been labeled at $4°$ C fluoresced uniformly. When these sperm were then warmed to $37°$ C, a redistribution of the label occurred so that bright patches were formed over the acrosome. This lateral movement failed to occur on *in vivo* capacitated sperm and the label remained diffusely distributed. These results were interpreted as evidence for a loss in membrane fluidity when sperm are capacitated.

Seminal Plasma Factors Associated with Capacitation

Though the existence of a seminal plasma component(s) that decapacitates sperm has been known for many years, its nature, mode of action, and method of action remain disputed. Early work has shown the decapacitation factor (DF) to be stable to both heat and cold, precipitable by ethanol, and pelleted by ultracentrifugation (Bedford and Chang, 1962). The factor pelleted by ultracentrifugation was reported resistant to Pronase but destroyed by β-amylase (Dukelow *et al.*, 1965, 1966). However, highly purified preparations of β-amylase have no effect on this activity (Williams *et al.*, 1967, 1970), nor do lysozyme, hyaluronidase, glucose oxidase, galactose oxidase, or neuraminidase (Williams *et al.*, 1967).

The Pronase digest of the high-speed pellet reportedly contained decapacitating activity of low molecular weight (500–1000), which was believed to be carbohydrate because of its Pronase resistance (Williams *et al.*, 1967). However, later experiments in the same laboratory showed that the low-molecular-weight DF was destroyed by Pronase and therefore probably a peptide (Robertson *et al.*, 1971); possibly this peptide may be the active site of a larger molecule. This small peptide has been designated *decapacitation factor*.

DF has been described as an inhibitor of neuraminidase (Srivastava *et al.*, 1970) and of the corona-penetrating enzyme (Zaneveld and Williams, 1970), which has been identified as an esterase (Bradford *et al.*, 1976), but DF has no effect on hyaluronidase or acrosin (Zaneveld and Williams, 1970).

A large seminal plasma glycoprotein of approximately 170,000 mol. wt.

has been identified but not isolated by Hunter and Nornes (1969) as a sperm-coating antigen of possible decapacitating activity and has been found to be absent from epididymal fluid. Reyes *et al.* (1975) found that reversible decapacitation activity was eluted in two of five fractions when rabbit seminal plasma was chromatographed on Sephadex G-200 and was completely precipitated by treatment of seminal plasma with cetylpyridinium chloride (CPC). When the CPC precipitate and the two peaks from gel chromatography were subjected to SDS gel electrophoresis, only one component (Coomassie blue and PAS positive; 115,000 mol. wt.) was common to these active fractions. Recently, a large (355,000 mol. wt.) glycoprotein (Table III) with reversible decapacitation activity, as shown by bioassays similar to those used by Chang (1957), has been isolated. This product of seminal plasma also prevents the follicular fluid-induced acrosome reaction (Eng and Oliphant, 1978). This glycoprotein has been designated *acrosome-stabilizing factor* (ASF) to suggest its mechanism of decapacitating sperm and to avoid confusion with the small peptide known as DF. Using the ability of ejaculated human sperm to penetrate hamster ova, the presence of an ASF-like substance in human seminal plasma has been demonstrated (Kanwar *et al.*, 1979).

Recently, Koehler *et al.* (1980) have shown that a component is added to the surface of rabbit sperm during ejaculation that is immunologically cross-reactive with antiserum against mouse 3T3 cell fibronectin. Upon capacitation

Table III
Characteristics of the Acrosome-Stabilizing Factor
Purified from Rabbit Seminal Plasma

Biological activity	Prevents follicular fluid-induced acrosome reaction
	Has reversible decapacitation activity
Native molecular weight	
Gel filtration	370,000
Disc electrophoresis	355,000
Subunit size	
SDS electrophoresis	121,000
Chemical composition	
mg Neutral hexose/mg protein	1/1.6
Lipid	0
Stability	
Stored frozen in seminal plasma	Stable for months
Heating at 56° C for 20 min	Stable
Solubility	
After purification	28 ± 5 μg/ml
Eluted from sperm surface	HIS medium (380 mOsM)

in utero this material is removed, and the authors speculate that because ASF and fibronectin have similar subunit molecular weights there may be a connection between ASF and the sperm-bound fibronectin they observed.

Methods Used to Induce Capacitation of Ejaculated Sperm

Ejaculated sperm from different species collected for use in *in vitro* fertilization have been capacitated by various methodologies. Cat sperm were incubated *in utero* for 2 hr before acquiring the capacity to fertilize ova *in vitro* (Hammer *et al.*, 1970), whereas human and canine require a preincubation of 6–7 hr in a defined medium (Kanwar *et al.*, 1979; Mahi and Yanagimachi, 1978). Rabbit sperm have been capacitated by incubation 6 hr *in utero* (Oliphant and Brackett, 1973a).

Although the conditions for the *in vitro* capacitation of rabbit sperm have been most difficult to achieve, this exaggerated difficulty may allow the dissection of the components of capacitation more readily than in species where capacitation occurs readily. Brackett and Oliphant (1975) established that treatment of rabbit sperm with media of high ionic strength (HIS) for 20 min produced sperm with the capacity to fertilize ova *in vitro*. Koehler (1976) showed that rabbit sperm treated with HIS had "cleared" areas in the plasma membrane over the acrosome similar to rabbit sperm incubated *in utero* or hamster sperm (Kinsey and Koehler, 1978) capacitated in defined medium. Oliphant and Singhas (1979) have demonstrated that ASF is rapidly removed from sperm by HIS treatment but will dissociate slowly if sperm are incubated in isotonic solutions. Recently, bovine sperm have been capacitated by a similar HIS treatment (Brackett *et al.*, 1980), and Triana *et al.* (1980) have demonstrated that HIS treatment of bovine sperm is an absolute prerequisite to follicular fluid-induced Ca^{2+} uptake into the sperm. As Ca^{2+} has been shown to be required for the acrosome reaction in all species examined (Yanagimachi and Usui, 1974; Oliphant *et al.*, 1977), the subsequent release of hyaluronidase after Ca^{2+} uptake by bovine sperm would suggest the completion of the acrosome reaction.

Recently, two other laboratories have attempted to use HIS-treated sperm for tubal insemination *in vivo;* both have indicated poor success (Akruk *et al.*, 1979; Bedford, personal communication). Our laboratory has reexamined these results and found that when $3–5 \times 10^5$ HIS-treated sperm were inseminated into the ostium of the oviduct at 12 hr post hCG, little or no fertilization occurred. This was the time used for insemination by the two laboratories. However, when the same amount of HIS-treated sperm were inseminated at 10 or 11 hr post hCG, 46 and 13% fertilization occurred (Table IV). Insemination of untreated sperm into the contralateral tube resulted in significantly fewer ($p < 0.02$) ova fertilized at 10 hr post hCG. These results

Table IV
Fertilization after Tubal Insemination with Treated Sperm

Time after hCG (hr)	No. of experiments	Ejaculated	High salt treated	*In vivo* capacitated
10	5	2/36 (6%)	24/52 (46%)	—
11	5	0/53 (0%)	5/39 (13%)	14/24 (58%)

compare favorably with those of Chang (1951). His classical work showed that no fertilization occurred when does were inseminated with washed ejaculated sperm 8 hr after an ovulating dose of hormone was given. He also found that 75% of the ova were fertilized with sperm that had been capacitated *in utero*.

Since Koehler (1976) had already established the similarity of membrane changes between HIS- and *in utero*-treated sperm, we examined oxygen utilization of sperm after HIS treatment. Pooled ejaculated sperm were treated for 20 min with either HIS or control medium. After this incubation sperm were resuspended in control medium and oxygen utilization measured. Dilution effects (Mann, 1964) were avoided by always using 10^8 sperm per milliliter. No significant increase above ejaculated controls was observed in oxygen utilized immediately after HIS treatment (Table V) or after an additional 2 hr. These data indicate that HIS treatment does not totally mimic the entire capacitation process. It would seem possible that after HIS treatment, sperm may acquire an increased respiration in the oviduct fluid; indeed, *in vitro* experiments have been reported that demonstrate this fact (Foley and Williams, 1967; Iritani *et al.*, 1969). These results indicate that membrane events here can be studied separately from metabolic (oxygen-utilization) changes associated with capacitation.

Table V
Sperm Respiration and Motility

	Ejaculated			High salt treated		
Time (hr):	0	1	2	0	1	2
Number of determinations:	17	16	14	17	17	12
ZO_2[a]	4.13	3.16	3.38	3.85	3.66	4.04
±S.E.	0.21	0.24	0.21	0.29	0.26	0.22
% motility	81.6	75.3	67.5	72.7	54.7	54.1
±S.E.	2.8	4.5	4.3	4.14	5.4	5.4

[a] Microliters of O_2 utilized by 10^8 cells in 1 hr at 37° C.

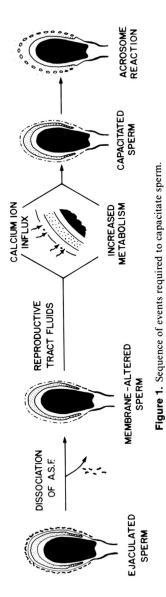

Figure 1. Sequence of events required to capacitate sperm.

A scheme of events associated with the preparation of sperm for fertilization can now be presented. Figure 1 indicates a likely sequence of events required to capacitate sperm and thus prepare them to undergo the acrosome reaction and fertilize the ova.

References

Akruk, S. R., Humphreys, W. J., and Williams, W. L., 1979, *In vitro* capacitation of ejaculated rabbit spermatozoa, *Differentiation* **13**:125-131.

Aonuma, S., Mayumi, T., Suzuki, K., Noguchi, T., Iwai, M., and Okabe, M., 1973, Studies on sperm capacitation. I. The relationship between a guinea-pig sperm-coating antigen and a sperm capacitation phenomenon, *J. Reprod. Fertil.* **35**:425-432.

Austin, C. R., 1952, "Capacitation" of the mammalian sperm, *Nature (London)* **170**:326.

Barros, C., and Austin, C. R., 1967, *In vitro* fertilization and the sperm acrosome reaction in the hamster, *J. Exp. Zool.* **166**:317-323.

Barros, C., Berrios, M., and Herrera, E., 1973, Capacitation *in vitro* of guinea pig spermatozoa in a saline solution, *J. Reprod. Fertil.* **34**:547-549.

Bedford, J. M., and Chang, M. C., 1962, Removal of decapacitation factor from seminal plasma by high speed centrifugation, *Am. J. Physiol.* **202**:179-181.

Brackett, B. G., 1968, Respiration of spermatozoa after *in utero* incubation in estrus and pseudopregnant rabbits, *Proc. 6th Int. Congr. Animal Reprod.* **1**:43-45.

Brackett, B. G., and Oliphant, G., 1975, Capacitation of rabbit spermatozoa *in vitro*, *Biol. Reprod.* **12**:260-274.

Brackett, B. G., and Server, J. B., 1970, Capacitation of rabbit spermatozoa in the uterus, *Fertil. Steril.* **21**:687-695.

Brackett, B. G., and Williams, W. L., 1965, *In vitro* fertilization of rabbit ova, *J. Exp. Zool.* **160**:271-274.

Brackett, B. G., Hall, J. L., and Oh, Y. K., 1978, *In vitro* fertilizing ability of testicular, epididymal and ejaculated rabbit spermatozoa, *Fertil. Steril.* **29**:571-582.

Brackett, B. G., Oh, Y. K., Evans, J. F., and Donawick, W. J., 1980, Fertilization and early development of cow ova, *Biol. Reprod.* **23**:189.

Bradford, M. M., McRorie, R. A., and Williams, W. L., 1976, A role for esterases in the fertilization process, *J. Exp. Zool.* **197**:297-301.

Chang, M. C., 1951, Fertilizing capacity of spermatozoa deposited in the fallopian tube, *Nature (London)* **168**:697-698.

Chang, M. C., 1957, A detrimental effect of seminal plasma on the fertilizing capacity of sperm, *Nature (London)* **179**:258-259.

Dukelow, W. R., Chernoff, H. N., and Williams, W. L., 1965, Properties of decapacitation factor and presence in various species, *J. Reprod. Fertil.* **14**:393-399.

Dukelow, W. R., Chernoff, H. N., and Williams, W. L., 1966, Enzymatic characterization of decapacitation factor, *Proc. Soc. Exp. Biol. Med.* **121**:396-398.

Edwards, R. G., Steptoe, P. C., and Purdy, J. M., 1970, Fertilization and cleavage *in vitro* of preovulatory human oocytes, *Nature (London)* **227**:307-309.

Eng, L. A., and Oliphant, G., 1978, Rabbit sperm reversible decapacitation by membrane stabilization with a highly purified glycoprotein from seminal plasma, *Biol. Reprod.* **19**:1083-1094.

First, N. L., 1971, Collection and preservation of spermatozoa, in: *Methods in Mammalian Embryology* (J. C. Daniel, ed.), Freeman, San Francisco, pp. 15-36.

Foley, C. W., and Williams, W. L., 1967, Effect of bicarbonate and oviduct fluid on preparation of spermatozoa, *Proc. Soc. Exp. Biol. Med.* **126**:634–638.

Fugimoto, S., Pahlavan, N., and Dukelow, W. R., 1974, Chromosome abnormalities in rabbit preimplantation blastocysts induced by superovulation, *J. Reprod. Fertil.* **40**:177–181.

Fussell, E. N., Roussel, J. D., and Austin, C. R., 1967, Use of the rectal probe method for electrical ejaculation of apes, monkeys and a prosimian, *Lab. Anim. Care* **17**:528–534.

Gordon, M., Dandekar, P. V., and Bartoszewicz, W., 1974, Ultrastructural localization of surface receptors for concanavalin A on rabbit spermatozoa, *J. Reprod. Fertil.* **36**:211–214.

Gould, K. G., Cline, E. M., and Williams, W. L., 1973, Observations on the induction of ovulation and fertilization *in vitro* in the squirrel monkey (*Saimiri sciurens*), *Fertil. Steril.* **24**:260–268.

Greep, R. O., and Koblinsky, M. A., 1977, *Frontiers in Reproduction and Fertility Control*, MIT Press, Cambridge, Mass., pp. 434–452.

Hamner, C. E., and Williams, W. L., 1963, Effect of the female reproductive tract on sperm metabolism in the rabbit and fowl, *J. Reprod. Fertil.* **5**:143–150.

Hamner, C. E., Jennings, L. L., and Sojka, N. J., 1970, Cat spermatozoa require capacitation, *J. Reprod. Fertil.* **23**:477–480.

Herr, J. C., and Eddy, E. M., 1980, Evidence for a sperm component acquired in the vas deferens, *Anat. Rec.* **146**:77A.

Hunter, A. G., and Nornes, H. O., 1969, Characterization and isolation of a sperm-coating antigen from rabbit seminal plasma with capacity to block fertilization, *J. Reprod. Fertil.* **20**:419–427.

Iritani, A., Gomes, W. R., and VanDemark, N. L., 1969, The effect of whole, dialysed and heated female genital tract fluids on respiration of rabbit and rat spermatozoa, *Biol. Reprod.* **1**:77–82.

Iwamatsu, T., and Chang, M. C., 1969, *In vitro* fertilization of mouse eggs in the presence of bovine follicular fluid, *Nature (London)* **224**:919–920.

Johnson, W. L., and Hunter, A. G., 1972, Immunofluorescent evaluation of the male rabbit reproductive tract for sites of secretion and absorption of seminal antigens, *Biol. Reprod.* **6**:13–22.

Kanwar, K. C., Yanagimachi, R., and Lopata, A., 1979, Effects of human seminal plasma on fertilizing capacity of human spermatozoa, *Fertil. Steril.* **31**:321–327.

Kinsey, W. H., and Koehler, J. K., 1978, Cell surface changes associated with *in vitro* capacitation of hamster sperm, *J. Ultrastruct. Res.* **64**:1–13.

Koehler, J. K., 1976, Changes in antigenic site distribution of rabbit spermatozoa after incubation in capacitating media, *Biol. Reprod.* **15**:444–456.

Koehler, J. K., Nudelman, E. D., and Hakomori, S., 1980, A collagen-binding protein on the surface of ejaculated rabbit spermatozoa, *J. Cell Biol.* **86**:529–536.

Kuehl, T. J., and Dukelow, W. R., 1975, Fertilization *in vitro* of *Saimiri sciurens* follicular oocytes, *J. Med. Primatol.* **4**:209–216.

Mahi, C. A., and Yanagimachi, R., 1978, Capacitation, acrosome reaction and egg penetration by canine spermatozoa in a single defined medium, *Gamete Res.* **1**:101–109.

Mann, T., 1964, *Biochemistry of the Semen*, Wiley, New York, pp. 343–352.

Mastroianni, L., and Mason, W. A., 1963, Collection of monkey semen by electroejaculation, *Proc. Soc. Exp. Biol. Med.* **112**:1025–1027.

Maudlin, I., and Fraser, L. R., 1977, The effect of PMSG dose on the incidence of chromosomal anomalies in mouse embryos fertilized *in vitro*, *J. Reprod. Fertil.* **50**:272–280.

Mills, J. A., Jeitles, G. G., and Brackett, B. G., 1973, Embryo transfer following *in vitro* and *in vivo* fertilization of rabbit ova, *Fertil. Steril.* **24**:602–608.

Mounib, M. S., and Chang, M. C., 1964, Effect of *in utero* incubation on the metabolism of rabbit spermatozoa, *Nature (London)* **201**:943–944.

Murdoch, R. N., and White, I. G., 1967, The metabolism of labelled glucose by rabbit spermatozoa after incubation *in utero*, *J. Reprod. Fertil.* **14**:213–223.

Nicolson, G. L., and Yanagimachi, R., 1972, Terminal saccharides on sperm plasma membranes: Identification by specific agglutinins, *Science* **177**:276–279.

Nicolson, G. L., Usui, N., Yanagimachi, R., Yanagimachi, H., and Smith, J. R., 1977, Lectin binding on the plasma membranes of rabbit spermatozoa, *J. Cell Biol.* **74**:950–962.

Noske, I. G., 1972, *In vitro* fertilization of the Mongolian gerbil egg, *Experientia* **28**:1348–1350.

Oliphant, G., 1976, Removal of sperm-bound seminal plasma components as a prerequisite to induction of the rabbit acrosome reaction, *Fertil. Steril.* **27**:28–38.

Oliphant, G., and Brackett, B. G., 1973a, Immunological assessment of surface changes of rabbit sperm undergoing capacitation, *Biol. Reprod.* **9**:404–414.

Oliphant, G., and Brackett, B. G., 1973b, Capacitation of mouse spermatozoa in media with elevated ionic strength and reversible decapacitation with epididymal extracts, *Fertil. Steril.* **24**:948–955.

Oliphant, G., and Singhas, C. A., 1979, Iodination of rabbit sperm plasma membranes: Relationship of specific surface proteins to epididymal function and sperm capacitation, *Biol. Reprod.* **21**:937–944.

Oliphant, G., Cabot, C. L., and Singhas, C. A., 1977, Nature of the rabbit acrosome reaction-inducing activity of follicular fluid, *J. Reprod. Fertil.* **50**:245–250.

O'Rand, M. G., 1977, Restriction of a sperm surface antigen's mobility during capacitation, *Dev. Biol.* **55**:260–270.

Oswald, C., and Zaneveld, L. J. D., 1980, Analysis of electroejaculated mouse semen, Abstracts of the Society for Study of Reproduction, No. 165.

Pavlok, A., and McLaren, A., 1972, The role of cumulus cells and the zona pellucida in fertilization of mouse eggs *in vitro*, *J. Reprod. Fertil.* **29**:91–97.

Pickworth, S., and Chang, M. C., 1969, Fertilization of Chinese hamster eggs *in vitro*, *J. Reprod. Fertil.* **19**:371–374.

Reyes, A., Oliphant, G., and Brackett, B. G., 1975, Partial purification and identification of a reversible decapacitation factor from rabbit seminal plasma, *Fertil. Steril.* **26**:148–157.

Robertson, R. T., Bhalla, V. K., and Williams, W. L., 1971, Purification and the peptide nature of decapacitation factor, *Biochem. Biophys. Res. Commun.* **45**:1331–1336.

Rogers, B. J., and Yanagimachi, R., 1975, Retardation of guinea pig sperm acrosome reaction by glucose: The possible importance of pyruvate and lactate metabolism in capacitation and the acrosome reaction, *Biol. Reprod.* **13**:568–575.

Scott, J. V., and Dziuk, P. J., 1959, Evaluation of the electroejaculation technique and the spermatozoa thus obtained from rats, mice, and guinea pigs, *Anat. Rec.* **31**:655–664.

Snider, D. R., and Clegg, E. D., 1972, Alteration of porcine sperm phospholipids during *in vivo* oviduct and uterus incubation, *Fed. Proc.* **31**:277.

Srivastava, P. N., Zaneveld, L. J. D., and Williams, W. L., 1970, Mammalian sperm acrosomal neuraminidases, *Biochem. Biophys. Res. Commun.* **39**:575–582.

Toyoda, Y., and Chang, M. C., 1974, Fertilization of rat eggs *in vitro* by epididymal spermatozoa and the development of eggs following transfer, *J. Reprod. Fertil.* **36**:9–22.

Triana, L. R., Babcock, D. F., Lorton, S. P., First, N. L., and Lardy, H. A., 1980, Release of acrosomal hyaluronidase follows increased membrane permeability to calcium in the presumptive capacitation sequence of spermatozoa of the bovine and other mammalian species, *Biol. Reprod.* **23**:47–59.

Turner, T. T., 1979, On the epididymis and its function, *Invest. Urol.* **16**:311–321.

Vaidya, R. A., Glass, R. H., Dandekar, P., and Johnson, K., 1971, Decrease in the electrophoretic mobility of rabbit spermatozoa following intra-uterine incubation, *J. Reprod. Fertil.* **24**:299–301.

Weil, A. J., and Rodenburg, J. M., 1962, The seminal vesicle as the source of the spermatozoa coating antigen of seminal plasma, *Proc. Soc. Exp. Biol. Med.* **109**:567–570.

Williams, W. L., Abney, T. O., Chernoff, H. N., Dukelow, W. R., and Pinsker, M. C., 1967, Biochemistry and physiology of decapacitation factor. *J. Reprod. Fertil. Suppl.* **2**:11–23.

Williams, W. L., Robertson, R. T., and Dukelow, W. R., 1970, Decapacitation factor and capacitation, in: *Advances in the Biosciences.* Vol. 4 (G. Raspe, ed.), Pergamon Press, New York, pp. 61–72.

Yanagimachi, R., 1969, *In vitro* capacitation of hamster spermatozoa by follicular fluid, *J. Reprod. Fertil.* **18**:275–286.

Yanagimachi, R., 1972, Fertilization of guinea pig eggs *in vitro, Anat. Rec.* **174**:9–20.

Yanagimachi, R., 1975, Acceleration of the acrosome reaction and activation of guinea pig spermatozoa by detergents and other reagents, *Biol. Reprod.* **13**:519–526.

Yanagimachi, R., and Chang, M. C., 1963, Fertilization of hamster eggs *in vitro, Nature (London)* **200**:281–282.

Yanagimachi, R., and Usui, N., 1974, Calcium dependence of the acrosome reaction and activation of guinea-pig spermatozoa, *Exp. Cell Res.* **89**:161–174.

Zaneveld, L. J. D., and Williams, W. L., 1970, A sperm enzyme that disperses the corona radiata and its inhibition by decapacitation factor, *Biol. Reprod.* **2**:363–368.

2

OVUM COLLECTION AND INDUCED LUTEAL DYSFUNCTION IN PRIMATES

OLIVIER KREITMANN, WILBERT E. NIXON, and GARY D. HODGEN

Recent advances in extracorporeal (*in vitro*) fertilization (IVF) and embryo transfer (ET) have demonstrated the applicability of this technique for the treatment of human infertility due to irreparable tubal dysfunction (Lopata *et al.*, 1980; Steptoe and Edwards, 1979). However, the rate of success remains extremely limited. The reasons for frequent failures are difficult to identify and overcome because stepwise laboratory research from human gamete collection to implantation of the embryo is constrained ethically and legally in many societies (Walters, 1979). Clearly, experimental studies that consider separately each step in the sequence of IVF and ET provide maximal opportunities for improved success rates for infertile couples.

Accordingly, we have undertaken an orderly sequence of laboratory studies in nonhuman primates, each experiment being designed for independent assessment of conditions affecting succeeding steps. This series of evaluations includes: (1) timing aspiration of the preovulatory follicle; (2) effects on corpus luteum function; (3) spontaneous versus induced folliculogenesis; (4) estimating oocyte fertilizability; (5) semen preparation; (6) conditions for sperm–egg interaction and IVF; (7) extracorporeal embryonic development; (8) the contemporaneous sequelae of ovarian and endometrial changes in the maternal milieu; and (9) embryo transfer and implantation. In addition, we have pursued development of alternatives to IVF and ET,

OLIVIER KREITMANN, WILBERT E. NIXON, and GARY D. HODGEN • Pregnancy Research Branch, National Institute of Child Health and Human Development, National Institutes of Health, Bethesda, Maryland 20205.

specifically, low tubal ovum transfer, to preserve the inherent biological and ethical advantages of *in vivo* fertilization. As indicated by the results presented here, the hominoid anatomical and endocrine characteristics inherent to the menstrual cycles of these surrogate primates [rhesus (*Macaca mulatta*) and cynomolgus (*Macaca fascicularis*) monkeys] establish their relevance. Here, we present observations on ovum collection from the preovulatory follicle and induced luteal dysfunction in nonhuman primates.

Ovum Collection

Theoretically, oocytes for IVF may be obtained from three sources: (1) maturation *in vitro* of immature oocytes from small follicles; (2) the "ripe" oocyte in the single, spontaneous preovulatory follicle of the normal menstrual cycle; and (3) multiple oocytes from follicles induced to grow after human menopausal gonadotropin (hMG) or clomiphene therapy. The present discussion emphasizes ovum collection from the single spontaneous dominant follicle.

Typically, only a few hours before ovulation the oocyte achieves maturation; that is, a status conducive to its subsequent fertilization in the fallopian tube is acquired. Premature removal of the oocyte from this intrafollicular environment drastically reduces the fertilizability of the ovum. Although techniques for successful and timely aspiration of the preovulatory oocyte have been developed in women (Edwards, 1973; Lopata *et al.*, 1980; Soupart and Morgenstern, 1973), extensive similar studies have not been reported for rhesus and cynomolgus monkeys.

Among the reasons for frequent failures of IVF is the difficulty of timely ovum collection; that is, how to obtain a fertilizable egg while avoiding imminent spontaneous rupture of the preovulatory follicle. Further, aspiration of the preovulatory follicle necessarily requires removal of follicular fluid, granulosa cells, and, it is hoped, the ovum. Indeed, when greater vigor is applied at aspiration to enhance the prospects of ovum retrieval, the potential for dysfunctional sequelae is also increased. Earlier reports have warned of potential consequences of removing follicular fluid and granulosa cells on subsequent corpus lutem function (Steptoe and Edwards, 1970).

In an earlier report employing a primate model (Kreitmann and Hodgen, 1980), we noted that among the effects of aspiration of the dominant follicle was an increased incidence of luteal phase defects in monkeys, manifest as abnormalities in patterns of progesterone in circulation. As spontaneous luteal dysfunction described in women (Askel, 1980) and monkeys (Wilks *et al.*, 1976) is often associated with infertility (Jones, 1979; Batzer, 1980; Rosenberg *et al.*, 1980), the apparent induction of luteal phase defects in some monkeys, as a result of follicular aspiration, suggests this too may be a contributing factor to failures in achieving and maintaining pregnancy after IVF and ET.

Aspiration of the Spontaneous Preovulatory Follicle

We began monitoring the progression of follicular phase hormonal events on Day 8 of the menstrual cycle by rapid radioimmunoassay (RIA) of serum E_2 (Goodman *et al.*, 1977; Hodgen *et al.*, 1974) and eventually LH. Laparoscopy was performed when two consecutive daily values of serum E_2 had exceeded 150 pg/ml and was confirmed by an LH surge usually 12–20 hr earlier, indicating the presence of a near-ovulatory follicle. More recently, we have found it necessary to measure serum LH more frequently, such as at 6-hr intervals. This markedly improved the predictability of follicular status. When the visual assessment was consistent with these hormonal indices of imminent ovulation, the dominant follicle was aspirated using a 22-gauge needle mounted on a 12-cc syringe containing 2–3 ml of warm, equilibrated (5% CO_2, 95% air) BWW medium (Biggers *et al.*, 1971) without bovine serum albumin (BSA). In most instances, the antral cavity was gently flushed two to three times in order to maximize the rate of ovum recovery. The contents of the aspirate were examined under a dissecting microscope immediately thereafter. The oocyte, when present, was classified as apparently mature, intermediate, or immature on the basis of morphological criteria (Soupart and Morgenstern, 1973; Edwards and Steptoe, 1975; Kreitmann and Hodgen, 1980); that is, the surrounding corona—cumulus investment, the presence or absence of a germinal vesicle in the ooplasm, or the first polar body in the perivitelline space.

At laparoscopy, we collected 31 oocytes from among 40 aspirates (recovery rate of 77.5%). By our subjective assessments 12 were fully mature (38.7%), 6 intermediate (19.3%), 10 immature (32.2%), and 3 atretic (9.6%). These differences in apparent ovum maturity reflect at least two primary sources of variation: (1) our limited ability to accurately assess (predict) the status of the preovulatory follicle and (2) inherent disparities between serum hormonal indices, oocyte maturity, and time of spontaneous follicular rupture.

In order to quantify the number of granulosa cells removed in the aspirate from the preovulatory follicle, the specimen was gently spun in a clinical centrifuge and incubated (37°C, 10 min) in Ham's F10 medium containing 25 mM Hepes buffer, 2% BSA, and 0.2% collagenase (Millipore Corp., 183 U/mg). After dissociation of the granulosa cells, an aliquot was used for cell counting in a hemocytometer.

Low Tubal Ovum Transfer and *in Vivo* Fertilization

That some of the eggs aspirated from these preovulatory follicles were fertilizable was demonstrated by a new experimental procedure, *low tubal ovum transfer*, developed in rhesus and cynomolgus monkeys and having

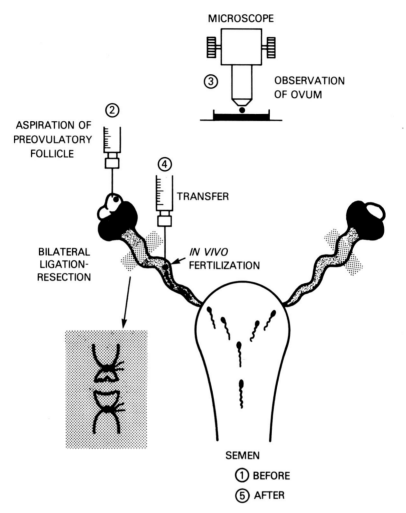

MICROSCOPE

③ OBSERVATION OF OVUM

② ASPIRATION OF PREOVULATORY FOLLICLE

④ TRANSFER

BILATERAL LIGATION-RESECTION

IN VIVO FERTILIZATION

SEMEN

① BEFORE

⑤ AFTER

Figure 1. Diagram of primate model for *low tubal ovum transfer*. The sequence of events is as follows: (1) Female copulates with fertile male; (2) laparoscopy for collection of the oocyte by aspiration of the preovulatory follicle; (3) microscopic examination of the ovum; (4) injection of the ovum into proximal region of the fallopian tube, beyond the point of obstruction; and (5) female copulates with fertile male again. (From Kreitmann and Hodgen, 1980.)

potential as a partial alternative to IVF. The ovum was aspirated from the dominant follicle of the monkey during laparoscopy immediately preceding the expected time of ovulation, as described, and injected into the lumen of the fallopian tube 1.0 to 2.0 cm above the utero-tubal junction (Figure 1). Previously, at laparotomy these monkeys underwent bilateral tubal resection and litigation of the ampullary region to simulate upper tubal obstruction.

After being mated the day before and after low tubal ovum transfer, several monkeys became pregnant (Table I), thereby preserving the efficiency and safety inherent to *in vivo* fertilization and confirming the quality of these ova collected from the near-ovulatory follicle.

Evaluation of Corpus Luteum Function

The normalcy of the luteal phase was examined in three ways: (1) progesterone secretion *in vivo*, as measured by the integrated area under the curves of peripheral levels during the 15 days following follicular aspiration; (2) *in vivo* response of the progesterone secretory pattern to exogenous human chorionic gonadotropin (hCG) (25 IU of hCG i.m. for 3 days in the midluteal phase); and (3) response of luteal cells to hCG *in vitro* (luteectomy being performed 4–6 days following follicular aspiration). For *in vitro* studies, luteal cells were dissociated with collagenase (Stouffer *et al.*, 1976) and counted. The dilution of dispersed luteal cells (Ham's F10, 25 mM Hepes, 1% BSA) was constant at 10^6 cells/ml, and progesterone production over approximately 4.30 hr with or without added hCG (100 ng/ml CR119) was determined by RIA (Stouffer *et al.*, 1977).

Induced Corpus Luteum Dysfunction

Among 21 complete menstrual cycles, where it was possible to thoroughly assess the consequences of aspirating the preovulatory follicle, two types of luteal phase defects were observed; that is, overt aberrations in patterns of serum progesterone. Necessarily, we had to assign arbitrary criteria to identify those cycles in which progesterone levels in circulation were

Table I
Pregnancies after *Low Tubal Ovum Transfer* in Monkeys[a]

Number of monkeys successful/total	Percent	Progression of events from follicular maturation through pregnancy
40/55	72.7	Avoidance of spontaneous rupture of the dominant follicle
31[b]/40	77.5	Ovum collected during aspiration of the preovulatory follicle
5[c]/31	16.1	Positive pregnancy tests for mCG[d]

[a]From Kreitmann and Hodgen (1980).
[b]Twenty of these oocytes were judged to be immature on the basis of morphological criteria. Larger numbers of granulosa cells on the oocyte were associated with immaturity and varying degrees of progesterone-deficient luteal dysfunction.
[c]Tubal resection and ligation was not performed on one monkey, but the ovum was transferred to the contralateral fallopian tube.
[d]In none of these five pregnancies was the site of implantation ectopic (tubal).

profoundly abnormal in the pattern of secretion and/or diminished integrated areas under the curve throughout the luteal phase. Accordingly, corpus luteum dysfunction was defined here as less than 50% of the normal serum progesterone concentrations during 7 or more successive days of the luteal phase.

As illustrated in Figure 2, several monkeys displayed defective patterns of progesterone in circulation, such that the curve was heavily skewed to the right as compared to normal (Edwards and Steptoe, 1975; Kreitmann *et al.*, 1981; Hodgen *et al.*, 1976). Although the mean levels of progesterone secretion ultimately attained in the late luteal phase did reach normal

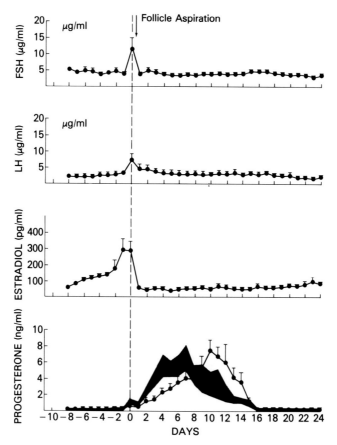

Figure 2. Peripheral serum levels of FSH, LH, E₂, and P in monkeys (N = 5) after aspiration of the spontaneous preovulatory follicle. Each value is the mean ± S.E. Data are normalized to the day of gonadotropin surge. The shaded area illustrates the normal pattern of serum P concentrations as previously reported (Hodgen *et al.*, 1976).

maxima, serum progesterone concentrations were consistently below those expected through the initial 7 to 8 days following aspiration of the preovulatory follicle. The patterns of pituitary gonadotropins and ovarian steroids in the antecedent follicular phase and the length of the luteal phase were normal. Following injection of hCG in the late luteal phase, to mimic "rescue" of the corpus luteum by endogenous chorionic gonadotropin in fertile menstrual cycles, serum progesterone levels were markedly enhanced and the coming menses was transiently deferred (Figure 4, 377J and 937G in upper panels).

A second type of luteal phase defect was seen in several cycles and is depicted in Figure 3. Here, the pattern of progesterone secretion remained uniformly low (inadequate) throughout the luteal phase defect. Some of these luteal phases tended to be slightly foreshortened as well, when the ensuing menses resumed within 11 or 12 days after follicular aspiration. The foregoing follicular phases were uneventful. Despite hCG administration in the late luteal phase to monkeys manifesting inadequate luteal function, the corpus luteum was unresponsive (Figure 4, 950G and 356J in lower panels).

Assessment of Luteal Cell Function *in Vitro*

Among monkeys manifesting the early phase aberration (shown in Figure 2), luteectomy was performed in the early- to midluteal phase of five such cycles to permit *in vitro* evaluation of luteal cell function. As expected, surgical ablation of the corpus luteum led to an abrupt decline in serum progesterone and early onset of menstruation (Kreitmann *et al.*, 1981). Except for the low progesterone concentrations in the early luteal phase prior to luteectomy, antecedent hormonal indices of these cycles were compatible with normal ovulatory menstrual cycles. When these dispersed luteal cells were incubated with and without hCG, progesterone production was low under basal conditions and strikingly elevated ($p < 0.05$) by hCG. Our findings suggest near-normal functional integrity of these luteal cells under hCG stimulation, despite earlier subnormal progesterone production.

Correlation between Granulosa Cell Loss and Luteal Phase Progesterone Deficiencies

The number of granulosa cells in the aspirate varied widely from 10×10^3 to 1710×10^3 ($491 \times 10^3 \pm 69 \times 10^3$; $\bar{x} \pm$ S.E.). This number can represent as much as 20% of the total number of luteal cells found in the monkey corpus luteum, although usually a lesser portion is lost during aspiration of the preovulatory follicle (Kreitmann *et al.*, 1981). Further, we notice extensive morphological heterogeneity among these granulosa cells; that is, the size and

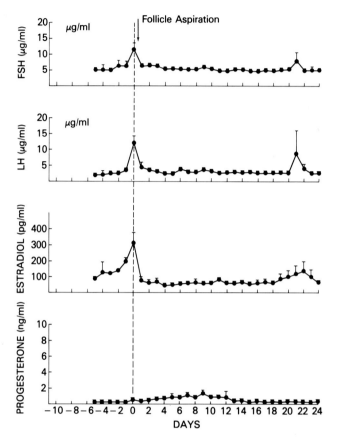

Figure 3. Peripheral serum levels of FSH, LH, E₂, and P in monkeys (N = 7) after aspiration of the spontaneous preovulatory follicle. Each value is the mean ± S.E. Data are normalized to the day of gonadotropin surge. (From Kreitmann *et al.*, 1981.)

density of granulations on their cell surfaces varied. Clearly, among follicles most susceptible to granulosa cell loss, progesterone secretion was lowest (r = 0.86). Conversely, overall progesterone secretion from the corpus luteum was greater when the preovulatory follicle yielded fewer granulosa cells at the time of aspiration. However, this relationship was not absolute, in that some monkeys displayed normal or near-normal luteal function despite loss of relatively large number of granulosa cells. Also, hCG-stimulated progesterone production by dispersed luteal cells *in vitro* was inversely related to the number of granulosa cells aspirated (Kreitmann *et al.*, 1981).

Induced Folliculogenesis

An alternative approach to ovum collection has been induction of multiple follicular maturation by exogenous gonadotropin or clomiphene

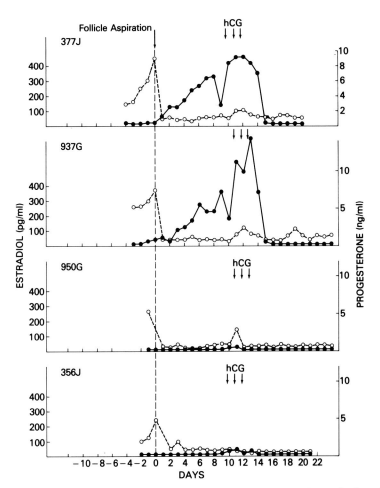

Figure 4. Peripheral serum levels of FSH, LH, E$_2$, and P in monkeys after aspiration of the spontaneous preovulatory follicle. Data are normalized to the day of follicle aspiration. (From Kreitmann *et al.*, 1981.)

treatment (Lopata *et al.*, 1978; Steptoe and Edwards, 1970). Numerous related studies have been conducted in nonhuman primates; these were recently reviewed by ʹKraemer (Kraemer *et al.*, 1979). Most efforts were directed toward achieving superovulation. For instance, an enhanced ovulation rate was obtained in rhesus monkeys given nMG for 10–12 days (total dose 750–900 IU FSH, i.m.), followed by hCG (2000 IU, i.m.) (Breckwoldt *et al.*, 1971). In cynomolgus monkeys, pregnant mare's serum gonadotropins (PMSG) and hCG have been used with success (Jainudeen and Hafez, 1973). In squirrel monkeys (*Saimiri sciureus*), PMSG or porcine FSH, and hCG were used (Bennett, 1967; Dukelow, 1970a,b). Also, baboons (*Papio cynocephalus*) were stimulated to superovulation by PMSG and hMG

(Kraemer et al., 1979), and oocytes collected from the oviducts after ovulation. Generally, these treatments result in a wide variability of responses between individuals and little control over the number of follicles stimulated into maturational development and ovulation. Further, these treatments are notoriously associated with progressive ovarian refractoriness to gonadotropins (Batta et al., 1978; Kraemer et al., 1979) and development of antibodies to heterologous gonadotropins (Batta et al., 1978; Bennett et al., 1973). Both the poor fertilizability of monkey eggs and the high rate of aberrant luteal function after induced ovulations illustrate the need for more study on these problems.

Discussion and Conclusions

The data presented indicate that overt luteal dysfunction can be introduced as a consequence of ovum collection by aspiration of the dominant follicle even after the preovulatory gonadotropin surges. The induced luteal phase defects varied both in degrees and the manner of their manifestation of deficiencies in progesterone secretion. Further, we noted a strong correlation ($r = -0.86$) between the number of granulosa cells removed, along with the ovum and follicular fluid, and subsequent aberrant luteal function.

Several issues deserve individual attention. First, although the incidence of corpus luteum dysfunction was apparently increased following aspiration of the near-ovulatory follicle, overt aberrations were found in less than one-half of the monkeys studied. Further, we cannot exclude from these observations the possibility of spontaneous corpus luteum dysfunction (Wilks et al., 1976; Aksel, 1980; Jones, 1979; Seppala et al., 1976; Strott et al., 1970). Second, the degree and type of luteal phase defect manifest may depend in part on both the timeliness of the aspiration and the vigor applied to enhance the rate of ovum collection; that is, premature and/or thorough evacuation of antral components may remove granulosa cells in greater numbers and/or preclude adequate exposure to the follicular fluid milieu of those cells remaining in situ. Among monkeys manifesting the lag in establishing full corpus luteum function, we offer two interpretations: (1) that the granulosa cells most vulnerable to loss in the aspirate were "destined" to be the principal source of progesterone secretion in the early luteal phase, and (2) that premature denial of the intraantral milieu may have delayed potentiation of luteal cell secretory potential, particularly when the changes mediated by the LH/FSH surge were incomplete at the time of follicular aspiration. Third, except when the serum progesterone pattern was grossly inadequate, luteal cells remained highly responsive to hCG both in vivo and in vitro, suggesting that marginal progesterone deficiences arising after ovum collection from the preovulatory follicle may be treatable by administration of either exogenous chorionic gonadotropin or progesterone. This is in striking constrast to spontaneous luteal dysfunction as a sequel to aberrant endogenous gonadotropin stimulation during follicular maturation (Stouffer and Hodgen, 1980; Wilks *et al.*, 1976; Aksel, 1980; Strott *et al.*, 1970), where progesterone rather than hCG has been more efficacious (Jones, 1979; Rosenberg *et al.*, 1980).

This primate model suggests that aspiration of the preovulatory follicle for ovum collection and IVF increases the incidence of luteal phase defects sufficiently to threaten fertility rates. Indeed, we do not know the minimal serum progesterone threshold necessary to initiate and maintain pregnancy in these nonhuman primates or women. The findings presented indicate the necessity for similar clinical investigations to scrutinize thoroughly the effects of follicular aspiration on corpus luteum function as a potential contributing factor in failures to achieve and sustain pregnancy after IVF and ET in humans.

ACKNOWLEDGMENTS

We gratefully acknowledge the expert technical assistance of Ms. Lydia Yuan, Mr. Don Barber, Mr. Arthur Tanner, Mr. James Lewis, Mr. Webster Coleman, Mr. Rudy Reid, and Mr. Charles Turner and the skillful secretarial assistance of Ms. Linda Baldwin.

The work was supported by the Délégation Générale à la Recherche Scientifique et Technique, Paris.

References

Askel, S., 1980, Sporadic and recurrent luteal phase defects in cyclic women: Comparison with normal cycles, *Fertil. Steril.* **33**:372.

Batta, S. K., Stark, R. A., and Brackett, B. G., 1978, Ovulation induction by gonadotropin and prostaglandin treatments of rhesus monkeys and observations of the ova, *Biol. Reprod.* **18**:264.

Batzer, F. R., 1980, Hormonal evaluation of early pregnancy, *Fertil. Steril.* **34**:1.

Bennett, J. P., 1967, The induction of ovulation in the squirrel monkey (*Saimiri sciureus*) with pregnant mares serum (PMS) and human chorionic gonadotropin (HCG), *J. Reprod. Fertil.* **13**:357.

Bennett, W. I., Dufau, M. L., Catt, K. J., and Tullner, W. W., 1973, Effect of human menopausal gonadotropin upon spermatogenesis and testosterone production in juvenile rhesus monkeys, *Endocrinology* **92**:813.

Biggers, J. D., Whitten, W. K., and Whittingham, D. G., 1971, The culture of mouse embryos *in vitro*, in: *Methods in Mammalian Embryology* (J. C. Danile, ed.), Academic Press, New York, p. 86.

Breckwoldt, M., Bettendorf, G., and Garcia, C. R., 1971, Induction of ovulation in noncycling and hypophysectomized rhesus monkeys with various human gonadotropins, *Fertil. Steril.* **22**:7.

Dukelow, W. R., 1970a, Induction and timing of single and multiple ovulations in the squirrel monkey (*Saimiri sciureus*), *J. Reprod. Fertil.* **22**:303.

Dukelow, W. R., 1970b, Reproductive physiology of primates, *Mich. Agric. Exp. Stn. J.* article No. 5262.

Edwards, R. G., 1973, Studies on human conception, *Am. J. Obstet. Gynecol.* **117**:587.

Edwards, R. G., and Steptoe, P. C., 1975, Induction of follicular growth, ovulation and luteinization in the human ovary, *J. Reprod. Fertil. Suppl.* **22**:121.

Goodman, A. L., Nixon, W. E., Johnson, D. K., and Hodgen, G. D., 1977, Regulation of folliculogenesis in the cycling rhesus monkey: Selection of the dominant follicle, *Endocrinology* **100**:155.

Hodgen, G. D., Tullner, W. W., Vaitukaitis, J. L., Ward, D. N., and Ross, G. T., 1974, Specific radioimmunoassay of chorionic gonadotropin during implantation in rhesus monkeys, *J. Clin. Endocrinol. Metab.* **39**:457.

Hodgen, G. D., Wilks, J. W., Vaitukaitis, J. L., Chen, H., Papkoff, H., and Ross, G. T., 1976, A new radioimmunoassay for follicle-stimulating hormone in macaques: Ovulatory menstrual cycles, *Endocrinology* **99**:137.

Jainudeen, M. R., and Hafez, E. S. E., 1973, Gonadotropin-induced multiple ovulation in the crab-eating monkey, *Macaca fascicularis, J. Reprod. Fertil.* **33**:151.

Jones, G. S., 1979, The luteal phase defect, in: *Modern Trends in Infertility and Conception Control,* Volume 1 (E. E. Wallach and R. D. Kempers, eds.), Waverly Press, Baltimore, p. 151.

Kraemer, D. C., Flow, B. L., Schriver, M. D., Kinney, G. M., and Pennycook, J. W., 1979, Embryotransfer in the non-human primate, feline and canine, *Theriogenology* **11**:51.

Kreitmann, O., and Hodgen, G. D., 1980, Low tubal ovum transfer: An alternative to *in vitro* fertilization, *Fertil. Steril.* **34**:375.

Kreitmann, O., Nixon, W. E., and Hodgen, G. D., 1981, Induced corpus luteum dysfunction after aspiration of the preovulatory follicle in monkeys, *Fertil. Steril.* **35**:671.

Lopata, A., McMaster, R., McBain, J. C., and Johnston, W. I. H., 1978, *In vitro* fertilization of preovulatory human eggs, *J. Reprod. Fertil.* **52**:339.

Lopata, A., Johnston, W. H., Hoult, I. J., and Speirs, A. I., 1980, Pregnancy following intrauterine implantation of an embryo obtained by *in vitro* fertilization of a preovulatory egg, *Fertil. Steril.* **33**:117.

Rosenberg, S. M., Luciano, A. A., and Riddick, D. H., 1980, The luteal phase defect: The relative frequency of, and encouraging response to, treatment with vaginal progesterone, *Fertil. Steril.* **34**:17.

Seppala, M., Hirvonen, E., and Rauta, T., 1976. Hyperprolactinemia and luteal insufficiency, *Lancet* **1**:229.

Soupart, P., and Morgenstern, L. L., 1973, Human sperm capacitation and *in vitro* fertilization, *Fertil. Steril.* **24**:462.

Steptoe, P. C., and Edwards, R. G., 1970, Laparoscopic recovery of preovulatory human oocytes after priming of ovaries with gonadotropins, *Lancet* **1**:683.

Steptoe, P. C., and Edwards, R. G., 1979, Report on human *in vitro* fertilization and embryotransfer, Meeting of the Royal College of Obstetricians and Gynecologists, London, January 26.

Stouffer, R. L., and Hodgen, G. D., 1980, Induction of luteal phase defects in rhesus monkeys by follicular fluid administration at the onset of the menstrual cycle, *J. Clin. Endocrinol. Metab.* **51**:669.

Stouffer, R. L., Nixon, W. E., Gulyas, B. J., Johnson, D. K., and Hodgen, G. D., 1976, *In vitro* evaluation of corpus luteum function of cycling and pregnant rhesus monkeys: Progesterone production by dispersed luteal cells, *Steroids* **27**:543.

Stouffer, R. L., Nixon, W. E., Gulyas, B. J., and Hodgen, G. D., 1977, Gonadotropin-sensitive progesterone production by rhesus monkey luteal cells *in vitro*: A function of age of the corpus luteum during the menstrual cycle, *Endocrinology* **100**:506.

Strott, C. A., Cargille, C. M., Ross, G. T., and Lipsett, M. B., 1970, The short luteal phase, *J. Clin. Endocrinol. Metab.* **30**:256.

Walters, L., 1979, Ethical issues in human *in vitro* fertilization and research involving early human embryos, in: *Ethics Advisory Board on Research involving human in vitro fertilization and embryotransfer*, May 4, Washington, D.C.

Wilks, J. W., Hodgen, G. D., and Ross, G. T., 1976, Luteal phase defects in the rhesus monkey: The significance of serum FSH:LH ratios, *J. Clin. Endocrinol. Metab.* **43**:3699.

3

ANALYSIS OF CULTURE MEDIA FOR *IN VITRO* FERTILIZATION AND CRITERIA FOR SUCCESS

BARRY D. BAVISTER

In mammals, fertilization takes place in a protected and well-controlled environment within the oviduct. Due to the obvious difficulty of studying fertilization *in situ*, *in vitro* fertilization techniques have been utilized in an attempt to understand this crucial stage of embryonic development. In these procedures, the male and female gametes are brought together in a suspending medium that is intended to provide satisfactory conditions for sperm penetration, fertilization, and cleavage to occur.

We should be able to derive useful information on these topics from the study of animal models; after all, *in vitro* fertilization in animal species has been possible for the past 25 years (see Blandau, 1980), stemming from the breakthrough discovery of the need for sperm capacitation (Austin, 1951; Chang, 1951). However, *in vitro* fertilization procedures are not as well defined, nor as successful in general, as might be expected after all this time. From the viewpoint of successful fertilization *in vitro* (and subsequent development as evidence of its normalcy), species may be divided into four categories, as follows.

1. Fertilization *in vitro* proven successful. Substantial or complete preimplantation development *in vitro*; proof of the normalcy of fertilization by birth of normal offspring after transfer of embryos (usually at an early cleavage stage). To date, only the rabbit, mouse, rat, and human are included in this category. Culture conditions for fertilization and development *in vitro* in the rat are less well defined

BARRY D. BAVISTER • Wisconsin Regional Primate Research Center, Madison, Wisconsin 53706.

than in the rabbit and mouse; little is known of optimal conditions for the human.

2. Fertilization apparently successful. High degree of reproducibility obtained in some instances; insufficient evidence of the normalcy of fertilization because of lack of data on the developmental potential of the embryos *in vitro*; no reported success with embryos transferred to recipient females. The hamster, guinea pig, cat, and dog are in this category.

3. Success with *in vitro* fertilization sporadic. Procedures not yet well defined; limited embryonic development *in vitro*; no successful embryo transfers following *in vitro* fertilization attempts. *Examples:* bovine, pig, nonhuman primates, and sheep.

4. No success reported at all. *Examples:* goat, horse.

Summarizing these observations, it seems reasonable to conclude that, at present, the "art" of fertilizing mammalian oocytes *in vitro* and subsequently obtaining full, normal development is not in a highly advanced state. This situation might be improved by critically analyzing each of the basic components of the *in vitro* fertilization system, in an attempt to uncover those areas in need of investigation. These basic components are obvious: the investigators, the spermatozoa and oocytes, and the culture media. The investigator is a variable component: different investigators often obtain different results, even when using the same technique. Moreover, there is no doubt that an individual investigator's expertise improves (sometimes dramatically) with time and experience, and in some undefinable way (probably the speed of handling the gametes is a major factor), the success rate with *in vitro* fertilization increases proportionately. Other contributors to this volume will address the involved questions of how to collect and treat spermatozoa and oocytes in ways most conducive to successful fertilization *in vitro*. I will attempt to describe some of the difficulties involved in (and raised by) the use of culture media to support fertilization.

Culture Media

The culture medium provides the milieu for essential changes to occur in spermatozoa (i.e., capacitation and the acrosome reaction) and supports the fertilization process itself. Several different techniques have been described for the accomplishment of fertilization *in vitro*, but a simple and successful one consists of placing a drop (50 μl) of culture medium in a plastic petri dish, covering it with a layer of mineral oil, equilibrating with 5% CO_2 in air, and then adding eggs and spermatozoa. The dish is incubated at 37°C for several hours and the eggs then examined for morphological evidence of fertilization (see the section Criteria for Success and Figures 2 and 5). This technique is borrowed from the method first described by Brinster (1963) for the culture of mouse embryos.

Most of the available information on culture media for *in vitro* fertilization comes from studies with four species: the rabbit, mouse, hamster, and guinea pig. By analyzing the conditions that permit successful fertilization *in vitro* and making suitable modifications, we could most probably increase the reliability and effectiveness of these methods. In addition, we might then be able to achieve fertilization *in vitro* with some of the "difficult" species referred to above. Last, but not least, we might gain some insight into the mechanisms involved in mammalian fertilization.

In a few studies, complex culture media were used for *in vitro* fertilization, e.g., TC 199, Ham's F10, or media were supplemented with

Table I

Simple Culture Media Used for *in Vitro* Fertilization

Species	Culture medium	Investigator(s)
Mouse	Toyoda[a]	Toyoda *et al.* (1971)
	BWW[a]	Miyamoto and Chang (1972, 1973b)
	Toyoda[a]	Miyamoto and Chang (1973a)
	Cross-Brinster[a]	Oliphant and Brackett (1973)
	Whitten[a]	Hoppe and Pitts (1973)
	Whittingham[a]	Fraser and Drury (1975)
	Brinster[a]	Wolf *et al.* (1976)
Rat	Toyoda[a]	Toyoda and Chang (1974a)
	Shalgi[a]	Shalgi *et al.* (1980)
Guinea pig	BWW[a]	Yanagimachi (1972)
	BWW[a]	Rogers and Yanagimachi (1975)
	MCM	Rogers and Yanagimachi (1975)
	Tyrode[b]	Rogers and Yanagimachi (1975)
Rabbit	Brackett	Fraser *et al.* (1971)
	Brackett	Brackett and Oliphant (1975)
Dog	BWW[a]	Mahi and Yanagimachi (1976)
	CCM	Mahi and Yanagimachi (1978)
Hamster	Tyrode	Yanagimachi and Chang (1964)
	Bavister[b]	Bavister (1969)
	Toyoda[a]	Parkening and Chang (1976)
	TALP[b]	Bavister and Yanagimachi (1977)
	BWW[a]	Hirao and Yanagimachi (1978)
Human	Bavister[b,c]	Edwards *et al.* (1969)
	Bavister[b,c]	Soupart and Morgenstern (1973)
	Lopata	Lopata *et al.* (1978)

[a] Modification of KRB.
[b] Modification of Tyrode's solution.
[c] Modified from original medium.

blood serum or with follicular fluid. It is very difficult to analyze the significance of different parameters under these complex conditions. The most common types of culture media, however, are simple balanced salt solutions (so called because they contain the major ions found in blood in approximately the correct proportions), supplemented with energy substrates and with protein (serum albumin). All subsequent comments are restricted to these varieties of simple culture media.

Many different culture medium formulations have been used successfully for *in vitro* fertilization of mammalian oocytes (Table I). In all, 14 apparently different culture media are listed here, and these have been used to fertilize oocytes of seven species. However, closer inspection reveals that many of these media are slight modifications of Krebs–Ringer bicarbonate solution (KRB) and several more are based on Tyrode's solution. Both of these solutions were formulated on the ions in human blood serum. Table II shows the results of an analysis of the culture media in Table I. Four parameters of extracellular fluid that are known to be important for somatic cell function have been studied in these media: ionic composition, energy sources, osmotic pressure, and protein component. These parameters are discussed below.

Ionic Composition. The ratios of the principal physiological cations [and ionic concentrations (not shown)] and the concentrations of chloride and bicarbonate all appear to be spread over a wide range, but this impression is due to one or two unusual formulations; values for the majority of the culture media fall within a narrow range, as shown by the small standard errors (Table

Table II
Analysis of 14 Culture Media Used for *in Vitro* Fertilization[a]

	Component	Range[b]	Mean ± S.E.M.[b]
Ions	Na^+/K^+ ratio	20–53	29.3 ± 2.9
	Ca^{2+}/Mg^{2+} ratio	1.4–5.6	2.76 ± 0.42
	Chloride concn.	77–138	110.0 ± 5.2
	Bicarbonate concn.	11–38	25.5 ± 2.1
Energy sources	Glucose	5.6 mM[c]	
	Lactate	10–25 mM[d]	
	Pyruvate	0.1–1.25 mM	
Other	Osmotic pressure	285–310 mOsM	
	pH	7.2–7.8	
	Protein (bovine serum albumin)	1–5 mg/ml[c]	

[a]See culture media listed in Table I.
[b]Ranges and means for ions from concentrations in meq/liter.
[c]Two exceptions.
[d]Three exceptions.

Table III
Ionic Composition of Mammalian Blood Serum[a]

Species	Component			
	Na^+/K^+	Ca^{2+}/Mg^{2+}	Cl^-	HCO_3^-
Mouse	NR[b]	3.8	NR	NR
Rabbit	25.6	1.5	105	28
Rat	25.7	4.8	118	21
Monkey	33.4	NR	115	NR
Human	34.4	2.7	103	26
Sheep	28.9	3.0	116	NR
·Pig	24.0	4.3	NR	NR
Bull	24.6	3.25	NR	NR

[a] Data from Altman (1961). Values for ionic ratios calculated from ion concentrations in meq/liter; values for Cl^- and HCO_3^- are meq/liter.
[b] NR, not reported.

II). For comparative purposes, the ionic composition of mammalian blood sera is shown in Table III. It is evident that for the parameters shown, culture media used for *in vitro* fertilization are similar in composition to blood serum.

The importance of bicarbonate concentration, which is a major component of the pH buffering system, will be discussed later. Culture media with the ionic characteristics described in Table II have been used successfully to fertilize oocytes of seven species (rabbit, mouse, guinea pig, hamster, rat, dog, and human) representing four orders of mammals. It is therefore tempting to assume that the mean ionic composition shown in Table II is the optimal one for mammalian fertilization *in vitro*. This is a dangerous conclusion, however, for the following reasons:

1. Very little is known about the effects of different ionic ratios and concentrations on fertilization, and there is a real need to investigate this in a critical manner. Values different from those shown in Table II might give higher or more consistent results. The demonstrated success with fertilization (in several species) in these media may simply reflect the tolerance of the gametes to these conditions; the gametes of some other species may not be able to tolerate the narrow range of ionic composition that is commonly used (Table II). This difference could at least partly explain the difficulty in fertilizing oocytes of some species *in vitro*.

2. A study in the rat showed that a low Na^+/K^+ ratio (3.1) enhanced the ability of the culture medium to support fertilization (Toyoda and Chang, 1974b). The concentration of K^+ ions in the culture medium was shown to be an important determinant of the ability of hamster

spermatozoa to undergo acrosome reactions (Mrsny and Meizel, 1980).

3. Comparison of culture media compositions with oviduct fluid is difficult, due to species variations and to technical problems inherent in fluid sampling methods. Reported values for ionic components of oviduct fluid from several mammalian species are shown in Table IV. Clearly, there is considerable species variability in the ionic composition of oviduct fluid. In some respects (Table IV) oviduct fluid is markedly different from blood serum (Table III). If the values given in Table IV represent the ideal ionic environment for the gametes of different species, then commonly used culture media (Table II), which are based on the ionic composition of human blood serum, may not provide the optimal ionic conditions for fertilization to take place.

Energy Sources. The results of several studies have shown that glucose alone is inadequate as an energy source for supporting fertilization *in vitro* and may even be inhibitory (Rogers and Yanagimachi, 1975; Rogers *et al.*, 1979). Addition of lactate and pyruvate increases the incidence of spermatozoa undergoing an acrosome reaction, and enhances success with *in vitro* fertilization (Miyamoto and Chang, 1973a; Bavister and Yanagimachi, 1977). Judging from the low amounts of glucose reported to be present in oviduct fluid of several species ($<$ 1–1.6 mM; Holmdahl and Mastroianni,

Table IV
Ionic Composition of Oviduct Fluid from Different Species

Species	Na$^+$/K$^+$	Ca^{2+}/Mg^{2+}	Cl$^-$	HCO$_3^-$	Reference[b]
		Component[a]			
Mouse	5.4	1.5	167	NR[c]	1
Rabbit	16–26[d]		104–119[d]		2–6
		76.6			2
		57.1		28.9	3
				43.5	5
Sheep	16.6	3.8	119	21.8	7
Pig	10.9	10.8	106	NR	8
Monkey	24.2	NR	118	NR	9, 10
Human	18.1	NR	117.2	NR	11
	16.9	NR	109.4	NR	12

[a]Values for Cl$^-$ and HCO$_3^-$ are meq/liter.
[b]References: (1) Borland *et al.* (1977); (2) Iritani *et al.* (1971); (3) Hamner and Williams (1965); (4) Holmdahl and Mastroianni (1965); (5) Brunton and Brusilow (1972); (6) Mastroianni and Wallach (1961); (7) Restall and Wales (1966); (8) Iritani *et al.* (1974); (9) Mastroianni *et al.* (1969); (10 Mastroianni *et al.* (1972); (11) Lippes *et al.* (1972); (12) David *et al.* (1973).
[c]NR, not reported.
[d]Range of values reported.

1965; Iritani *et al.*, 1969, 1971, 1974; Mastroianni *et al.*, 1969), the level of glucose almost universally used in culture media (Table II) may be excessive.

Osmotic Pressure. A wide range of osmotic pressure seems to be acceptable for fertilization *in vitro*. According to Miyamoto and Chang (1973b), hamster and mouse oocytes can be fertilized in culture media with osmotic pressures of 177–496 and 250–388 mOsM, respectively. The ranges for optimal results were 270–402 and 299–365 mOsM for hamster and mouse, respectively. There are almost no data on the optimal osmotic pressures for fertilization in other species. However, no sharply defined osmotic pressure optimum has been demonstrated for *in vitro* fertilization in any mammalian species.

Protein. This may be a very important component of the culture medium. In some species (e.g., hamster, mouse), serum albumin plays an essential (but as yet undefined) role in the achievement of fertilization *in vitro* (Miyamoto and Chang, 1973a; Hoppe and Whitten, 1974; Bavister, unpublished work). It seems that protein does not simply sustain the viability of spermatozoa in culture, but also plays some specific part in the acrosome reaction (Meizel, 1978). With some other species (e.g., guinea pig), serum albumin is not essential in the culture solution, but its presence is undoubtedly beneficial (Yanagimachi, 1972). It is possible that proteins leaking from spermatozoa into the culture medium play a clandestine role in these cases. There is an obvious need for greater understanding of the way in which proteins contribute to the development of the sperm acrosome reaction; this could lead to elucidation of the mechanisms of this event, about which little is known.
Total protein levels in oviduct fluid near the time of ovulation are low compared with blood serum protein concentrations (60–80 mg/ml for most species: Altman, 1961): levels between 3 and 14 mg/ml have been reported for oviduct fluid of the pig, monkey, rabbit, sheep, and human (Hamner and Williams, 1965; Restall and Wales, 1966; Iritani *et al.*, 1969, 1971, 1974; Mastroianni *et al.*, 1969, 1972). This range is somewhat higher than the commonly used levels of protein (albumin) in culture media for *in vitro* fertilization (1–5 mg/ml). Whether or not proteins in oviductal secretions have any specific role in fertilization *in vivo* is unknown at present.

pH. The pH of the culture medium does seem to be critical. About 10 years ago, I found that increasing the pH of the culture medium was an important factor in obtaining *in vitro* fertilization in the hamster (Bavister, 1969). This approach was also helpful in achieving fertilization of human oocytes *in vitro* (Edwards *et al.*, 1969). In the hamster system, the optimum pH was found to be between 7.6 and 7.8; higher pH levels led to high incidences of polyspermic fertilization (Bavister, 1969). Later, several different pH buffers were evaluated, in an endeavor to avoid using bicarbonate–CO_2 and the inconveniences of a CO_2 atmosphere (Bavister, unpublished work). The results of this study (Table IV) showed that phosphate buffer, as might be expected, was quite useless for *in vitro* fertilization. By contrast, TES and HEPES (Good *et al.*, 1966) were efficient pH buffers, but anomalies were noted in the formation of pronuclei. Tris-citrate was an excellent buffer, and even stimulated sperm motility, but no fertilization was ever obtained with this buffer. Perhaps, in retrospect, this was due to chelation of Ca^{2+} ions. The bicarbonate–CO_2 buffer system yielded the best overall results, and although unwieldy, it has been used in my studies ever since.

In the experiments referred to above, in which a high optimal pH was found for hamster *in vitro* fertilization, the culture conditions were crude: the sperm concentration required was about $10^6/ml$, and the cumulus cells (surrounding the oocytes) and their matrix material were also needed in order to sustain sperm viability. These features contributed to a culture environment that was somewhat uncontrolled and certainly chemically undefined. It would be difficult to learn much about the mechanisms of fertilization in this situation. The discovery in follicular fluid of substances beneficial to sperm motility and fertilization by Yanagimachi (1969a,b), and the subsequent characterization of these sperm motility factors by Meizel, Bavister, and their colleagues (Bavister, 1975; Bavister *et al.*, 1979; Mrsny *et al.*, 1979; Meizel *et al.*, 1980), have led to the development of a greatly improved culture medium and procedures for *in vitro* fertilization of hamster oocytes (Bavister and Yanagimachi, 1977; Leibfried and Bavister, 1981). The culture medium is a modified Tyrode's solution containing lactate and pyruvate, and chemically defined sperm motility factors (hypotaurine and isoproterenol). No cumulus

Table V

Comparison of pH Buffers for *in Vitro* Fertilization of Hamster Oocytes

Buffer system	No. of experiments	No. of eggs seminated	No. of eggs fertilized (mean % ± S.E.)	pH control[a]
$NaHCO_3$ (25 mM)/ CO_2 (5%)	3	138	127 (99 ± 15)	−0.1
Phosphate (25 mM)	2	98	2 (0 ± 4.7)	−0.4
TES (42 mM)	5	155	51 (55.8 ± 13.3)	−0.2
HEPES (42 mM)	4	86	37 (64.2 ± 16.2)	−0.2
Tris-citrate (25 mM)	4	207	0	−0.2

[a]pH decrease over duration of experiment from starting value of 7.6.

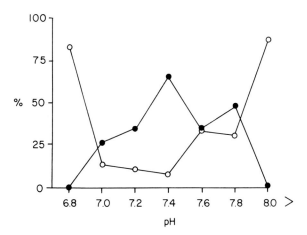

Figure 1. Optimum pH for *in vitro* fertilization of hamster oocytes. Values shown are overall percentages of totals of six experiments (three replicates); 33–37 oocytes examined at each pH level. (○) Unpenetrated oocytes are percentage of total eggs inseminated; (●) oocytes showing large, well-formed pronuclei (together with sperm tail and two polar bodies) as percentage of total eggs inseminated.

components are present, and the only significant undefined constituent is serum albumin (crystalline, fatty acid free, 3 mg/ml). Use of the sperm motility factors permits the sperm concentration to be reduced routinely to 10^4/ml, which is only 1% of the level used previously. However, fertilization can be obtained at sperm concentrations as low as 10^2/ml (Bavister, 1979). The key feature of this culture system is that the very low sperm concentration and absence of cumulus components permit a stable culture environment to be maintained for the duration of the experiment.

Preliminary data on the pH optimum for fertilization with the improved system are shown in Figure 1. Hamster epididymal spermatozoa were preincubated for 3 hr and then incubated with freshly ovulated, cumulus-free oocytes for a further 3 hr. Different pH levels were obtained in the same experiment by varying the concentrations of bicarbonate used. Criteria for assessing fertilization to be in progress were the presence of two large pronuclei of equal size, a sperm tail in the vitellus, and two polar bodies (an example is shown in Figure 2). It can be seen (Figure 1) that fertilization took place over a wide pH range (7.0–7.8), but the optimum was at pH 7.4. At pH 7.6 and above, the incidence of nonpenetrated eggs increased sharply. In this recent series of experiments with a well-defined and controlled culture environment, pH was still a crucial factor in obtaining fertilization; however, the optimum pH is now 7.4 rather than 7.6 or 7.8 as in previous work. One interpretation of these results is that the pH optimum in earlier studies was distorted by the crude culture conditions necessary at that time. The lower pH

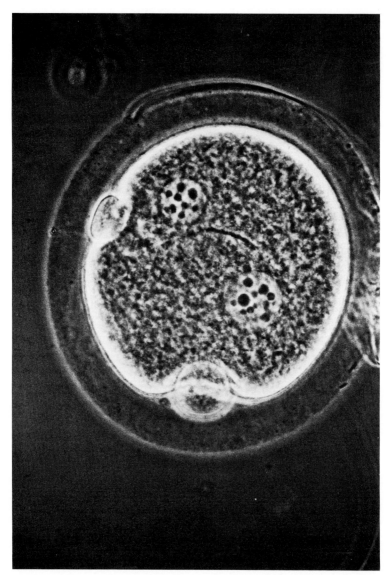

Figure 2. Typical hamster oocyte inseminated *in vitro* showing evidence of fertilization. Note large pronuclei, each with many nucleoli, in vitellus, with tail of fertilizing spermatozoon running between them, and two polar bodies at the periphery of the oocyte. Phase-contrast, unfixed, × 500.

optimum now revealed may be more compatible with continued development of *in vitro*-fertilized oocytes; it is very puzzling why hamster embryos will not undergo the second cleavage division in culture. A high pH was suggested as one reason for this failure (Whittingham and Bavister, 1974).

The hamster *in vitro* fertilization system developed in my laboratory now yields very reproducible results: we have consistently obtained at least 90% monospermic fertilization of hamster oocytes (see Figure 2) in over 25 consecutive experiments. A detailed description of the procedures used is in preparation. Approximately 80% of the inseminated oocytes will cleave to the two-cell stage in culture (Figure 3) but no further, for unknown reasons. Because it is possible to use very small numbers of spermatozoa in this system, comparable to those present at the site of fertilization *in vivo* (Bavister, 1979), we may be close to achieving optimal conditions for *in vitro* fertilization in the hamster. Unfortunately, we have no information on the normalcy and viability of the zygotes because of the two-cell block in this species.

I would like to suggest that the systematic approach of first defining the important variables in the culture system (for example, pH and sperm motility factors in the case of the hamster) and then controlling them can lead to substantial improvements in *in vitro* fertilization technology. This approach can produce increases in the percentage of fertilized oocytes and in the reliability (efficiency) of the method, and may also contribute to a reduction in anomalies of embryonic development that otherwise might arise.

Criteria for Success

The criteria employed to assess the occurrence and normalcy of fertilization *in vitro* are most important. The use of suitably stringent criteria should be considered an integral part of the *in vitro* fertilization technique. Most of the reports of successful *in vitro* fertilization of mammalian oocytes made prior to 1954 are now believed to be based on inadequate criteria. There are two principal reasons why great care needs to be exercised in evaluating the outcome of *in vitro* fertilization experiments. First, there is the susceptibility of mammalian oocytes to undergo, within a short time after ovulation, degenerative changes that may suggest the occurrence of fertilization. These changes may involve spontaneous activation (with formation of pronuclei or cleavage of oocytes) or cytoplasmic fragmentation (an example of this is described later). The actual time interval between ovulation and the beginning of degeneration of oocytes varies from 9 to 36 hr, depending on the species (see Marston and Chang, 1964). Second, there is the likelihood that abnormal conditions *in vitro* exacerbate this situation. A wide variety of different factors that may be associated with *in vitro* fertilization conditions have been implicated at one time or another in encouraging parthenogenesis or

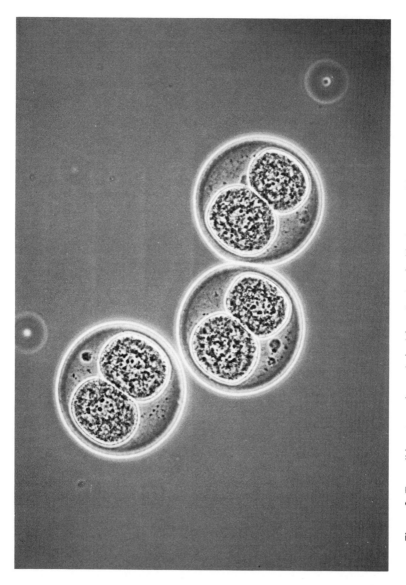

Figure 3. Two-cell hamster embryos derived from *in vitro*-fertilized oocytes. Phase-contrast, unfixed, × 125.

fragmentation of oocytes. One of the most serious problems is the effect of aging on oocytes (see Kaufman, 1975). If the interval between semination of oocytes and examination for signs of fertilization is very long, the possibility of spontaneous activation (parthenogenesis) may be greatly increased. Such aged oocytes might still be capable of undergoing fusion with spermatozoa but nevertheless be incapable of normal development. This problem can be reduced, if not eliminated, by examining oocytes as soon as possible after semination. A practical way to accomplish this, now used by many investigators, is to preincubate spermatozoa to allow capacitation to occur in the absence of oocytes. Penetration of eggs should then occur very soon after mixing the gametes together.

The difficulties referred to above may be more readily appreciated by examining a typical *in vitro* fertilization system (Figure 4). In marked contrast to the in vivo situation, many *in vitro* fertilization techniques necessitate the use of very large numbers of spermatozoa, which may rapidly demolish the cumulus oophorus present (in most species) around the freshly ovulated

IN VIVO   IN VITRO

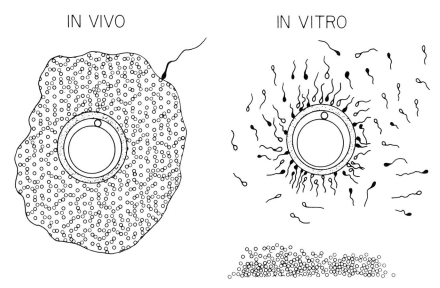

Figure 4. Diagrammatic representation of fertilization conditions *in vivo*, and in a typical *in vitro* system. Oocyte *in vivo* is shown surrounded by granulosa cell mass (cumulus oophorus); a single spermatozoon is shown at the periphery. Under *in vitro* conditions, large numbers of spermatozoa are usually present, and the cumulus matrix is dissolved; cumulus cells are dispersed and many spermatozoa attach to the zona pellucida. Spermatozoa in this situation are represented as acrosome-reacted (hollow heads) or with intact acrosomes (solid heads); it is not certain in which category the fertilizing sperm belongs. Many spermatozoa undergo an acrosome reaction at a distance from the oocyte, and may not take part in fertilization. Note: cumulus disruption may only be partial in some species *in vitro*, e.g., rabbit.

oocyte. The oocytes thus become exposed directly to many spermatozoa and to their breakdown products. Incidentally, the likelihood of polyspermic fertilization may be considerably enhanced under these conditions.

In order to guard against the possibility that degenerative changes in the oocyte (or cleaving embryo) have influenced the results of *in vitro* fertilization experiments, stringent criteria should be applied. These criteria may be morphological, developmental, or genetic. One scheme of such criteria for assessing fertilization and development is shown in Figure 5. This scheme is neither all-inclusive nor is it intended to deny the potential value of other criteria, such as biochemical analyses. Ideally, use of the criteria in Figure 5 will convincingly demonstrate that fertilization has indeed taken place in a

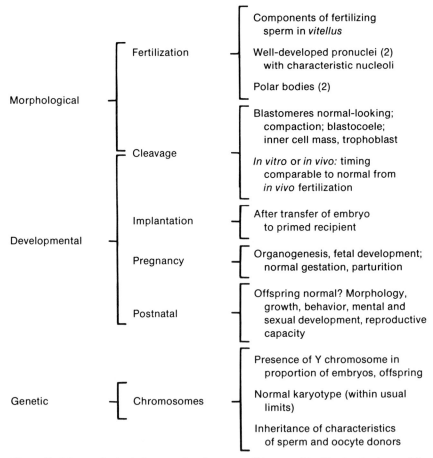

Figure 5. Scheme of criteria for assessing the accomplishment of fertilization *in vitro* and for evaluating the normalcy and viability of embryos.

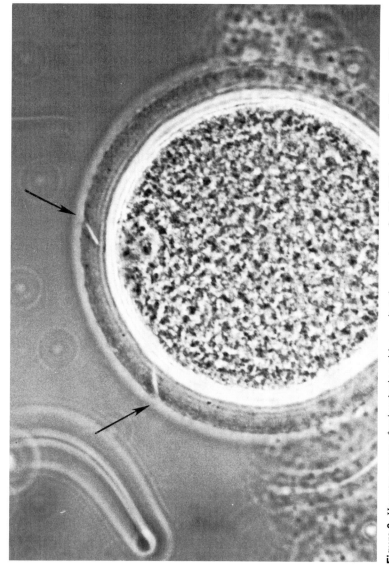

Figure 6. Hamster oocyte after incubation with capacitated spermatozoa for 3 hr. Slits in zona pellucida resembling sperm penetration slits can be seen (arrows), but no spermatozoa were found in this oocyte. Other oocytes from same experiment were penetrated. Phase-contrast, unfixed, × 500.

normal manner. However, it is not always possible to apply such a wide range of criteria. In the hamster, for example, no development of fertilized oocytes in culture has been reported beyond the two-cell stage. In this case, the use of appropriate criteria should at least demonstrate that oocytes have been activated by sperm penetration and may have the potential to develop further (see "Fertilization," Figure 5). It is particularly important to establish that development of sperm and oocyte components (pronuclei) is synchronous.

From the foregoing discussion, it is evident that the mere association of spermatozoa with oocytes *in vitro*, even the presence of sperm within the perivitelline space, does not constitute unequivocal evidence that fertilization is in progress, even if the ooctye is seen to be undergoing activation. The events of sperm penetration and oocyte activation can sometimes proceed independently or asynchronously. The cleavage of seminated ooctyes, without accompanying evidence that spermatozoa gained access to the vitellus, may actually be misleading (Blandau, 1980). Obviously, all of the criteria shown in Figure 5 cannot be demonstrated in a single oocyte, but in attempts to produce viable embryos by *in vitro* fertilization, we should ensure as far as possible that each stage of development has been accomplished before we can confidently proceed to the next. This cautious approach may save much time and frustration in the long run.

Two examples of potentially misleading situations are shown in Figures 6 and 7. The fertilizing mammalian spermatozoon leaves a characteristic curved slit in the zona pellucida. The presence of such a slit in the zona might thus be taken as an indication of sperm penetration. Figure 6 shows a hamster oocyte with two of these slits in the zona pellucida, suggesting the entry of two spermatozoa; careful inspection, however, revealed that no spermatozoa were present in this egg (the hamster spermatozoon is so large as to be quite unmistakable within the vitellus). The slits shown in Figure 6 are therefore artifacts. Figure 7 appears to show an embryo at about the 32-cell stage, although some blastomeres are clearly degenerating. Such an appearance might be taken as evidence of successful fertilization. However, no compaction of the embryo is seen, which would be expected by this stage of development. Moreover, this particular object was recovered from the oviduct of a mated hamster at a time (about 30 hr after ovulation) when all of its sibling embryos were at the 2-cell stage. Quite clearly, this object is the product of degenerative fragmentation of an oocyte.

Conclusions

A satisfactory culture milieu for mammalian fertilization can be provided by simple balanced salt solutions supplemented with appropriate energy sources and protein. However, we do not know if the composition of such culture media approximates the optimal (*in vivo*) conditions closely enough.

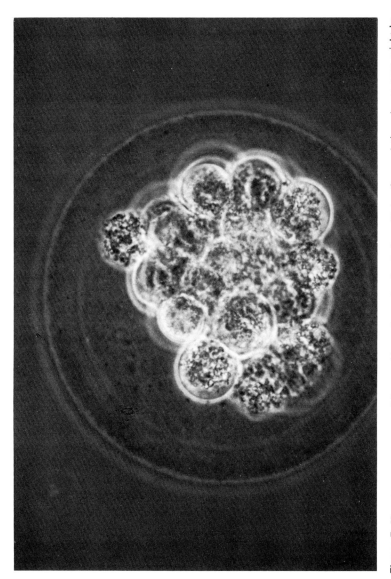

Figure 7. Hamster oocyte recovered from oviduct of mated animal about 30 hr after ovulation. Appearance might be mistaken for cleaving embryo, but this is actually a fragmented oocyte. Phase-contrast, unfixed, × 500.

A need for critical investigation of specific parameters of the culture environment is indicated. By refining culture media and techniques as a result of such analyses, it may be possible to increase the efficiency of *in vitro* fertilization and to accomplish this routinely in several important species that have resisted such attempts. The use of more precise culture techniques together with appropriate, stringent criteria will undoubtedly accelerate the accumulation of a pool of information on mammalian *in vitro* fertilization.

ACKNOWLEDGMENTS

Support during the preparation of this paper came from NIH Grant RR00167 to the Wisconsin Regional Primate Research Center and NIH Grant 7 R01 HD14235 to B. Bavister. I thank Dr. Ruth Shalgi for providing unpublished data. I am grateful to Sharon Paulsen for her help in researching material discussed in this presentation, to Debbie Torgerson for her excellent secretarial assistance, to Donna McConnell and Bob Dodsworth for artwork, and to Dr. Dorothy Boatman for helpful comments and suggestions. Wisconsin Regional Primate Research Center Publication No. 21-002.

References

Altman, P., 1961, in: *Blood and Other Body Fluids* (D. S. Dittmer, ed.), Federation of American Societies for Experimental Biology, Washington, D.C.

Austin, C. R., 1951, Observations on the penetration of the sperm into the mammalian egg, *Aust. J. Sci. Res. Ser. B* **4**:581–589.

Bavister, B. D., 1969, Environmental factors important for *in vitro* fertilization in the hamster, *J. Reprod. Fertil.* **18**:544–545.

Bavister, B. D., 1975, Properties of the sperm motility-stimulating component derived from human serum, *J. Reprod. Fertil.* **43**:363–366.

Bavister, B. D., 1979, Fertilization of hamster eggs *in vitro* at sperm: egg ratios close to unity, *J. Exp. Zool.* **210**:259–264.

Bavister, B. D., and Yanagimachi, R., 1977, The effects of sperm extracts and energy sources on the motility and acrosome reaction of hamster spermatozoa *in vitro*, *Biol. Reprod.* **16**:228–237.

Bavister, B. D., Chen, A. F., and Fu, P. C., 1979, Catecholamine requirement for hamster sperm motility *in vitro*, *J. Reprod. Fertil.* **56**:507–513.

Blandau, R. J., 1980, *In vitro* fertilization and embryo transfer, *Fertil. Steril.* **33**:3–11.

Borland, R. M., Hazra, S., Biggers, J. D., and Lechene, C. P., 1977, The elemental composition of the gametes and preimplantation embryo during the initiation of pregnancy, *Biol. Reprod.* **16**:147–157.

Brackett, B. G., and Oliphant, G., 1975, Capacitation of rabbit spermatozoa *in vitro*, *Biol. Reprod.* **12**:260–274.

Brinster, R. L., 1963, A method for *in vitro* cultivation of mouse ova from two-cell to blastocyst, *Exp. Cell Res.* **32**:205–208.

Brunton, W. J., and Brusilow, S., 1972, Microanalytical data for blood plasma and oviductal fluid of rabbit does. Cited by Brackett, B. G., and Mastroianni, L., 1974, in: *The Oviduct and Its Functions* (A. D. Johnson, and C. W. Foley, eds.), Academic Press, New York, p. 138.

Chang, M. C., 1951, Fertilizing capacity of spermatozoa deposited into the fallopian tubes, *Nature (London)* **168**:697.

David, A., Serr, D. M., and Czernobilsky, B., 1973, Chemical composition of human oviduct fluid, *Fertil. Steril.* **24**:435–439.

Edwards, R. G., Bavister, B. D., and Steptoe, P. C., 1969, Early stages of fertilization *in vitro* of human oocytes matured *in vitro*, *Nature (London)* **221**:632–635.

Fraser, L. R., and Drury, L. M., 1975, The relationship between sperm concentration and fertilization *in vitro* of mouse eggs, *Biol. Reprod.* **13**:513–518.

Fraser, L. R., Dandekar, P. V., and Vaidya, R. A., 1971, *In vitro* fertilization of tubal rabbit ova partially or totally denuded of follicular cells, *Biol. Reprod.* **4**:229–233.

Good, N. E., Winget, G. D., Winter, W., Connolly, T. N., Izawa, S., and Singh, R. M. M., 1966, Hydrogen ion buffers for biological research, *Biochemistry* **5**:467–477.

Hamner, C. E., and Williams, W. L., 1965, Composition of rabbit oviduct secretions, *Fertil. Steril.* **16**:170–176.

Hirao, Y., and Yanagimachi, R., 1978, Temperature dependence of sperm–egg fusion and post-fusion events in hamster fertilization, *J. Exp. Zool.* **205**:433–438.

Holmdahl, T. H., and Mastroianni, L., Jr., 1965, Continuous collection of rabbit oviduct secretions at low temperatures, *Fertil. Steril.* **16**:587–595.

Hoppe, P.C., and Pitts, S., 1973, Fertilization *in vitro* and development of mouse ova, *Biol. Reprod.* **8**:420–426.

Hoppe, P. C., and Whitten, W. K., 1974, An albumin requirement for fertilization of mouse eggs *in vitro*, *J. Reprod. Fertil.* **39**:433–436.

Iritani, A., Gomes, W. R., and VanDemark, N. L., 1969, Secretion rates and chemical composition of oviduct and uterine fluids in ewes, *Biol. Reprod.* **1**:72–76.

Iritani, A., Nishikawa, Y., Gomes, W. R., and VanDemark, N. L., 1971, Secretion rates and chemical composition of oviduct and uterine fluids in rabbits, *J. Anim. Sci.* **33**:829–835.

Iritani, A., Sato, E., and Nishikawa, Y., 1974, Secretion rates and chemical composition of oviduct and uterine fluids in sows, *J. Anim. Sci.* **39**:582–588.

Kaufman, M. H. 1975, The experimental induction of parthenogenesis in the mouse, in: *The Early Development of Mammals* (M. Balls, and A. E. Wild, eds.), Cambridge University Press, London, pp. 25–44.

Leibfried, M. L., and Bavister, B. D., 1981, The effects of taurine and hypotaurine on *in vitro* fertilization in the golden hamster, *Gamete Res.* **4**:57–63.

Lippes, J., Enders, R. G., Pragay, D. A., and Bartholomew, W. R., 1972, The collection and analysis of human fallopian tubal fluid, *Contraception* **5**:85–103.

Lopata, A., McMaster, R., McBain, J. C., and Johnston, W. I. H., 1978, *In-vitro* fertilization of preovulatory human eggs, *J. Reprod. Fertil.* **52**:339–342.

Mahi, C. A., and Yanagimachi, R., 1976, Maturation and sperm penetration of canine ovarian oocytes *in vitro*, *J. Exp. Zool.* **196**:189–196.

Mahi, C. A., and Yanagimachi, R., 1978, Capacitation, acrosome reaction, and egg penetration by canine spermatozoa in a simple defined medium, *Gamete Res.* **1**:101–109.

Marston, J. H., and Chang, M. C., 1964, The fertilizable life of ova and their morphology following delayed insemination in mature and immature mice, *J. Exp. Zool.* **155**:237–252.

Mastroianni, L., and Wallach, R. C., 1961, Effect of ovulation and early gestation on oviduct secretions in rabbit, *Am. J. Physiol.* **200**:815–818.

Mastroianni, L., Urzua, M., Avalos, M., and Stambaugh, R. 1969, Some observations on fallopian tube fluid in the monkey, *Am. J. Obstet. Gynecol.* **103**:703–709.

Mastroianni, L., Urzua, M., and Stambaugh, R., 1972, The internal environmental fluids of the oviduct, in: *The Regulation of Mammalian Reproduction* (S. S. Segal, R. Crozier, P. Corfman, and P. Condliffe, eds.), Thomas, Springfield, Ill., pp. 376–384.

Meizel, S., 1978, The mammalian sperm acrosome reaction, a biochemical approach, in:

Development in Mammals, Volume 3 (M. H. Johnson, ed.), North-Holland, Amsterdam, pp. 1–64.

Meizel, S., Lui, C. W., Working, P. K., and Mrsny, R. J., 1980, Taurine and hypotaurine: Their effects on motility, capacitation and acrosome reaction of hamster sperm *in vitro* and their presence in sperm and reproductive tract fluids of several mammals, *Dev. Growth Differ.* **22**:483–494.

Miyamoto, H., and Chang, M. C., 1972, Fertilization *in vitro* of mouse and hamster eggs after the removal of follicular cells, *J. Reprod. Fertil.* **30**:309–312.

Miyamoto, H., and Chang, M. C., 1973a, The importance of serum albumin and metabolic intermediates for capacitation of spermatozoa and fertilization of mouse eggs *in vitro*, *J. Reprod. Fertil.* **32**:193–205.

Miyamoto, H., and Chang, M. C., 1973b, Effect of osmolality on fertilization of mouse and golden hamster eggs *in vitro*, *J. Reprod. Fertil.* **33**:481–487.

Mrsny, R. J., and Meizel, S., 1980, K^+ influx is required for the hamster sperm acrosome reaction, *J. Cell Biol.* **87**:130a.

Mrsny, R. J., Waxman, L., and Meizel, S., 1979, Taurine maintains and stimulates motility of hamster spermatozoa during capacitation *in vitro*, *J. Exp. Zool.* **210**:123–128.

Oliphant, G., and Brackett, B. G., 1973, Capacitation of mouse spermatozoa in media with elevated ionic strength and reversible decapacitation with epididymal extracts, *Fertil. Steril.* **24**:948–955.

Parkening, T. A., and Chang, M. C., 1976, *In vitro* fertilization of ova from senescent mice and hamsters, *J. Reprod. Fertil.* **48**:381–383.

Restall, B. J., and Wales, R. G., 1966, The fallopian tube of the sheep. III. The chemical composition of the fluid from the fallopian tube, *Aust. J. Biol. Sci.* **19**:687–698.

Rogers, B. J., and Yanagimachi R., 1975, Retardation of guinea pig sperm acrosome reaction by glucose: The possible importance of pyruvate and lactate metabolism in capacitation and the acrosome reaction, *Biol. Reprod.* **13**:568–575.

Rogers, B. J., Chang, L., and Yanagimachi, R., 1979, Glucose effect on respiration: Possible mechanism for capacitation in guinea pig spermatozoa, *J. Exp. Zool.* **207**:107–112.

Shalgi, R., Kaplan, R., Kraicer, P., and Nebel, L., 1980, personal communication.

Soupart, P., and Morgenstern, L. L., 1973, Human sperm capacitation and *in vitro* fertilization, *Fertil. Steril.* **24**:462–478.

Toyoda, Y., and Chang, M. C., 1974a, Fertilization of rat eggs *in vitro* by epididymal spermatozoa and the development of eggs following transfer, *J. Reprod. Fertil.* **36**:9–22.

Toyoda, Y., and Chang, M. C., 1974b, Capacitation of epididymal spermatozoa in a medium with high K/Na ratio and cyclic AMP for the fertilization of rat eggs *in vitro*, *J. Reprod. Fertil.* **36**:125–134.

Toyoda, Y., Yokoyama, M., and Hosi, T., 1971, Studies on the fertilization of mouse eggs *in vitro*. I. *In vitro* fertilization of eggs by fresh epididymal sperm, *Jp. J. Anim. Reprod.* **16**:147–151.

Whittingham, D. G., and Bavister, B. D., 1974, Development of hamster eggs fertilized *in vitro* or *in vivo*, *J. Reprod. Fertil.* **38**:489–492.

Wolf, D. P., Inoue, M., and Stark, R. A., 1976, Penetration of zona-free mouse ova, *Biol. Reprod.* **15**:213–221.

Yanagimachi, R., 1969a, *In vitro* capacitation of hamster spermatozoa by follicular fluid, *J. Reprod. Fertil.* **18**:275–286.

Yanagimachi, R., 1969b, *In vitro* acrosome reaction and capacitation of golden hamster spermatozoa by bovine follicular fluid and its fractions, *J. Exp. Zool.* **170**:269–280.

Yanagimachi, R., 1972, Fertilization of guinea pig eggs *in vitro*, *Anat. Rec.* **174**:9–20.

Yanagimachi, R., and Chang, M. C., 1964, *In vitro* fertilization of golden hamster ova, *J. Exp. Zool.* **156**:361–376.

4

IN VITRO CULTURE OF THE ZYGOTE AND EMBRYO

BENJAMIN G. BRACKETT

Scientific investigations during the last three decades have led to the present capability of nurturing the embryonic development from zygote to blastocyst stages *in vitro* for several mammalian species including cow (Wright *et al.*, 1976b), ferrett (Whittingham, 1975), man (Edwards *et al.*, 1970), mouse (Whitten and Biggers, 1968; Mukherjee and Cohen, 1970), rabbit (Maurer *et al.*, 1969; Kane and Foote, 1971; Ogawa *et al.*, 1971; Kane, 1972), and sheep (Tervit *et al.*, 1972). As ova of several species (man, rabbit, sheep, cow, and ferret) are relatively large and thus have greater endogenous reserves, it was suggested by Biggers (1979) that they might be more independent of the oviductal and uterine environments before implantation than the relatively smaller ova of other species (rat, hamster, and vole). Successful culture to blastocysts of ferret, mouse, rabbit, and human zygotes has followed *in vitro* fertilization. Various aspects of preimplantational development of mammalian embryos in culture have been well reviewed previously (see Biggers *et al.*, 1971; Whittingham, 1971, 1975; Brinster, 1972, 1973; Seidel, 1977; Anderson, 1978; Maurer, 1978; Biggers, 1979; Brackett, 1979b; Brinster and Troike, 1979).

Several criteria have been taken as endpoints for assessing zygote (one-cell ovum undergoing fertilization) development, or embryo development in culture. These include: (1) development to morula or blastocyst stages; (2) normal cleavage taken to include symmetrical characteristic appearance of

BENJAMIN G. BRACKETT • Department of Clinical Studies–New Bolton Center, University of Pennsylvania School of Veterinary Medicine, Kennett Square, Pennsylvania 19348, and Department of Obstetrics and Gynecology, University of Pennsylvania School of Medicine, Philadelphia, Pennsylvania 19104.

the blastomeres of cleaved ova along with temporal development comparable to that normally observed when fertilization and development occur within the oviduct; (3) positive viability as reflected by fluorescent staining (Church and Raines, 1980) after successive cleavages in culture, also appropriate after storage of embryos in ways to arrest development, e.g., frozen storage; and (4) normal development following transfer of *in vitro*-cultured embryos to a recipient or surrogate dam. The latter endpoint represents the best way for assessing normalcy of development. It is important to bear in mind that, in the absence of sperm, parthenogenetic cleavage and blastocyst formation reportedly follow a variety of treatments (mouse: Graham, 1974; Kaufman and Sachs, 1976; rhesus monkey: Abramczuk *et al.*, 1977). Normalcy of development of rabbit *in vitro*-fertilized zygotes, first documented by Chang (1959), has been a part of many additional reports (see Brackett, 1979b, 1981). Although complete culture of *in vitro*-fertilized rabbit zygotes through oviductal stages has been achieved (Seidel *et al.*, 1976; Brackett, 1979b), successful term development following transfer of resulting blastocysts into uteri of recipient does has not been possible. In contrast, several reports of mouse *in vitro* fertilization and embryo culture have described successful gestational development following transfer of resulting morulae or early blastocysts to uteri of recipients. Thus, oviductal influences have apparently been adequately duplicated *in vitro* for this laboratory animal (Mukherjee and Cohen, 1970; Mukherjee, 1972; Hoppe and Pitts, 1973; Fraser and Drury, 1975; Whittingham, 1975; Parkening *et al.*, 1976; Whittingham, 1977). Successful development following uterine transfer of human *in vitro*-fertilized embryos reaching the eight-cell stage has been reported (Steptoe and Edwards, 1978; Lopata *et al.*, 1980). In the mouse and man, then, *in vitro*-fertilized embryos have developed into offspring without the usual passage through the oviductal environment.

In the mouse and the rabbit, development to late morulae or early blastocysts is a prerequisite to subsequent normal uterine development. In man, rhesus monkey, swine, and a few other species, the embryo normally reaches the uterus prior to the morula or blastocyst stages and if the goal of *in vitro* fertilization and embryo culture is to circumvent the oviductal environment, it becomes unnecessary to carry embryonic development so far in culture. In addition to practical and research applications of embryo culture when coupled with embryo transfer technology, the ability to sustain embryonic development *in vitro* presents an opportunity for basic investigations of many important aspects involved in early mammalian development. This chapter reviews some important observations that have contributed to the present level of success in the culture of mammalian zygotes and preimplantation embryos and points to some of the areas in which increased knowledge is desirable.

General Observations on Fertilization and
Early Development *in Vitro*

In developing an appropriate milieu to support *in vitro* fertilization and early embryonic development, the approach might involve initial efforts either with a very simple defined medium or with complex defined media and/or biological fluids (e.g., serum or oviductal fluids). In contrast to the classical microbiological approach involving complex media from which components can be systematically removed to ascertain their importance in bacterial growth, the paucity of mammalian ova and/or embryos coupled with early recognized inhibitory effects has led to emphasis on the experimental approach beginning with simple media and striving to enhance quality and/or quantity of embryonic development by the addition of promising ingredients. The problem of providing ova and/or embryos with optimal nutrients is confounded by their hardiness, which may reflect genetic or prior experimental influences, their stage of development, the physical conditions that prevail, and interacting influences of various constituents of culture media. The ovum and developing embryo obviously represent the total of many dynamic, constantly changing processes that are, in turn, frequently demanding changing conditions for their continued development. Insights regarding embryonic requirements for a changing milieu follow from studies of appropriately synchronous oviductal fluids.

Early efforts by Hammond (1949) to culture mouse ova in a medium composed of a simple salt solution supplemented with glucose and egg white resulted in survival of eight-cell but not of two-cell mouse embryos. Addition of the egg white proteins elevated the pH from less than 5.0 to somewhere between 7.5 and 7.8. Chang (1959) referred to the salt solution as acidic saline and supplemented it with glucose and serum in his best initial rabbit *in vitro* fertilization experiments. Acidic saline supplemented with glucose and 5 or 10% heat-treated (to destroy complement) rabbit serum (5 or 10% serum solution) was found to support the consistent accomplishment of fertilization *in vitro* when close attention was paid to maintaining gametes at body temperature and when uterine-capacitated spermatozoa were used for insemination (Brackett and Williams, 1965). In the best, early experiments, some uterine fluid was recovered along with the uterine-capacitated sperm used for insemination and this resulted in elevation of the pH to 7.8; this pH was also found for estrous oviductal fluid in the rabbit (Bishop, 1957). Further improvement followed efforts to duplicate, in a defined medium, the influences of the female reproductive tract deemed most important for the fertilization process (Brackett and Williams, 1968). In addition to glucose for energy, the simple fertilization medium included crystalline bovine serum albumin (BSA), substituted for the protein content of serum found to be adequate through earlier work, and bicarbonate to maintain a pH of 7.8 under a moist air atmosphere containing 5% CO_2 at 38° C. More consistent results follow maintaining the gametes at body temperature. In addition to a moist atmosphere, 4.0 ml of medium in a small tissue culture dish (30-mm diameter $\times$ 12-mm depth) with paraffin or silicone oil completely filling the space between medium and sealable top was found to afford consistent temperature control, and these conditions have been adopted for much work in the author's laboratory.

Early rabbit fertilization experiments suggested a relatively anaerobic environment under paraffin oil to favor sperm penetration (Moricard, 1950, 1954; Brackett and Williams, 1965, 1968). Consistent *in vitro* fertilization of rabbit ova followed equilibration of the fertilization medium and paraffin oil, used to cover it, with 5% CO_2 in N_2 prior to gamete incubation under an atmosphere of 5% CO_2 in moist air (Brackett and Williams, 1968; Brackett, 1969). The 8% O_2 content in the fertilization medium (Brackett and Williams, 1968) duplicated that reported for the rabbit oviductal lumen (Bishop, 1956; Mastroianni and Jones, 1965). These considerations led to adoption of a moist 5% CO_2, 8% O_2, and 87% N_2 atmosphere for many rabbit *in vitro* fertilization studies.

Although glucose is readily used by sperm cells and crystalline bovine albumin was reported to support development of two-cell to morula-stage rabbit embryos (Brinster, 1970), the simple defined fertilization medium was found inadequate for zygote culture; thus, ova were routinely transferred into a serum-supplemented medium following sperm penetration (Brackett and Williams, 1968; Brackett, 1969). When rabbit ova, recovered from the ovarian surface soon after ovulation, were added to uterine sperm suspended in the defined fertilization medium supplemented with 20% heated rabbit serum, the rate of ovum cleavage observed between 24 and 36 hr was retarded; however, at least some of the embryos were viable as evidenced by successful embryo transfer (Seitz *et al.*, 1970a). It was found that the cleavage lag could be overcome by transferring the ova from the sperm-containing fertilization medium after 5 hr into a 10% serum solution (Seitz *et al.*, 1970b). In addition to avoiding possible detrimental effects of the sperm cells, the effects of lowering the pH from approximately 7.6 to 7.2 and of lowering the osmolality from around 332 to 287 mOsM/kg quite likely favored utilization by the zygote of pyruvate provided by the serum to support normal temporal development through 2-, 4-, and 8-cell stages. Proportions of 2-cell-stage mouse embryos reaching the blastocyst stage in culture are known to depend on an interaction between energy source and pH, i.e., a decrease in the pH of the medium results in a decrease in the optimum concentration of pyruvate necessary for supplying energy for ovum development (Brinster, 1965b). The above observations suggest that different *in vitro* conditions are optimal for sperm penetration and for embryonic development. As is the case in the rabbit, mouse ova are routinely transferred from the sperm incubate before 8 hr after insemination for embryo culture (Hoppe and Pitts, 1973). Supplementation of the simple defined medium, pH 7.8, which allows sperm penetration of rabbit ova with a relatively high concentration of pyruvate (Brackett and Oliphant, 1975), enables fertilization and continued development to the 8- to 16-cell stages in a single defined medium.

Although fertilization of rabbit ova can take place under a gas phase with 0% O_2 or under 95% O_2, development of resulting embryos does not proceed following transfer to recipients, in contrast to continued development resulting from fertilization under 20% O_2 (Brackett, 1978). Mouse embryos can develop in an atmosphere with lowered oxygen tension (Whitten, 1957), but a definite requirement for at least 0.5% O_2 has been demonstrated (Auerbach and Brinster, 1968). Whitten (1971) reported that 5% O_2 allowed the development of one-cell mouse ova into blastocysts, whereas no blastocysts developed in 0 or 20% oxygen. More recently, C57 mouse zygotes were found to develop into blastocysts under either 5 or 20% O_2 when cultured in either Whitten's (1971) or Brinster's (1965b, 1972) media, with slightly better results following culture under 5% O_2 in Whitten's medium (Brinster and Troike, 1979). Bovine embryos have been found to develop better under 5% O_2 than under 20% O_2 (Wright *et al.*, 1976c), but a significant difference in development of ovine embryos was not found under the two conditions (Wright *et al.*, 1976a). Brinster and Troike (1979) concluded that various levels of oxygen quite likely influence development by altering the oxidation–reduction potential in the ovum and/or embryo. In earlier work, Brinster (1965d) found an enhancement of two-cell to blastocyst development when concentrations of pyruvate and lactate found to be optimal were combined. This effect was attributed to maintenance (via the lactate dehydrogenase reaction) of $NAD^+:NADH + H^+$ ratios within an appropriate physiological range. The favorable roles attributed to maintenance of body temperature, high pH, and low oxygen tension on fertilization taken with the central role of pyruvate as an energy source for the initiation of zygote development point to the importance of the sum of interacting influences and the resulting oxidation–reduction potential as important regulators of early development *in vitro*.

Fertilization and early development can take place over a wide range of osmolarity. Development of *in vitro*-fertilized rabbit zygotes to the eight-cell stage can occur at 221 mOsM (Brackett, 1969). The optimal osmolarity for culture of rabbit embryos was reported to be 270 mOsM (Naglee *et al.*, 1969). Appropriate atmospheric pressure during culture was found to improve the

viability of rabbit embryos (Elliott *et al.*, 1974), and the best development
occurred at an atmospheric pressure of 16 inches of water (3 cm Hg or 4052
N/m^2 at 352 ft above sea level).

A simple chemically defined medium with an osmolarity of 242 mOsM
supported development of certain F_1 hybrid mouse zygotes to blastocysts
(Whitten and Biggers, 1968). Slightly hypotonic conditions may favor early
embryonic development *in vitro*. The optimal osmolarity for development of
two-cell mouse embryos was found to be 276 mOsM (Brinster, 1965a).

The medium described by Whitten and Biggers (1968) with additional
pyruvate supported mouse zygote development after *in vitro* insemination in
lactate-supplemented Toyoda's medium (Toyoda *et al.*, 1971); the blastocyst
stage was reached by 10% of the fertilized ova (Miyamoto and Chang, 1972).
The same medium (Whitten and Biggers, 1968) when supplemented with 0.1
or 0.2% BSA was superior to several complex tissue culture media in
maintaining viability of sheep embryos *in vitro* (Wright *et al.*, 1976a). An
improvement in culture results for sheep embryos followed elevation of the
BSA content to 0.5%, which also yielded better results than 1.5% BSA (Peters
et al., 1977). Development from one-cell to blastocyst stage and from eight-
cell to hatching blastocyst stage was observed, but the results with embryos
earlier than the eight-cell stage were poor. Similar results have been reported
with swine embryos using the same medium but with 1.5% BSA and in a
humidified 5% CO_2, 5% O_2, 90% N_2 atmosphere (Wright, 1977; Lindner and
Wright, 1978). Whitten's medium (1971) is the same as that described by
Whitten and Biggers (1968) except it contains more NaCl to render it isotonic.
Good results followed use of Whitten's medium (1971) for *in vitro* fertilization
and culture of F_1 hybrid mouse ova to morulae or early blastocysts (Hoppe
and Pitts, 1973).

Metabolic Requirements for Embryonic Development in Vitro

Greatest progress in mammalian embryo culture has emanated from
experimentation involving the mouse (due to economic and genetic considerations). Variations of a medium for embryo culture consisting of a
modified Krebs Ringer bicarbonate solution with an energy source and a fixed
nitrogen source have been exploited to yield much of our present knowledge
(Brinster, 1963, 1965b, 1972). Ions found necessary for successful development
include Na^+, K^+, Ca^+, Mg^{2+}, Cl^-, PO_4^{3-}, and HCO_3^-. Optimum levels of
potassium, calcium, magnesium, and phosphate are similar to serum values
(Wales, 1970). Calcium is necessary for membrane stability, permeability, and
cell–cell interaction, especially at the time of compaction to form morulae

(Whitten, 1971; Ducibella and Anderson, 1975). Osmolality is maintained by the appropriate NaCl concentrations.

It is now clear from experiments with mouse embryos that during preimplantational development there is a gradual change in energy substrate requirements (see Brinster, 1973). In the beginning, the oocyte needs pyruvate (or oxaloacetate) in the culture medium, but the two-cell stage is able to develop when supplied pyruvate, oxaloacetate, lactate, or phosphoenol-pyruvate. After the eight-cell stage, the embryo is able to survive and develop using glucose or any of a number of other carbon chains, e.g., pyruvate, oxalocaetate, lactate, phosphoenolpyruvate, malate, α-ketoglutrate, acetate, or citrate (Brinster and Thomson, 1966). When the embryo reaches the blastocyst stage or at about the time of implantation, energy source requirements and energy metabolism are apparently similar to those of most adult cells.

Exceptions to such generalizations based on mouse (Brinster, 1965b) and rabbit studies (Daniel, 1967) have been reported. These include the inability of glucose to promote development of 8-cell sheep embryos or 16-cell cow embryos (Boone *et al.*, 1978) and the inhibition of development of 4-cell pig embryos by pyruvate (Davis and Day, 1978). In the latter work, pig embryonic development from 4-cell to blastocyst stage took place in a bicarbonate-buffered salt solution (as used in BMOC-2: Brinster, 1965a) supplemented with either glucose and BSA or BSA alone.

During the first 2 days of development in the mouse embryo, 90–100% of the oxygen consumption of the embryo can be attributed to pyruvate oxidation (Brinster, 1967b; Mills and Brinster, 1967). Carbon dioxide formed from pyruvate accounts for over 50% of the oxygen uptake throughout the rabbit embryo preimplantation period (Brinster, 1969a). Glucose oxidation is very low, accounting for less than 10% of the oxygen consumption by the mouse ovum, but glucose oxidation increases 100-fold during the pre-implantation period with major increases at fertilization and blastocyst formation; glucose is oxidized about as well as pyruvate by the blastocyst (Brinster, 1967a). As in the mouse, rabbit embryos oxidize glucose poorly initially; in the morula and blastocyst stages glucose oxidation becomes substantial (Brinster, 1968). Incorporation of pyruvate and glucose carbon increases as does oxidation of the two substrates (Brinster, 1969b); however, carbon from glucose is incorporated into the embryo to a much greater extent than is carbon from pyruvate. In contrast to glucose metabolism in the mouse embryo, which is by the Embden–Meyerhof and Krebs cycle pathways (Brinster, 1967a), the pentose shunt is active in glucose oxidation up to the morula stage in the rabbit (Friedhandler, 1961; Brinster, 1968) and rat (Sugawara and Takeuchi, 1973).

Although 2-cell mouse embryos can develop to blastocysts in media containing no amino acids or protein (Cholewa and Whitten, 1970), improvement follows inclusion of crystalline BSA in most experiments. The mechanism for such improvement is not completely clear. Several possibilities have been suggested including supplementation of amino acids, stabilization of the membranes, and reduction in leakage of endogenous amino acids from the embryos (Brinster, 1965c, 1971), removal of toxic metal ions present in the culture media (Cholewa and Whitten, 1970), or as a means for adding unidentified nutrients to the medium (Kane, 1979). Addition of an amino nitrogen source to a culture medium for rabbit embryos may be of greater importance than for the mouse. Kane and Foote (1970 a–c) found amino acids beneficial to the development of 2- and 4-cell-stage rabbit embryos; without BSA, few blastocysts formed in a simple synthetic medium. Incorporation of radioisotopically labeled amino acids into protein has been demonstrated throughout the preimplantation period in the mouse (Mintz, 1964) and rabbit (Manes and Daniel, 1969). The level of incorporation is generally low in the early cleavage stages but increases markedly between the 8- and 16-cell stages to reach high levels in the morula and blastocyst. A similar pattern was found with fatty acids, and it was concluded that exogenous fatty acids can be used by mouse embryos in culture both for incorporation into embryo lipids and for energy production (Flynn and Hillman, 1980). From a recent investigation of the role of commercial BSA preparations on rabbit zygote to blastocyst development *in vitro*, is was concluded that energy was provided by albumin-bound fatty acids and that blastocyst hatching was promoted by a non-albumin component (Kane and Headon, 1980).

Bicarbonate and CO_2 in equilibrium are most commonly employed to buffer media for embryo culture. However, the main effect of bicarbonate on embryo development is not regulation of pH, as development will not occur when other buffers (e.g., Tris, phosphate, HEPES, or TES) are substituted although pH is maintained constant (Brinster, 1972). Incubation of two-cell mouse embryos for only 2–4 hr in phosphate-buffered medium resulted in a permanent reduction in their subsequent ability to develop into blastocysts (Quinn and Wales, 1973). Serum-enriched phosphate-buffered saline with low bicarbonate content proved inferior for culture of viable sheep embryos to synthetic oviduct fluid, which is bicarbonate buffered (Tervit and Gould, 1978). The degree of mouse embryo development could not be experimentally related to graded concentrations of CO_2; development comparable to that afforded by the 5% level generally employed resulted with concentrations between 1 and 10% (Brinster, 1972). The preimplantation embryo uses carbon dioxide as a carbon source during development (Wales *et al.*, 1969; Graves and Biggers, 1970; Quinn and Wales, 1971). The greatest CO_2 fixation begins at the eight-cell stage and extends to the blastocyst when general metabolism is highest. Thus, in addition to its role in maintaining constant pH, bicarbonate is important in media for embryo culture to sustain embryo development, for blastocyst formation, and for blastocyst expansion. Condensation of CO_2 with pyruvate by pyruvate carboxylase and malate dehydrogenase may account for one of its important roles (Quinn and Wales, 1971). Additionally, *in vitro* development of mouse embryos requires bicarbonate for *de novo* pyrimidine biosynthesis, and this requirement is most pronounced at the morula to blastocyst transition, the period of increasing RNA synthesis (recently reviewed by Brinster and Troike, 1979). Rabbit zygotes developed to the morula stage in a HEPES-buffered medium without bicarbonate, but bicarbonate was necessary for progression to the blastocyst stages (Kane, 1975). Also, Cross (1974) demonstrated that the amount of bicarbonate necessary for blastocyst expansion in the rabbit is greater than the bicarbonate produced metabolically by the embryo and, therefore, must be supplied by the culture medium. High concentrations of bicarbonate are present in rabbit oviductal and uterine fluids (Vishwakarma, 1962; Hamner and Williams, 1964; David *et al.*, 1969).

Complex Media and Biological Fluids for Embryo Culture

In mammals other than the mouse, defined culture media apparently lack important constituents that ensure continued *in vivo* development of blastocysts even though the embryos can be cultured to this stage *in vitro*. Although fertilization of cow ova can take place *in vitro* in a simple defined medium, more complex media are necessary for cleavage (Brackett *et al.*, 1980). The best medium found by Wright *et al.* (1976a,c) for supporting cow embryo development *in vitro* is Ham's F10 (Ham, 1963) supplemented with 10% heat-treated fetal calf serum in a 5% CO_2, 5% O_2, 90% N_2 atmosphere; development progressed from the one-cell to the early blastocyst stage and from the two-cell to the expanded blastocyst stage after 155–165 hr *in vitro* and from the eight-cell to the hatched blastocyst stage after 165 hr *in vitro*. The viability of cow embryos recovered 5 days after estrus and cultured 24 hr was not statistically significantly different from the viability of embryos immediately transferred to recipients (Peters *et al.*, 1978). Similar conditions have been used for human zygote culture (Seitz *et al.*, 1971; Edwards and Steptoe, 1975; Lopata *et al.*, 1980).

Most consistent results for rabbit embryo culture have followed use of an extensively modified Ham's F10 medium developed by Kane and Foote (1970c) and Naglee *et al.* (1969) with modifications (Kane and Foote, 1971; Kane, 1972; Maurer, 1978). It consists of a basic salt solution, vitamins, amino acids, and trace elements. Kane (1972) reported 81% development of New Zealand White zygotes to the blastocyst stage with no glucose in the medium.

This represents a significant improvement over development of rabbit zygotes to blastocysts afforded by heat-treated bovine serum plus glucose (Maurer *et al.*, 1969). Maurer (1978) reported development of two- and four-cell rabbit embryos into hatched blastocysts with diameters up to 4 mm after 6 to 10 days in the complex defined medium when held under appropriate (16 or 32 inches water) atmospheric pressure. Only 6% of the cultured embryos developed into fetuses following embryo transfer 96 hr after initiation of culture (Maurer, 1978). Only 3.3 and 6.7% of the two- and four-cell rabbit embryos that developed into morula and blastocyst stages under similar *in vitro* conditions continued gestational development to term when transfers were made into uterine horns and oviducts, respectively, of recipients (Binkerd and Anderson, 1979). Ogawa *et al.*, (1971) reported 65% development of rabbit zygotes to blastocysts in a very complex medium consisting of several combined tissue culture media.

Efforts to sustain development of *in vitro*-fertilized rabbit embryos to the blastocyst stage have led to results comparable to those obtained with *in vivo*-fertilized embryos (Ogawa *et al.*, 1972; Seidel *et al.*, 1976; Brackett, 1979b). Also, as is the case for *in vivo*-fertilized zygotes, *in vitro*-fertilized embryos apparently require additional as yet unknown factors that ensure their continued development after *in vitro* culture (Mills *et al.*, 1973; Seidel *et al.*, 1976). That contributions from the female reproductive tract supply specific embryonic requirements follows from studies in the rabbit (Kendle and Telford, 1970; Beier *et al.*, 1972). The inability to culture *in vitro*-fertilized hamster ova beyond the two-cell stage (Yanagimachi and Chang, 1964) may be due to inappropriateness of the bicarbonate buffering system (Whittingham and Bavister, 1974). However, when considered along with the striking hormonally influenced changes in proteins within the female luminal fluids (Hall *et al.*, 1977, 1978), a role for such components in nurturing zygote development represents an alternative hypothesis. Development of mouse zygotes to blastocysts in cultured mouse oviducts reflected hormonal influences in previous work (Whittingham, 1968). Much is known of the composition of oviductal and uterine fluids under various hormonal conditions and in different sites within the tubular female reproductive tract (for review see Brackett and Mastroianni, 1974). Recently applied technology affords the opportunity to study microenvironmental influences (Borland *et al.*, 1977, 1980). Of paramount importance for additional study is the regulatory role played by the hormonally altered composition of oviductal and uterine fluids. Early efforts to obtain fertilization and/or embryonic development in oviductal fluids often led to failure. Rabbit embryonic development is not possible in estrogen-influenced oviductal fluids (Kille and Hamner, 1973; Cline *et al.*, 1977; Stone *et al.*, 1977). The latter contain a low-molecular-weight inhibitory factor (Stone *et al.*, 1977) that has recently been characterized as a small peptide (Richardson *et al.*, 1980).

Some success in prolonged culture of sheep and cow embryos has followed efforts to duplicate the known composition of sheep oviductal fluid (Restall and Wales, 1966) with a synthetic oviductal fluid medium (Tervit *et al.*, 1972; Tervit and Rowson, 1974; Tervit and Gould, 1978). This medium also supports cleavage of pig embryos and development from the four- to eight-cell stages to the blastocyst stage (Schneider *et al.*, 1975). Also, swine embryos in one- to four-cell stages have been successfully cultured for 2 days in the oviducts of rabbits (Polge *et al.*, 1972). Sheep and cow embryos continue to cleave and retain their viability following transfer to the rabbit oviduct for up to 4 days (Averill *et al.*, 1955; Hunter *et al.*, 1962; Adams *et al.*, 1968; Lawson *et al.*, 1972). Such results have followed use of estrous or pseudopregnant does. The pig oviduct can support the penetration of cow ova by bull sperm (Bedirian *et al.*, 1975), and recently the oviduct of pseudo-pregnant rabbit does has been found capable of supporting fertilization of the squirrel monkey and of the golden hamster (DeMayo *et al.*, 1980). In the latter work, the process was referred to as xenogenous fertilization. These lines of investigation point to a need to further explore gamete and early embryonic requirements normally provided by the oviduct, and they also emphasize the potential value of comparative studies from which demonstration of important similarities among species might be anticipated.

Conclusions

In efforts to advance knowledge in mammalian embryo culture, several factors must be borne in mind. The extent and quality of the *in vitro* development of zygotes and embryos can vary greatly even if the culture conditions are apparently comparable. Genetics, experimental treatments that precede embryo culture, and physiological variables are important considerations that greatly influence experimental results.

Iwamatsu and Chang (1971) reported sperm penetration and fertilization *in vitro* to vary according to the strain of mouse used, which confirmed previous *in vivo* observations. Strain differences have subsequently been shown to affect the fertilizing capacity of sperm (Fraser and Drury, 1976; Fraser, 1977), sperm–egg interaction (Parkening and Chang, 1976; Kaleta, 1977), and the fertilizability of eggs (Kasai *et al.*, 1978). Variation in timing of sperm penetration *in vitro*, events of fertilization, and significant differences in the proportion of eggs cleaved 20 hr after insemination were recently reported for four different strains of mice (Niwa *et al.*, 1980). Male parents of a certain mouse strain significantly influenced the timing of initial embryonic cleavage following *in vivo* fertilization, and the genetic determinants were autosomal rather than Y-linked (Shire and Whitten, 1980a). Also, the more rapidly cleaving embryos were more likely to form blastocysts in culture. Additional experiments revealed a similar influence of female parents on timing of first cleavage, and further predictable genetic influences on the success of embryo culture were described (Shire and Whitten, 1980b).

Experimental treatments preceding embryo culture might also be responsible for observed levels of development. For example, development of rabbit embryos to morula and blastocyst stages was similar after *in vitro* fertilization with high-ionic-strength-capacitated sperm and *in vivo*-capacitated sperm, but the levels of development were depressed when the capacitating treatment involved, in addition to high ionic strength, a brief sperm incubation with dibutyryl cAMP (Brackett, 1979b).

An example of physiological variables that are reflected by varying degrees of zygote and embryonic development after *in vitro* fertilization involves comparison of fertilizing ability of ejaculated and epididymal rabbit spermatozoa. When treated similarly, epididymal sperm were capable of more rapid penetration of ova as reflected by development of the fertilization process and cleavage through the four-cell stage (Brackett *et al.*, 1978; Brackett, 1979a). A possible explanation, though speculative, is that additional sperm membrane stabilizing factors are elaborated by the accessory glands, making *in vitro* capacitation (and perhaps pronuclear development also) of ejaculated sperm a slower process. Apparently, influences that retard the rate of embryonic development *in vitro* (when compared with that *in vivo*) serve to decrease the viability or the potential for continued embryonic development upon transfer into a suitable recipient. A harmless, reversible inhibitor of embryonic development that could be added to a culture medium might prove useful in short-term storage and as an aid in synchronizing embryos with surrogate dams. Efforts to enhance, or speed up, *in vitro* development by elimination of deterrents or by addition of promoting factors to a medium might result in more vigorous embryos with a higher degree of viability as reflected by consistently high proportions of embryos exhibiting continued gestational development following transfer. In mammalian species the state of the art points scientists toward the goal of consistent attainment following fertilization *in vitro* of complete preimplantational embryonic development *in vitro* that is comparable in all respects to that taking place *in vivo*.

The ability to maintain and culture embryos *in vitro* is crucial to the development of many innovative technologies of predicted utility in animal breeding (Brackett *et al.*, 1981). Comparative studies are indicated as are additional biochemical investigations that become feasible with development of better micromethods. With a better understanding of embryonic development in mammalian species in which embryos are not so readily available, prudent selection of mouse strains can be useful in providing appropriate model systems for resolution of basic reproductive mechanisms. The exploitation of such anticipated knowledge should enable significant advances in the efforts of animal agriculture to feed a hungry world.

ACKNOWLEDGMENTS

The author gratefully acknowledges the suggestions of R. L. Brinster in the preparation of this manuscript. This work was supported by Grant HD 09406 from the National Institute of Child Health and Human Development.

References

Abramczuk, J., Stark, R. A., Konwinski, M., Solter, D., Mastroianni, L., and Koprowski, H., 1977, Parthenogenetic activation of rhesus monkey follicular oocytes *in vitro*, *J. Embryol. Exp. Morphol.* **42**:115–126.

Adams, C. E., Moor, R. M., and Rowson, L. E. A., 1968, Survival of cow and sheep eggs in the rabbit oviduct, *Proc. 6th Int. Congr. Anim. Reprod. A.I.* **1**:573.

Anderson, G. B., 1978, Advances in large mammalian embryo culture, in: *Methods in Mammalian Reproduction* (J. C. Daniel, ed.), Academic Press, New York, pp. 273–283.

Auerbach, S., and Brinster, R. L., 1968, Effect of oxygen concentration on the development of two-cell mouse embryos, *Nature (London)* **217**:465.

Averill, R. L., Adams, C. E., and Rowson, L. E. A., 1955, Transfer of mammalian ova between species, *Nature (London)* **176**:167.

Bedirian, K. N., Shea, B. F, and Baker, R. D., 1975, Fertilization of bovine follicular oocytes in bovine and porcine oviducts, *Can. J. Anim. Sci.* **55**:251–256.

Beier, H. M., Mootz, U., and Kühnel, W., 1972, Asynchronous egg transfer during delayed uterine secretion in the rabbit, *Proc. 7th Int. Congr. Anim. Reprod. A.I.* **3**:1891–1896.

Biggers, J. D., 1979, Fertilization and blastocyst formation, in: *Animal Models for Research on Contraception and Fertility* (N. J. Alexander, ed.), Harper & Row, New York, pp. 223–252.

Biggers, J. D., Whitten, W. K., and Whittingham, D. G., 1971, The culture of mouse embryos *in vitro*, in: *Methods in Mammalian Embryology* (J. C. Daniel, ed.), Freeman, San Francisco, pp. 86–116.

Binkerd, P. E., and Anderson, G. B., 1979, Transfer of cultured rabbit embryos, *Gamete Res.* **2**:65–73.

Bishop, D. W., 1956, Oxygen concentrations in the rabbit genital tract, *Proc. 3rd Int. Congr. Anim. Reprod. A.I.* **2**:53.

Bishop, D. W., 1957, Metabolic conditions within the oviduct of the rabbit, *Int. J. Fertil.* **2**:11.

Boone, W. R., Dickey, J. F., Luszcz, L. J., Dantzler, J. R., and Hill, J. R., 1978, Culture of ovine and bovine ova, *J. Anim. Sci.* **47**:908–913.

Borland, R. M., Hazra, S., Biggers, J. D., and Lechene, C. P., 1977, The elemental composition of the environments of the gametes and preimplantation embryo during the initiation of pregnancy, *Biol. Reprod.* **16**:147–157.

Borland, R. M., Biggers, J. D., Lechene, C. P., and Taymor, M. L., 1980, Elemental composition of fluid in the human fallopian tube, *J. Reprod. Fertil.* **58**:479–482.

Brackett, B. G., 1969, Effects of washing the gametes on fertilization *in vitro*, *Fertil. Steril.* **20**:127–142.

Brackett, B. G., 1978, *In vitro* fertilization: A potential means for toxicity testing, *Environ. Health Perspect.* **24**:65–71.

Brackett, B. G., 1979a, *In vitro* assessment of sperm fertilizing ability, in: *Animal Models for Research on Contraception and Fertility* (N. J. Alexander, ed.), Harper & Row, New York, pp. 254–268.

Brackett, B. G., 1979b, *In vitro* fertilization and embryo culture, in : *Beltsville Symposium in Agricultural Research 3, Animal Reproduction* (H. W. Hawk, ed.), Allenheld, Osmun Co., New Jersey, pp. 171–193.

Brackett, B. G., 1981, Applications of *in vitro* fertilization, in: *New Technologies in Animal Breeding* (B. G. Brackett, G. E. Seidel, Jr., and S. M. Seidel, eds.), Academic Press, New York.

Brackett, B. G., and Mastroianni, L., Jr., 1974, Composition of oviductal fluid, in: *The Oviduct and Its Functions* (D. Johnson and W. Foley, eds.), Academic Press, New York, pp. 133–159.

Brackett, B. G., and Oliphant, G., 1975, Capacitation of rabbit spermatozoa *in vitro*, *Biol. Reprod.* **12**:260–274.

Brackett, B. G., and Williams, W. L., 1965, *In vitro* fertilization of rabbit ova, *J. Exp. Zool.* **160**:271–281.

Brackett, B. G., and Williams, W. L., 1968, Fertilization of rabbit ova in a defined medium, *Fertil. Steril.* **19**:144–145.

Brackett, B. G., Hall, J. L., and Oh, Y. K., 1978, *In vitro* fertilizing ability of testicular, epididymal, and ejaculated rabbit spermatozoa, *Fertil. Steril.* **29**:571–582.

Brackett, B. G., Oh, Y. K., Evans, J. F., and Donawick, W. J., 1980, Fertilization and early development of cow ova, *Biol. Reprod.* **23**:189–205.

Brackett, B. G., Seidel, G. E., Jr., and Seidel, S. M., (eds.), 1981, *New Technologies in Animal Breeding*, Academic Press, New York.

Brinster, R. L., 1963, A method for *in vitro* cultivation of mouse ova from two-cell to blastocyst, *Exp. Cell Res.* **32**:205.

Brinster, R. L., 1965a, Studies on the development of mouse embryos *in vitro*. I. The effect of osmolarity and hydrogen ion concentration. *J. Exp. Zool.* **158**:49–58.

Brinster, R. L., 1965b, Studies on the development of mouse embryos *in vitro*. II. The effect of energy source, *J. Exp. Zool.* **158**:59–68.

Brinster, R. L., 1965c, Studies on the development of mouse embryos *in vitro*. III. The effect of fixed-nitrogen source, *J. Exp. Zool.* **158**:69–78.

Brinster, R. L., 1965d, Studies on the development of mouse embryos *in vitro*. IV. Interaction of energy sources, *J. Reprod. Fertil.* **10**:227.

Brinster, R. L., 1967a, Carbon dioxide production from glucose by the preimplantation mouse embryo, *Exp. Cell Res.* **47**:271–277.

Brinster, R. L., 1967b, Carbon dioxide production from lactate and pyruvate by the preimplantation mouse embryo, *Exp. Cell Res.* **47**:634.

Brinster, R. L., 1968, Carbon dioxide production from glucose by the preimplantation rabbit embryo, *Exp. Cell Res.* **51**:330–334.

Brinster, R. L., 1969a, Radioactive carbon dioxide production from pyruvate and lactate by the preimplantation rabbit embryo, *Exp. Cell Res.* **54**:205–209.

Brinster, R. L., 1969b, The incorporation of carbon from glucose and pyruvate into the preimplantation mouse embryo, *Exp. Cell Res.* **58**:153–159.

Brinster, R. L., 1970, Culture of two-cell rabbit embryos to morulae, *J. Reprod. Fertil.* **21**:17–22.

Brinster, R. L., 1971, Uptake and incorporation of amino acids by the preimplantation mouse embryo, *J. Reprod. Fertil.* **27**:329–338.

Brinster, R. L., 1972, Cultivation of the mammalian egg, in: *Growth, Nutrition and Metabolism of Cells in Culture*, Volume II (G. Rothblat and V. Cristofalo, eds.), Academic Press, New York, pp. 251–286.

Brinster, R. L., 1973, Nutrition and metabolism of the ovum, zygote, and blastocyst, in: *Handbook of Physiology—Endocrinology II*, Section 7, Part 2 (R. O. Greep and E. A. Astwood, eds.), American Physiological Society, Washington, D.C., pp. 165-185.

Brinster, R. L., and Thomson, J. L., 1966, Development of eight-cell mouse embryos *in vitro*, *Exp. Cell Res.* **42**:308-315.

Brinster, R. L., and Troike, D. E., 1979, Requirements for blastocyst development *in vitro*, *J. Anim. Sci.* **49**:26-34.

Chang, M. C., 1959, Fertilization of rabbit ova *in vitro*, *Nature (London)* **184**:466-467.

Cholewa, J. A., and Whitten, W. K., 1970, Development of two-cell mouse embryos in the absence of a fixed-nitrogen source, *J. Reprod. Fertil.* **22**:553-555.

Church, R. B., and Raines, K., 1980, Biological assay of embryos utilizing fluorescein diacetate, *Theriogenology* **13**:91.

Cline, E. M., Randall, P. A., and Oliphant, G., 1977, Hormone mediated oviductal influence on mouse embryo development, *Fertil. Steril.* **28**:766-771.

Cross, M. H., 1974, Rabbit blastocoele bicarbonate accumulation rate, *Biol. Reprod.* **11**:654.

Daniel, J. C., 1967, The pattern of utilization of respiratory metabolic intermediates by preimplantation rabbit embryos *in vitro*, *Exp. Cell Res.* **47**:619-624.

David, A., Brackett, B. G., Garcia, C. R., and Mastroianni, L., Jr., 1969, Composition of rabbit oviduct fluid in ligated segments of the fallopian tube, *J. Reprod. Fertil.* **19**:285-289.

Davis, D. L., and Day, B. N., 1978, Cleavage and blastocyst formation by pig eggs *in vitro*, *J. Anim. Sci.* **46**:1043-1053.

DeMayo, F. J., Mizoguchi, H., and Dukelow, W. R., 1980, Fertilization of squirrel monkey and hamster ova in the rabbit oviduct (xenogenous fertilization), *Science* **208**:1468-1469.

Ducibella, T., and Anderson, E., 1975, Cell shape and membrane changes in the eight-cell mouse embryo: Prerequisites for morphogenesis of the blastocyst, *Dev. Biol.* **47**:45.

Edwards, R. G., and Steptoe, P. C., 1975, Physiological aspects of human embryo transfer, in: *Progress in Infertility* (S. J. Behrman and R. W. Kistner, eds.), Little, Brown & Co., Boston, pp. 377-409.

Edwards, R. G., Steptoe, P. C., and Purdy, J. M., 1970, Fertilization and cleavage *in vitro* of preovulator human oocytes, *Nature (London)* **227**:1307.

Elliott, D. S., Maurer, R. R., and Staples, R. E., 1974, Development of mammalian embryos *in vitro* with increased atmospheric pressure, *Biol. Reprod.* **11**:162-167.

Flynn, T. J., and Hillman, N., 1980, The metabolism of exogenous fatty acids by preimplantation mouse embryos developing *in vitro*, *J. Embryol. Exp. Morphol.* **56**:157-168.

Fraser, L. R., 1977, Differing requirements for capacitation *in vitro* of mouse spermatozoa from two strains, *J. Reprod. Fertil.* **49**:83-87.

Fraser, L. R., and Drury, L. M., 1975, The relationship between sperm concentration and fertilization *in vitro* of mouse eggs, *Biol. Reprod.* **13**:513-518.

Fraser, L. R., and Drury, L. M., 1976, Mouse sperm genotype and the rate of egg penetration *in vitro*, *J. Exp. Zool.* **197**:13-20.

Friedhandler, L., 1961, Pathways of glucose metabolism in fertilized rabbit ova at various pre-implantation stages, *Exp. Cell Res.* **22**:303-316.

Graham, C. F., 1974, The production of parthenogenetic mammalian embryos, *Biol. Rev.* **49**:393-442.

Graves, C. N., and Biggers, J. D., 1970, Carbon dioxide fixation by mouse embryos prior to implantation, *Science* **167**:1506.

Hall, J. L., Stephenson, R., Mathias, C., and Brackett, B. G., 1977, Hormonal dependence of cyclic patterns in hamster uterine fluid proteins, *Biol. Reprod.* **17**:738-774.

Hall, J. L., Stephenson, R. B., and Brackett, B. G., 1978, Protein patterns of hamster female reproductive tract fluids, *Fed. Proc.* **37**:282 (abstract no. 373).

Ham, R. G., 1963, An improved nutrient solution for diploid Chinese hamster and human cell lines, *Exp. Cell Res.* **29**:515-526.

Hammond, J., 1949, Recovery and culture of tubal mouse ova, *Nature (London)* **163**:28–29.

Hamner, C. E., and Williams, W. L., 1964, Identification of sperm stimulating factor of rabbit oviduct fluid, *Proc. Soc. Exp. Biol. Med.* **117**:240–243.

Hoppe, P. C., and Pitts, S., 1973, Fertilization *in vitro* and development of mouse ova, *Biol. Reprod.* **8**:420–426.

Hunter, G. L., Bishop, G. P., Adams, C. E., and Rowson, L. E. A., 1962, Successful long-distance aerial transport of fertilized sheep ova, *J. Reprod. Fertil.* **3**:33.

Iwamatsu, T., and Chang, M., 1971, Factors involved in the fertilization of mouse eggs *in vitro*, *J. Reprod. Fertil.* **26**:197–208.

Kaleta, E., 1977, Influence of genetic factors on the fertilization of mouse ova *in vitro*, *J. Reprod. Fertil.* **51**:375–381.

Kane, M. T., 1972, Energy substrates on culture of single cell rabbit ova to blastocysts, *Nature (London),* **238**:468.

Kane, M. T., 1975, Bicarbonate requirements for culture of one-cell rabbit ova to blastocysts, *Biol. Reprod.* **12**:552–555.

Kane, M. T., 1979, Fatty acids as energy sources for culture of one-cell rabbit ova to viable morulae, *Biol. Reprod.* **20**:323–332.

Kane, M. T., and Foote, R. H., 1970a, Fractionated serum dialysate and synthetic media for culturing 2- and 4-cell rabbit embryos, *Biol. Reprod.* **2**:356–362.

Kane, M. T., and Foote, R. H ., 1970b, Culture of two- and four-cell rabbit embryos to the blastocyst stage in serum and serum extracts, *Biol. Reprod.* **2**:245–250.

Kane, M. T., and Foote, R. H., 1970c, Culture of two- and four-cell rabbit embryos to the expanding blastocyst stage in synthetic media, *Proc. Soc. Exp. Biol. Med.* **133**:921–925.

Kane, M. T., and Foote, R. H., 1971, Factors affecting blastocyst expansion of rabbit zygotes and young embryos in the defined media, *Biol. Reprod.* **4**:41.

Kane, M. T., and Headon, D. R., 1980, The role of commercial bovine albumin preparations in the culture of one-cell rabbit embryos to blastocysts, *J. Reprod. Fertil.* **60**:469–475.

Kasai, K., Minato, Y., and Toyoda, Y., 1978, Fertilization and development *in vitro* of mouse eggs from inbred and F_1 hybrids, *Jpn. J. Anim. Reprod.* **24**:19–22.

Kaufman, M. H., and Sachs, L., 1976, Complete preimplantation development in culture of parthenogenetic mouse embryos, *J. Embryol. Exp. Morphol.* **35**:179–190.

Kendle, K. E., and Telford, J. M., 1970, Investigations into the mechanism of the antifertility action of minimal doses of megestrol acetate in the rabbit, *Br. J. Pharm.* **40**:759–774.

Kille, J. W., and Hamner, C. E., 1973, The influence of oviductal fluid on the development of one cell rabbit embryos *in vitro*, *J. Reprod. Fertil.* **35**:415–423.

Lawson, R. A. S., Rowson, L. E. A., and Adams, C. E., 1972, The development of cow eggs in the rabbit oviduct and their viability after re-transfer to heifers, *J. Reprod. Fertil.* **28**:313–315.

Lindner, M., and Wright, R. W., Jr., 1978, Morphological and quantitative aspects of the development of swine embryos *in vitro J. Anim. Sci.* **46**:711–718.

Lopata, A., Johnston, I. W. H., Hoult, I. J., and Speirs, A. I., 1980, Pregnancy following intrauterine implantation of an embryo obtained by *in vitro* fertilization of a preovulatory egg, *Fertil. Steril.* **33**:117–120.

Manes, C., and Daniel, J. C., 1969, Quantitative and qualitative aspects of protein synthesis in the preimplantation rabbit embryo, *Exp. Cell Res.* **55**:261–268.

Mastroianni, L., Jr., and Jones, R., 1965, Oxygen tension within the rabbit fallopian tube, *J. Reprod. Fertil.* **9**:99.

Maurer, R. R., 1978, Advances in rabbit embryo culture, in: *Methods in Mammalian Reproduction* (J. C. Daniel, ed.), Academic Press, New York, pp. 259–272.

Maurer, R. R., Whitener, R. H., and Foote, R. H., 1969, Relationship of *in vivo* gamete aging and exogenous hormones to early embryo development in rabbits, *Proc. Soc. Exp. Biol. Med.* **131**:882–885.

Mills, J. A., Jeitles, G. G., Jr., and Brackett, B. G., 1973, Embryo transfer following *in vitro* and *in vivo* fertilization of rabbit ova, *Fertil. Steril.* **24:**602–608.

Mills, R. M., and Brinster, R. L., 1967, Oxygen consumption of preimplanted mouse embryos, *Exp. Cell Res.* **47:**337–342.

Mintz, B., 1964, Synthetic processes and early development in the mammalian egg, *J. Exp. Zool.* **157:**85–100.

Miyamoto, H., and Chang, M. C., 1972, Development of mouse eggs fertilized *in vitro* by epididymal spermatozoa, *J. Reprod. Fertil.* **30:**135–137.

Moricard, R., 1950, Penetration of the spermatozoon *in vitro* in the mammalian oviduct (oxydo potential level), *Nature (London),* **165:**763.

Moricard, R., 1954, Observation of *in vitro* fertilization in the rabbit, *Nature (London)* **173:**1140.

Mukherjee, A. B., 1972, Normal progeny from fertilization *in vitro* of mouse oocytes matured in culture and spermatozoa capacitated *in vitro, Nature (London)* **237:**397–398.

Mukherjee, A. B., and Cohen, M. M., 1970, Development of normal mice by *in vitro* fertilization, *Nature (London)* **228:**472–473.

Naglee, D. L., Maurer, R. R., and Foote, R. H., 1969, Effect of osmolarity on *in vitro* development of rabbit embryos in a chemically defined medium, *Exp. Cell Res.* **58:**331.

Niwa, K., Araki, M., and Iritani, A., 1980, Fertilization *in vitro* of eggs and first cleavage of embryos in different strains of mice, *Biol. Reprod.* **22:**1155–1159.

Ogawa, S., Satoh, K., and Hashimoto, H., 1971, *In vitro* culture of rabbit ova from the single cell to the blastocyst stage, *Nature (London)* **233:**422–424.

Ogawa, S., Satoh, K., Hamada, M., and Hashimoto, H., 1972, *In vitro* culture of rabbit ova fertilized by epididymal sperm in chemically defined media, *Nature (London)* **238:**270–271.

Parkening, T. A., and Chang, M. C., 1976, Strain differences in the *in vitro* fertilizing capacity of mouse spermatozoa as tested in various media, *Biol. Reprod.* **15:**647–653.

Parkening, T. A., Tsunoda, Y., and Chang, M. C., 1976, Effects of various low temperatures, cryoprotective agents and cooling rates on the survival, fertilizability and development of frozen-thawed mouse eggs, *J. Exp. Zool.* **197:**369–374.

Peters, D. F., Anderson, G. B., and Cupps, P. T., 1977, Culture and transfer of sheep embryos, *J. Anim. Sci.* **45:**350–354.

Peters, D. F., Anderson, G. B., BonDurant, R., Cupps, P. T., and Drost, M., 1978, Transfer of cultured bovine embryos, *Theriogenology* **10:**337–342.

Polge, C., Adams, C. E., and Baker, R. D., 1972, Development and survival of pig embryos in the rabbit oviduct, *Proc. 7th Int. Congr. Anim. Reprod. A.I.* **4:**60.

Quinn, P., and Wales, R. G., 1971, Fixation of carbon dioxide by preimplantation mouse embryos *in vitro* and the activities of enzymes involved in the process, *Aust. J. Biol. Sci.* **24:**1277.

Quinn, P., and Wales, R. G., 1973, Growth and metabolism of preimplantation mouse embryos cultured in phosphate-buffered medium, *J. Reprod. Fertil.* **35:**289.

Restall, B. J., and Wales, R. G., 1966, The fallopian tube of the sheep. III. The chemical composition of the fluid from the fallopian tube, *Aust. J. Biol. Sci.* **19:**687.

Richardson, L. L., Hamner, C. E., and Oliphant, G., 1980, Some characteristics of an inhibitor of embryonic development from rabbit oviductal fluid, *Biol. Reprod.* **22:**553–559.

Schneider, H. J., Jr., Krug, J. L., and Olds, D., 1975, Observations of recovery and culture of cow ova, *J. Anim. Sci.* **40:**187.

Seidel, G. E., Jr., 1977, Short-term maintenance and culture of embryos, in: *Embryo Transfer in Farm Animals* (Monograph 16) (K. J. Betteridge, ed.), Canada Department of Agriculture, pp. 20–24.

Seidel, G. E., Jr., Bowen, R. A., and Kane, M. T., 1976, *In vitro* fertilization, culture and transfer of rabbit ova, *Fertil. Steril.* **27:**862–870.

Seitz, H. M., Jr., Brackett, B. G., and Mastroianni, L., Jr., 1970a, *In vitro* fertilization of ovulated rabbit ova recovered from the ovary, *Biol. Reprod.* **2**:262–267.

Seitz, H. M., Jr., Rocha, G., Brackett, B. G., and Mastroianni, L., Jr., 1970b, Influence of the oviduct on sperm capacitation in the rabbit, *Fertil. Steril.* **21**:325–328.

Seitz, H. M., Jr., Rocha, G., Brackett, B. G., and Mastroianni, L., Jr., 1971, Cleavage of human ova *in vitro*, *Fertil. Steril.* **22**:255–262.

Shire, J. G. M., and Whitten, W. K., 1980a, Genetic variation in the timing of first cleavage in mice: Effect of paternal genotype, *Biol. Reprod.* **23**:363–368.

Shire, J. G. M., and Whitten, W. K., 1980b, Genetic variation in the timing of first cleavage in mice: Effect of maternal genotype, *Biol. Reprod.* **23**:369–376.

Steptoe, P. C., and Edwards, R. G., 1978, Brith after the re-implantation of a human embryo, *Lancet* **2**:366.

Stone, S. L., Richardson, L. L., Hamner, C. E., and Oliphant, G., 1977, Partial characterization of hormone-mediated inhibition of embryo development in rabbit oviduct fluid, *Biol. Reprod.* **16**:647–653.

Sugawara, S., and Takeuchi, S., 1973, On glycolysis in rat eggs during preimplantation stages, *Tohoku J. Agric. Res.* **24**:76–85.

Tervit, H. R., and Gould, P. G., 1978, The culture of sheep embryos in either a bicarbonate-buffered medium or a phosphate-buffered medium enriched with serum, *Theriogenology* **9**:251–257.

Tervit, H. R., and Rowson, L. E. A., 1974, Birth of lambs after culture of sheep ova *in vitro* for up to 6 days, *J. Reprod. Fertil.* **38**:177–179.

Tervit, H. R., Whittingham, D. G., and Rowson, L. E. A., 1972, Successful culture *in vitro* of sheep and cattle ova, *J. Reprod. Fertil.* **30**:493–497.

Toyoda, Y., Yokoyama, M., and Hosi, T., 1971, Studies on the fertilization of mouse eggs *in vitro*. I. *In vitro* fertilization of eggs by fresh epididymal sperm, *Jpn. J. Anim. Reprod.* **16**:147–151.

Vishwakarma, P., 1962, The pH and bicarbonate ion content of the oviduct and uterine fluids, *Fertil. Steril.* **13**:481–485.

Wales, R. G., 1970, Effects of ions on the development of the preimplantation mouse embryo *in vitro*, *Aust. J. Biol. Sci.* **23**:421.

Wales, R. G., Quinn, P., and Murdoch, R. N., 1969, The fixation of carbon dioxide by the 8-cell mouse embryo, *J. Reprod. Fertil.* **20**:541.

Whitten, W. K., 1957, Culture of tubal ova, *Nature (London)* **179**:1081.

Whitten, W. K., 1971, Nutrient requirements for the culture of preimplantation embryos *in vitro*, in: *Advances in the Biosciences*, Volume 6, (G. Raspe, ed.), Pergamon Press, Oxford pp. 129–141.

Whitten, W. K., and Biggers, J. D., 1968, Complete development *in vitro* of the pre-implantation stages of the mouse in a simple chemically defined medium, *J. Reprod. Fertil.* **17**:399–401.

Whittingham, D. G., 1968, Development of zygotes in cultured mouse oviducts. II. The influence of the estrous cycle and ovarian hormones upon the development of the zygote, *J. Exp. Zool.* **169**:399–406.

Whittingham, D. G., 1971, Culture of mouse ova, *J. Reprod. Fertil. Suppl.* **14**:7–21.

Whittingham, D. G., 1975, Fertilization, early development and storage of mammalian ova, in: *The Early Development of Mammals* (M. Balls and A. E. Wilds, eds.), Cambridge University Press, London, pp. 1–24.

Whittingham, D. G., 1977, Fertilization *in vitro* and development to term of unfertilized mouse oocytes previously stored at $-196°C$, *J. Reprod. Fertil.* **49**:89–94.

Whittingham, D. G., and Bavister, B. D., 1974, Development of hamster eggs fertilized *in vitro* or *in vivo*, *J. Reprod. Fertil.* **38**:489–492.

Wright, R. W., 1977, Successful culture *in vitro* of swine embryos to the blastocyst stage, *J. Anim. Sci.* **44**:854.

Wright, R. W., Anderson, G. B., Cupps, P. T., Drost, M., and Bradford, G. E., 1976a, *In vitro* culture of embryos from adult and prepuberal ewes, *J. Anim. Sci.* **42**:912.

Wright, R. W., Anderson, G. B., Cupps, P. T., and Drost, M., 1976b, Blastocyst expansion and hatching of bovine embryos cultured *in vitro*, *J. Anim. Sci.* **43**:170.

Wright, R. W., Anderson, G. B., Cupps, P. T., and Drost, M., 1976c, Successful culture *in vitro* of bovine embryos to the blastocyst stage, *Biol. Reprod.* **14**:157.

Yanagimachi, R., and Chang, M. C., 1964, *In vitro* fertilization of golden hamster ova, *J. Exp. Zool.* **156**:361–376.

5

MECHANISMS OF FERTILIZATION IN MAMMALS

R. YANAGIMACHI

The spermatozoa of most invertebrates (e.g., sea urchins) and nonmammalian vertebrates (e.g., fishes and amphibians) have full capacity to fertilize eggs upon leaving the testis. Testicular spermatozoa of mammals, on the other hand, do not possess the ability to do so. Their fertilizing capacity develops as they pass through the epididymis (Young, 1931; Nishikawa and Waide, 1952; Blandau and Rumery, 1964; Bedford, 1966; Orgebin-Crist, 1967). This process, apparently "unique" to mammals, is referred to as the epididymal *maturation* of spermatozoa. Even after their maturation, however, spermatozoa require an additional phase of maturation or *capacitation* within the female genital tract before they are able to fertilize eggs (Austin, 1951, 1952; Chang, 1951a). Thus, epididymal maturation and capacitation are two extra steps that mammaliam spermatozoa must take before they can effect fertilization. In this chapter, I will discuss how mammalian spermatozoa prepare themselves for fertilization and how the spermatozoa and eggs interact during fertilization. The process and mechanisms of sperm transport in the female genital tract will not be dealt with extensively here. Readers are referred to Bishop (1961, 1969), Blandau (1969), Bedford (1970b, 1972b), Thibault (1972, 1973a), Zamboni (1972), Blandau and Gaddum-Rosse (1974), Hafez and Thibault (1975), Overstreet and Katz (1977), Overstreet and Cooper (1978, 1979b), Overstreet *et al.* (1978), Shalgi and Kraicer (1978), Cooper *et al.* (1979) and Hunter (1975, 1980). The rejection or elimination of extra spermatozoa by the fertilized egg, one of the most fascinating events in

R. YANAGIMACHI • Department of Anatomy and Reproductive Biology, University of Hawaii School of Medicine, Honolulu, Hawaii 96822.

fertilization, will not be discussed here. Instead, readers are referred to the chapter by Dr. Wolf in this volume. The physiology of egg activation has been described and discussed to some extent by Gwatkin (1977) and Yanagimachi (1978a). There are numerous reviews dealing with general aspects of mammalian fertilization. The following are recommended to aid in grasping the outline of mammalian fertilization: Austin and Bishop (1957), Austin and Walton (1960), Austin (1961, 1968), Blandau (1961), Pikó (1969), Thibault (1969), Bedford (1970a,b, 1972b), Gwatkin (1976, 1977), Yanagimachi (1977, 1978a), Bedford and Cooper (1978) and Hunter (1980).

Epididymal Maturation and Capacitation of Spermatozoa

To the best of our knowledge, spermatozoa of all mammalian species require epididymal maturation (Bedford, 1979). Epididymal maturation includes various morphological as well as physiological and biochemical changes in the sperm components (for reviews, see Orgebin-Crist, 1969; Bedford, 1975; Hamilton, 1977). One of the most readily recognizable changes is the development of the sperm's potential to move. Although the characteristics of the motor apparatus itself may change during maturation, changes in the properties of the plasma membrane seem to be largely responsible for it (Mohri and Yanagimachi, 1980). In fact, the plasma membrane is the site of the most prominent changes during epididymal maturation. Table I lists some of the changes that occur on or in the plasma membrane during maturation.

It is well established that the sperm plasma membrane has the property of adsorbing a variety of substances from its environment. Some of them come from the seminiferous tubule, epididymis, and vas deferens (Table I). Upon ejaculation, the sperm surface is further coated with seminal plasma components (Table II). Some of these surface-coating materials are so tightly bound to the spermatozoa that they cannot be readily eluted by simple washings with physiological saline or common organic solvents (Weil, 1965; Scacciati and Mancini, 1975). The notion that the removal or alteration of the coating materials constitutes a part of capacitation (Weinman and Williams, 1964; Pikó, 1967, 1969; Hunter and Nornes, 1969; Bedford, 1970a; Johnson, 1975) has been popular. According to Oliphant and Brackett (1973), antibodies raised against rabbit seminal plasma strongly agglutinate ejaculated rabbit spermatozoa even after the spermatozoa are incubated for 18 hr in a noncapacitating medium. When the spermatozoa are incubated in the uterus of the estrous female (an environment known to induce capacitation), they gradually become incapable of agglutination by the antibodies, with complete loss by 12 hr. This clearly indicates that the seminal plasma components on the sperm surface are gradually removed or altered as capacitation proceeds. Removal (or alteration) of the seminal plasma components from the sperm

Table I
Changes on or in the Sperm Plasma Membrane during Maturation

Phenomena	Site	References[a]
Adsorption of antigens, glycoproteins, sialic acid, and others	Testis	1-6
	Epididymis	1, 3, 7-20
	Vas deferens	1, 3
Changes in net negative surface charge	Testis-epididymis	21-29
Changes in distribution pattern of intramembranous particles	Epididymis	20
Changes in lipid composition and integrity[b]	Testis-epididymis	28, 30-45
Possible adsorption or integration of carnitine, acetylcarnitine, glycerylphosphoryl choline, and lipids[b]	Epididymis	46-53
Changes in activity of surface ATPase	Epididymis	54
Reduction in surface SH groups	Epididymis	55

[a] (1) Hunter and Hafs (1964); (2) Baker and Amann (1970, 1971), (3) Killian and Amann (1973); (4) Millette and Bellve (1977); (5) O'Rand and Romrell (1977); (6) Romrell and O'Rand (1978); (7) Martan and Risley (1963); (8) Martan et al. (1964); (9) Weinman and Williams (1964); (10) Rajalakshmi and Prasad (1969); (11) Baker and Amann (1971); (12) Fléchon (1975); (13) Lea et al. (1978); (14) Olson and Hamilton (1978); (15) Nicolson and Yanagimachi (1979); (16) Nicolson et al. (1977, 1979); Lewin et al. (1979); (17) Kohane et al. (1980a); (18) Moore (1980); (19) Wenstrom and Hamilton (1980); (20) Suzuki and Nagano (1980); Olson (1980); (21) Bedford (1963); (22) Cooper and Bedford (1971); (23) Yanagimachi et al. (1972); (24) Bedford et al. (1973); (25) Fléchon (1975); (26) Fléchon and Morstin (1975); (27) Temple-Smith and Bedford (1976); (28) Hammerstedt et al. (1979); (29) Moore (1979); Holt (1980); (30) Dawson and Scott (1964); (31) Grogan et al. (1966); (32) Quinn and White (1967); (33) Scott et al. (1967); (34) Hamilton and Fawcett (1970); (35) Lavon et al. (1970, 1971); (36) Poulos et al. (1973); (37) Poulos et al. (1975); (38) White (1973); (39) Terner et al. (1975); (40) Voglmayr (1975); (41) Davis (1978); (42) Legault et al. (1978); (43) Legault et al. (1979a); (44) Legault et al. (1979b); (45) Evans and Setchell (1979); (46) Crabo et al. (1967); (47) Brooks et al. (1974); (48) Back et al. (1974) (49) Brooks (1979); (50) Casillas and Chaipayungpan (1979); (51) Teichman et al. (1974); (52) Cummins et al. (1974); (53) Cummins and Teichman (1974); (54) Chulavatnatol and Yindipit (1976); (55) Reyes et al. (1976).

[b] Whether these events occur on/in the sperm plasma membrane or in other components of the spermatozoa is not clear.

surface, however, cannot be considered to represent the entire process of capacitation because in the rabbit, both ejaculated spermatozoa (exposed to seminal plasma) and spermatozoa from the distal corpus or cauda epididymis (not exposed to seminal plasma) are functionally capacitated at the same rate (Cummins and Orgebin-Crist, 1971; Overstreet and Bedford, 1974a; Bedford and Cooper, 1978). Apparently, the removal or alteration of materials that coat the sperm surfaces before spermatozoa are exposed to seminal plasma is equally or even more important in terms of capacitation.

The plasma membrane over the sperm head is believed to be the major site for coating during epididymal maturation and at ejaculation. However,

Table II

Changes on or in the Sperm Plasma Membrane upon Contact with
Seminal Plasma

Phenomena	References[a]
Adsorption of macromolecules including the so-called decapacitation factor	1–4
Adsorption of ABO blood group substances	5, 6
Adsorption of HL-A antigen	7
Adsorption of lactoferrin	8
Adsorption of collagen-binding protein	10
Alteration of membrane surface charge	9
Alteration of lectin-binding sites	11, 12
Reduction in the ability to adsorb extracellular substances	13
Exposure to lipids, phospholipids, and phospholipases	14–19
Integration of lipoproteins	20

[a](1) Weil and Rodenburg (1962); (2) Herrmann and Uhlenbruck (1972); (3) Killian and Amann (1973); (4) Oliphant and Singhas (1979); Vierula and Rajaniemi (1980); (5) Edwards et al. (1964); (6) Boettcher (1968); (7) Kerek et al. (1973); (8) Hekman and Ruemke (1969); (9) Moore and Hibbitt (1975); Moore (1979); (10) Koehler et al. (1980); (11) Nicolson and Yanagimachi (1972); (12) Nicolson et al. (1977); (13) Blank et al. (1974); (14) Hartree and Mann (1960); (15) Clegg and Foote (1973); (16) Poulos et al. (1973); (17) Jain and Anand (1976); (18) Darin-Benett et al. (1977); (19) Kunze and Bohn (1978); (20) Davis (1978).

coating may also occur on other parts of the spermatozoon. According to Hamilton and Gould (1980), a galactosyltransferase in the rete testis fluid forms a galactose-bearing glycoprotein coat predominantly along the sperm tail. Thus, removal or alteration of the surface coat might occur over the entire surface of the spermatozoon during capacitation, although the rate, degree, and manner of removal or alteration may differ in different regions of the spermatozoon.

Spermatozoa of some species (e.g., mouse, rat, guinea pig, and human) are known to gain the ability to fertilize eggs when incubated in relatively simple chemically defined media (see Rogers, 1978, for references). This might indicate that sperm surface-coating materials in these species are readily eluted or modified by simply exposing them to artificial media. Spermatozoa of some other species (e.g., rabbit, pig, bull, and monkey), which less readily gain their fertilizing capacity in artificial media, may require some more specific conditions for the removal or modification of surface coats. According to Brackett and Oliphant (1975), briefly exposing ejaculated rabbit spermatozoa to a hypertonic medium (380 mOsM) enhances the removal of the surface coat, thus facilitating capacitation of spermatozoa. This, however, may not be the mechanism by which rabbit spermatozoa are normally capacitated *in vivo*. The idea that special enzymes within the female genital tract are involved in the removal or modification of sperm surface coats (Kirton and Hafs, 1965; Johnson and Hunter, 1972; Johnson, 1975; Oliphant, 1976; Talbot and Franklin, 1978a,b) is certainly attractive, but requires confirmation. Neutrophils (Ericsson, 1970; Soupart, 1970), eosinophils (Ericsson, 1969), and cumulus cells (Gwatkin *et al.*, 1972; Gwatkin, 1977) have been implicated in capacitation of spermatozoa in some species, but whether these cellular components actually play an essential role in capacitation *in vivo* has not been well established. Suggestions that *in vivo* capacitation requires cell-to-cell contact between spermatozoa and the endometrium (Soupart and Orgebin-Crist, 1966; Hamner and Sojka, 1967) have been largely ignored in the past, but do deserve serious attention. When I mated estrous hamster females and examined the distribution of spermatozoa at various time intervals, I found that the heads of spermatozoa become temporarily associated with the epithelium of the uterotubal junction and the lowermost segment of the isthmic portion of the oviduct before they begin to ascend toward the ampulla (Yanagimachi, unpublished data). Although the biological significance of sperm–epithelium association is unknown, it is tempting to speculate that the epithelium in specific regions of the female genital tract induces an alteration in the sperm surface coats by means of enzymatic or other actions.

The site where capacitation begins and where it is completed may vary from species to species. In species in which semen is deposited directly into the uterus at coitus (e.g., many rodents, the dog, and pig), capacitation may start in the uterus, but the principal site for capacitation is believed to be the oviduct (Hunter, 1968; Zamboni, 1972; Hunter and Hall, 1974). In species in which semen is deposited in the vagina (e.g., the rabbit and human), capacitation may start in the vagina or as soon as the spermatozoa migrate into the cervix. In the rabbit, spermatozoa can be fully capacitated in either the uterus or the oviduct after the two are surgically separated (Adams and Chang, 1962), but capacitation seems to be most efficient when spermatozoa are sequentially exposed to both the uterus and the oviduct (Bedford, 1969a). In other words, the uterus and oviduct (possibly the cervix as well), each with its own specific environmental characteristics, seem to work synergistically in capacitating spermatozoa. As the sperm surface is coated with a variety of materials of different origins, it is unlikely that all the coating materials are removed or altered simultaneously. Rather, they are probably removed or modified in more than one step under normal conditions. Bedford (1969a), Bavister (1973), and Mahi and Yanagimachi (1973) have all provided circumstantial evidence that capacitation is not a single-step phenomenon.

In vivo, there is a close temporal correlation between the migration of *fertilizing* spermatozoa to the ampulla (the usual site of fertilization) and the commencement of ovulation. When animals (the rabbit, rat, and guinea pig) are mated before ovulation, fertilizing spermatozoa stay in the isthmic region of the oviduct until ovulation commences (Harper, 1973; Yanagimachi and Mahi, 1976; Shalgi and Kraicer, 1978; Overstreet et al., 1978; Overstreet and Cooper, 1979b). The entry of eggs into the ampulla and the ascent of fertilizing spermatozoa to the ampulla seem to occur synchronously. As spermatozoa entering the ampulla almost immediately fertilize the eggs, these spermatozoa must have completed at least the major part of capacitation by the time they left the isthmus.

It is probable that the genital tract of the estrous female provides the most favorable conditions for capacitation of spermatozoa of the same species. However, it is unlikely that the conditions the female tract provides are strictly species specific, for the female tract of one species can capacitate spermatozoa of some other species. For instance, the rabbit oviduct is apparently capable of inducing capacitation of squirrel monkey and hamster spermatozoa (DeMayo et al., 1980), although it may be less effective than monkey and hamster oviducts (cf. Bedirian et al., 1975, for possible capacitation of bovine spermatozoa in porcine oviduct). Capacitation may not even be strictly organ specific: rabbit spermatozoa, for instance, can be capacitated in such ectopic sites as the colon, bladder, and anterior chamber of the eye (Noyes et al., 1958; Hamner and Sojka, 1967), although capacitation under these conditions may be "partial" rather than complete (Bedford, 1970a).

How quickly spermatozoa are capacitated in vivo and in vitro seems to be a much more complex problem than generally thought. First of all, spermatozoa in the same region of the epididymis or in the same ejaculate may not be (most probably are not) in the same physiological state. Some spermatozoa might well be in more advanced stages of maturation than others (Orgebin-Crist, 1965). Thus, it is quite possible that individual spermatozoa are capacitated at different rates (Dziuk, 1965). If this is the case, then there must be a median time at which the largest proportion of spermatozoa are completing capacitation. The median capacitation time would, of course, vary according to species. Even within the same species, the median capacitation time may vary according to strain (Braden, 1958; Fraser and Drury, 1976; Fraser, 1977a; Hoppe, 1980; Niwa et al., 1980) and depend on the physiological (e.g., nutritional or seasonal) state of the male. The physiological (e.g., hormonal) state of the female (Chang, 1958, 1969; Soupart, 1967, 1972; Bedford, 1970a; Chang and Hunter, 1977), the site of sperm deposition (Adams and Chang, 1962; Bedford, 1969b), and the composition and condition of the medium (Rogers and Yanagimachi, 1975; McMaster et al., 1978) must also influence the rate of capacitation. The flexibility of the capacitation time can be readily understood if we assume that capacitation involves removal or alteration of the sperm surface coat. Although the chemical properties of sperm surface-coating materials must be genetically

Table III

Changes Associated with Sperm Capacitation

Site	Detected or suspected phenomena	References[a]
Plasma membrane	Loss or alteration of surface-adsorbed materials	1–12
	Changes in properties of protein	13
	Partial (or localized) loss of lectin-binding sites	14–20
	Reduction of net negative surface charge	20, 21
	Reduction of free surface SH and NH_2 groups	56
	Changes in phospholipids	22, 23
	Changes in fluidity	24
	Changes in distribution pattern of intramembranous particles	19, 25–28
	Changes in permeability and osmotic properties	29
	Removal or alteration of cholesterol	26–28, 30, 31
	Removal of Zn^{2+}	32–34
	Increased susceptibility to heterologous globulin	35
	Increased susceptibility to follicular fluid	36, 37
	Increased susceptibility to leukocytes	38
	Exposure or activation of Ca^{2+} uptake sites	39, 40
Acrosomal membrane	Changes in molecular configuration	41
Others	Increase in O_2 uptake	42–47
	Changes in or involvement of intracellular cAMP	48–53
	Changes in intracellular choline plasmalogen	54, 55

[a] (1) Weinman and Williams (1964); (2) Pikó (1967); (3) Pikó (1969); (4) Bedford (1970a); (5) Hunter and Nornes (1969); (6) Johnson and Hunter (1972); (7) Aonuma et al. (1973); Oliphant and Brackett (1973); (8) Brackett and Oliphant (1975); (9) Johnson (1975); (10) Schill et al. (1975); (11) Koehler (1976); Koehler et al. (1980); (12) Oliphant (1976); Ericsson (1967); Vaidya et al. (1969); Iritani et al. (1975); Byrd et al. (1979); Oliphant and Singhas (1979); Kohane et al. (1980b); (13) Esbenshade and Clegg (1977); (14) Gordon et al. (1974); (15) Gordon et al. (1975); (16) Gordon (1977); (17) Talbot and Franklin (1978a); (18) Talbot and Franklin (1978b); (19) Kinsey and Koehler (1978); (20) Courtens and Fournier-Delpech (1979); Lewin et al. (1979); (21) Vaidya et al. (1971); (22) Clegg et al. (1975); Snider and Clegg (1975); (23) Langlais et al. (1980); Bearer and Friend (1980); (24) O'Rand (1977a, 1979); (25) Koehler and Gaddum-Rosse (1975); (26) Friend (1977); (27) Friend (1980); (28) Friend et al. (1977); (29) Bedford (1964); (30) Davis (1976); (31) Davis (1978); Davis et al. (1979, 1980); (32) Huacuja et al. (1973); (33) Delgado et al. (1976a); (34) Johnson and Eliasson (1978); (35) O'Rand and Metz (1976); (36) Bedford (1969b); (37) Oliphant (1976); (38) Bedford (1965); (39) Yanagimachi and Usui (1974); (40) Babcock et al. (1979); (41) Delgado et al. (1976b); (42) Hamner and Williams (1963); (43) Mounib and Chang (1964); (44) Murdoch and White (1967); (45) Iritani et al. (1969, 1975); (46) Grotjan et al. (1974); (47) Stone et al. (1973); (48) Hicks et al. (1972a); (49) Hicks et al. (1972b); (50) Rogers and Morton (1973); (51) Rosado et al. (1974); (52) Hoskins and Casillas (1975); (53) Huacuja et al. (1977); (54) Cummins and Teichman (1974); (55) Soupart et al. (1979); (56) Rosado et al. (1973).

determined, the rate of removal or alteration of these materials is probably greatly influenced by the environment to which the spermatozoa are exposed. Any conditions that accelerate the removal or alteration of the materials would reduce the capacitation time, whereas those that retard or prevent it would prolong or inhibit capacitation. However, we must be aware that the removal or alteration of the surface-coating materials is merely a part of the complex process of capacitation. There are many other phenomena associated with capacitation (Table III). Any of these phenomena or changes, if they are really involved in capacitation, could be limiting factors controlling capacitation time.

Acrosome and Acrosome Reaction

Acrosomal Enzymes and Their Intraacrosomal Distributions

The acrosome is a membrane-bound, caplike structure covering the anterior portion of the sperm nucleus. Fawcett (1975) divided the acrosome into three segments; the apical, principal, and equatorial segments. As the apical and principal segments behave in the same manner at the time of the acrosome reaction, subdivision of the anterior part of the acrosome into two segments is probably unnecessary in terms of acrosomal function. I will therefore consider the acrosome as consisting of two segments, the anterior segment (acrosomal cap) and the posterior segment (equatorial segment) (Figure 1).

The term *equatorial segment* (which denotes the segment of the acrosome located in the equatorial region of the sperm head) is appropriate for spermatozoa of many species, but is certainly not suitable for spermatozoa of some species such as the mouse and rat (Figure 2; also cf. Phillips, 1977). However, as the purpose of this article is not to discuss terminology, to avoid confusion the term equatorial segment will be used.

Classical cytochemical studies of developing acrosomes have revealed that the acrosomal contents are glycoprotein or glycolipid in nature (Wislocki, 1949; Leblond and Clermont, 1952; Onuma and Nishikawa, 1963). More recent biochemical studies have demonstrated that the acrosome is a structure analogous to a lysosome (Allison and Hartree, 1970; Hartree, 1975) or a zymogen granule of pancreatic cells (Friend, 1977). It contains a variety of hydrolyzing enzymes such as hyaluronidase, proteinase, esterase, neuraminidase, acid phosphatase, phospholipase, arylsulfatase, β-N-acetylglucosaminidase, and collagenase (cf. Stambaugh, 1978). Although some of these enzymes may be localized in or on the acrosomal membrane, rather than in the acrosomal contents, the existence of a variety of hydrolytic enzymes within the acrosome has been unequivocally established. In intact acrosomes, some of these enzymes, notably acrosin, are not in a biologically active state (Meizel

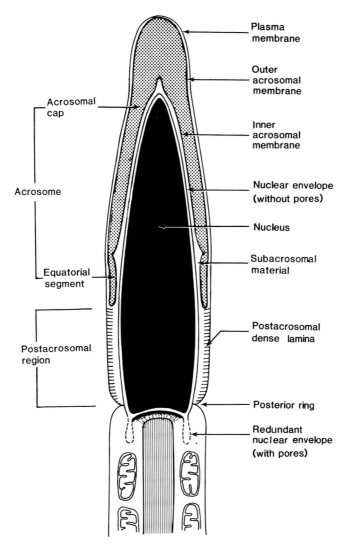

Figure 1. Diagram of a sagittal section of a mammalian sperm head showing its structural elements.

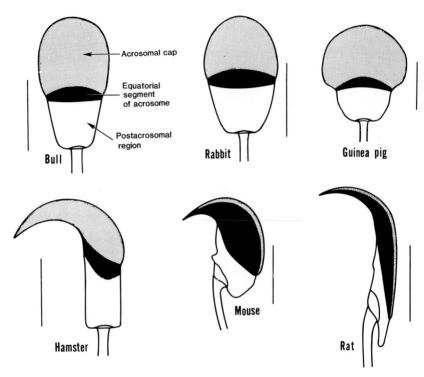

Figure 2. Diagrams illustrating the relative size and topographical relationship between the acrosomal cap and the equatorial segment of the spermatozoa of six different species. Scale bars all equal 5μm.

and Mukerji, 1975, 1976) and the acrosomal contents exhibit, at least in some species, fine striations with regular periodicity, suggesting a paracrystalline state of the enzymes within the acrosome (Phillips, 1972).

Hyaluronidase and acrosin are the two acrosomal enzymes that have been most extensively studied and well characterized (for reviews, see McRorie and Williams, 1974; Morton, 1976, 1977; Stambaugh, 1978). The literature concerning the intraacrosomal distributions of these two enzymes is, however, still somewhat confusing. While cytochemical studies utilizing antihyaluronidase antibodies have demonstrated that hyaluronidase is located predominantly within the matrix of the acrosomal cap (Mancini *et al.*, 1964; Fléchon and Dubois, 1975; Morton, 1975; Gould and Bernstein, 1975), Morton (1975) believes that at least some residual hyaluronidase is bound to the inner acrosomal membrane. The literature is even more confusing with regard to the intraacrosomal distribution of acrosin. Morton (1975, 1977) and Green and Hockaday (1978), who labeled spermatozoa with antiacrosin antibodies or soybean trypsin inhibitor, maintain that acrosin is localized on the inner acrosomal membrane. This seems to support the notion that the bulk of acrosin activity is located on the inner acrosomal membrane (Brown and Hartree, 1974; Multamaki and Suominen, 1976; Anand *et al.*, 1977; Fritz *et al.*, 1975). However, we must be aware that Morton (1975) examined his specimens by light microscopy, which is not suitable for subcellular localization of enzyme activity. Although Green and Hockaday (1978) used electron microscopy and demonstrated some acrosin activity over the inner acrosomal membrane, their published micrographs clearly demonstrate that the bulk of acrosin activity is in the matrix of the acrosome, and not on the inner acrosomal membrane. One gains the impression that the acrosin activity Green and Hockaday reported on the inner acrosomal membrane is a result of secondary deposition of the reaction products. Using an identical technique for bull spermatozoa, Shams-Borhan *et al.* (1979) were unable to demonstrate any acrosin activity on the inner acrosomal membrane. Instead, they detected acrosin activity over the outer acrosomal membrane (in my interpretation, the outer aspect of acrosomal matrix, not over the outer acrosomal membrane). Yanagimachi and Teichman (1972) and Gaddum-Rosse and Blandau (1977), who used less specific cytochemical techniques for proteinases, failed to demonstrate significant proteinase activity on the inner acrosomal membrane; the bulk of proteinase activity appeared to be in the acrosomal matrix.

Little is known about the intraacrosomal distribution of other acrosomal enzymes except for a nonspecific esterase that is localized in the acrosomal cap of mouse spermatozoa (Bryant and Unnithan, 1973). The only conclusion we can draw at the present time about the intraacrosomal distribution of enzymes is that all the enzymes, the distributions of which have thus far been examined (i.e., hyaluronidase, acrosin, and esterase), are confined to the acrosomal cap. How other acrosomal enzymes are distributed within the acrosome and whether the equatorial segment is enzymatically "empty" must be determined by future studies.

Morphology and Biological Significance of the Acrosome Reaction

The acrosome, a relatively unstable structure, may be spontaneously disrupted during the senescence and death of spermatozoa, or as a result of harsh treatment. Such degenerative changes are called a "false" acrosome reaction and should be clearly distinguished from the "true" acrosome reaction that occurs in actively motile spermatozoa capable of fertilizing eggs (Bedford, 1970a; Meizel, 1978).

The importance of the acrosome reaction in mammalian fertilization was first recognized by Austin and Bishop (1958). They reported that the acrosomal caps of highly motile spermatozoa of the guinea pig and hamster were modified, and then lost, before spermatozoa began to penetrate zonae pellucidae. The observation that the acrosome reaction in mammalian spermatozoa involves membrane vesiculation or multiple fusions between the plasma and the underlying outer acrosomal membranes was first made by Pikó and Tyler (1964) for the rat followed by Barros *et al.* (1967) and for the hamster and rabbit. These and subsequent studies using electron microscopy have demonstrated that the morphological pattern of the acrosome reaction is fundamentally the same in all mammalian species thus far studied (Figure 3). Russell *et al.* (1979a) published results of work in which they labeled the plasma membrane of boar spermatozoa with filipin (a polyen antibody that specifically binds to membrane cholesterol and produces characteristic deformations of the membrane) before inducing the acrosome reaction with Ca^{2+} ionophore. Their micrographs of acrosome-reacted spermatozoa convincingly demonstrated that the membrane vesicles that appear during the acrosome reaction are truly mosaics of both the plasma and the outer acrosomal membranes.

The membrane vesiculation is usually confined to the acrosomal cap region (Barros *et al.*, 1967; Bedford and Cooper, 1978), but the equatorial segment can also participate in vesiculation (cf. Figures 2 and 3 of Bedford, 1967a; Figures 6, 9, and 10 of Bedford, 1968; cf. also Yanagimachi and Noda,

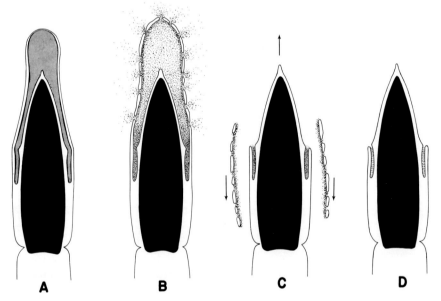

Figure 3. Diagrams showing the progression of the acrosome reaction. (A) Before the reaction. (B) The reaction is in progress; multiple fusions between the plasma and outer acrosomal membranes allow escape of the acrosomal contents (enzymes). (C, D) The reaction is complete; visiculated membranes held together by a "sticky" material may be left behind as the spermatozoon moves forward.

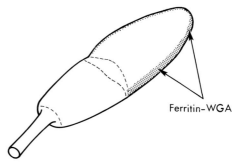

Figure 4. Diagram of the head of a rabbit cauda epididymal spermatozoon labeled with ferritin-conjugated wheat germ agglutinin. The lateral periphery of the acrosomal region is labeled (dots), indicating that the surface characteristics of the plasma membrane of this region are different from those of the remaining areas. The acrosome reaction may start in this peripheral region.

Ferritin–WGA

1970a; Barros *et al.*, 1973b; Szollosi and Hunter, 1973, 1978; Soupart and Strong, 1974; and McMaster *et al.*, 1978).* One thing that seems to be certain is that the membrane vesiculation occurs much more readily in the cap region than in the equatorial region of the acrosome. Although Yanagimachi and Noda (1970a) maintained that the equatorial segment of the acrosome vesiculates while spermatozoa pass through the zona pellucida, the vesiculations they observed could have been due to aging of supernumerary spermatozoa trapped within the zona. Fertilizing spermatozoa probably do not undergo extensive vesiculation of the equatorial segment under normal conditions (Bedford, 1972a; Bedford and Cooper, 1978).

Whether the membrane vesiculation in the acrosomal cap region occurs simultaneously over its entire area or starts from a certain point is not known. Bedford (1974) noted that the frontal margin of the acrosomal cap (rabbit) is closely applied to the overlying plasma membrane and surmised that this could be the point where the membrane vesiculation (the acrosome reaction) begins. When I labeled rabbit cauda epididymal spermatozoa with ferritin-conjugated wheat germ agglutinin, the peripheral margin of the sperm head membrane had a specific affinity to the agglutinin (unpublished data; Figure 4). Although this only informs us that the peripheral margin of the sperm head membrane has different characteristics from membranes elsewhere on the head, it is tempting to speculate that this region represents the site where membrane vesiculation starts. Friend (1977) noted two distinct regions where calcium is highly concentrated in the acrosomal cap of the guinea pig spermatozoon (Figure 5). As calcium has been implicated in the acrosome reaction (see p. 98), Friend surmised that these two regions could be the sites for the initiation of membrane vesiculation.

*Roomans (1975) studied the affinity of human sperm membranes to Ca^{2+} by incorporating Ca^{2+} in fixatives and examining the thickness of the membranes by electron microscopy. According to him, the outer acrosomal membrane, not the plasma and inner acrosomal membranes, has a strong affinity to Ca^{2+}. There seems to be no difference in Ca^{2+} affinity between the outer acrosomal membranes of the acrosomal cap and the equatorial segment.

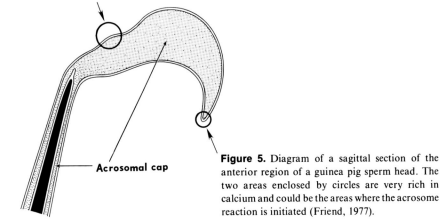

Figure 5. Diagram of a sagittal section of the anterior region of a guinea pig sperm head. The two areas enclosed by circles are very rich in calcium and could be the areas where the acrosome reaction is initiated (Friend, 1977).

The speed of the acrosome reaction probably varies according to species and the conditions of the medium surrounding the spermatozoa. When guinea pig spermatozoa were preincubated in Ca^{2+}-free medium and later exposed to Ca^{2+}, "vesiculation" of the acrosomal caps was seen (by electron microscopy) as early as 1 min after exposure to Ca^{2+}; the acrosome reactions of many spermatozoa were completed within the next 2 min (Yanagimachi and Usui, 1974). Talbot and Franklin (1976) estimated that hamster spermatozoa require about 20 min to complete the acrosome reaction *in vitro*. When hamster spermatozoa were first preincubated in K^+-deficient medium before K^+ and nigericin were added, 50% of the spermatozoa completed acrosome reactions within 15 min (Mrsny and Meizel, 1980a). The amount of time required for fertilizing spermatozoa to undergo the acrosome reaction *in vivo* is unknown.

The biological function of the acrosome reaction is at least twofold. First, it provides for the release or exposure of acrosomal enzymes believed to assist the passage of spermatozoa through the egg investments. Second, the reaction triggers, through some unknown mechanisms, a physiological change in the plasma membrane covering the equatorial segment and/or the postacrosomal region, which renders the sperm plasma membrane capable of fusing with the egg plasma membrane (Yanagimachi and Noda, 1970b; Yanagimachi, 1977, 1978a).

Site and Cause of Initiation of the Acrosome Reaction in Vivo

As the acrosome reaction results in the release or exposure of acrosomal enzymes, it is reasonable to assume that the reaction normally begins in the vicinity of the egg or upon contact with the cumulus oophorus surrounding the egg. In the rabbit (Bedford, 1969b) and mouse (Bryant, 1974), spermatozoa lying freely in the oviduct have intact acrosomes. In the guinea pig, spermatozoa flushed from the lower half of the oviduct seldom show the acrosome reaction, whereas those flushed from the upper half of the oviduct show a significantly high incidence of the acrosome reaction (Yanagimachi and Mahi, 1976). According to Austin and Bishop (1958), most of the actively motile spermatozoa flushed from the oviducts of hamsters and guinea pigs have intact acrosomes, while those found within the cumulus oophorus often have altered (swollen) or no acrosomal caps. Yanagimachi and Noda (1970a) observed several actively motile hamster spermatozoa within the cumulus oophorus, all of which had either altered (swollen or wrinkled) or no acrosomal caps. These observations seem to support the notion that the acrosome reaction *in vivo* does not start until spermatozoa reach the vicinity of the cumulus or come into contact with the cumulus. This, however, should not be taken as an indication that spermatozoa are incapable of initiating the acrosome reaction *in vivo* in the absence of eggs or egg investments. Overstreet and Cooper (1979a) have reported that some rabbit spermatozoa undergo the acrosome reaction within the isthmic region of the oviduct several hours before ovulation commences, indicating that spermatozoa can initiate the acrosome reaction *in vivo* without participation of eggs and/or egg investments.

It is well known that sea urchin spermatozoa do not require capacitation. They initiate the acrosome reaction upon contact with the jelly coat of the egg or with a substance emanating from the jelly (Dan, 1952, 1956, 1967). The active components of the jelly material are known to be glycoproteins (Vasseur, 1949). According to SeGall and Lennarz (1979) and Kopf and Garbers (1980), the fucose sulfate polysaccharide moiety of the jelly material is responsible for induction of the acrosome reaction. Because jellyless eggs, as well as simple physical or chemical stimuli such as high alkalinity of the medium and contact with a glass surface, can also induce the acrosome reaction (Dan, 1952, 1967; Decker *et al.*, 1976), it seems that any conditions or agents that cause "perturbance" or increased "excitability" of the membrane trigger the acrosome reaction. The matrix of the cumulus oophorus surrounding the mammalian egg may be analogous to the jelly coat of the sea urchin egg. This matrix may well be the natural acrosome reaction-triggering substance. This, however, does not imply that the cumulus material is the only substance capable of inducing the acrosome reaction *in vivo*. The material of the zona pellucida itself, or substances associated with the zona, as well as physical conditions or substances within the oviduct may all have some potency to induce or facilitate the acrosome reaction. Mother nature may provide more than one means of triggering the acrosome reaction *in vivo*.

In marsupials, eggs are completely devoid of follicle (cumulus and corona) cells at the time of ovulation (Harding *et al.*, 1976; Rodger and Bedford, 1980). Therefore, the acrosome reaction of fertilizing spermatozoa in these species must occur on the surface of the zona.

Site of Acrosome Reaction in Fertilizing Spermatozoa in Vitro

In vitro fertilization may be achieved by mixing epididymal or ejaculated spermatozoa with eggs in suitable media without preincubation of spermatozoa. The spermatozoa then must undergo capacitation and the acrosome reaction after being mixed with the eggs. In most *in vitro* experiments, a large number of spermatozoa (>3000–6000 per egg; e.g., Niwa and Chang, 1974) are deposited around the eggs. Under these conditions, the cumulus oophorus will partially or completely disperse (most probably due to hyaluronidase released from dead or moribund spermatozoa) and spermatozoa with intact acrosomes may reach the surface of the zona shortly after insemination; spermatozoa undergoing acrosome reactions will be seen on the zona sometime thereafter (e.g., Yanagimachi and Noda, 1970a; Thompson *et al.*, 1974). When eggs are freed from the cumulus prior to insemination, acrosome-intact spermatozoa may bind to the zona immediately after insemination and begin their acrosome reactions on the zona surface sometime thereafter (e.g., Saling *et al.*, 1979). Thus, under certain *in vitro* conditions, spermatozoa can undergo both capacitation and the acrosome reaction directly on the zona surface before penetrating it. Although capacitation and the acrosome reaction on the zona are certainly possible, we must be aware that this is most probably not what happens under ordinary *in vivo* conditions. Under ordinary *in vivo* conditions, fertilizing spermatozoa probably complete their capacitation before contact with the cumulus oophorus and begin acrosome reactions shortly before their contact with the cumulus or while they are passing through the cumulus. If the cumulus has already disintegrated extensively or is completely absent (e.g., due to postovulatory aging prior to fertilization), capacitated spermatozoa with intact acrosomes may reach the zona where they initiate their acrosome reaction. Such situations should be considered exceptional rather than the rule *in vivo*.

Sperm Surface and Membrane Components Involved in the Acrosome Reaction

As stated previously, the surface of mature epididymal or freshly ejaculated spermatozoa is coated with macromolecular substances. These substances seem to protect or stabilize the sperm plasma membrane and prevent spermatozoa from undergoing "premature" acrosome reactions (Bedford, 1970a). During capacitation some or all of these surface molecules must be removed or modified, rendering the sperm plasma membrane capable of fusing with the underlying outer acrosomal membrane. If removal or alteration of the surface-coating substances is prevented or if high concentrations of the coating substances are present in the medium surrounding the spermatozoa, acrosome reaction would be prevented. According to Eng and Oliphant (1978), a seminal plasma component (glycoprotein) added to the medium prevents rabbit spermatozoa from initiating acrosome reactions. Kanwar *et al.* (1979) presented indirect evidence that the continuous presence of seminal plasma components in the medium prevents human spermatozoa from undergoing the acrosome reaction. Tung *et al.* (1980) observed that bivalent (IgG) autoantibodies to guinea pig spermatozoa or testicular cells completely inhibited acrosome reaction (without sperm agglutination) in an immunologically specific manner; the study based on monovalent (Fab) antibodies was inconclusive, as they caused dispersal of sperm rouleaux and loss of sperm viability. This study thus indicates that antisperm antibodies may have blocked the membrane molecules involved in the acrosome reaction, and that these molecules are both sperm-specific and autoimmunogenic. How the seminal plasma and other extrinsic macromolecular components inhibit the acrosome reaction is unknown. It is possible that these components cross-link intramembranous particles within the sperm plasma membrane, preventing the particles from freely moving laterally within the membrane phospholipid bilayers (Johnson, 1975). Friend *et al.* (1977) have shown that prior to the acrosome reaction some intramembranous particles in the plasma membrane migrate laterally leaving patchlike particle-free areas in the membrane, which are believed to be the initiating sites for membrane fusion (the acrosome reaction). The seminal plasma components or substances adsorbed to the sperm surface during epididymal maturation may prevent this rearrangement of intramembranous particles and thus block an essential step in the acrosome reaction.

Changes in the composition and spatial arrangement of membrane lipids may be important for the acrosome reaction. Davis (1976, 1978) maintains that the cholesterol content of the rat sperm plasma membrane decreases (due to absorption by extracellular albumin) during capacitation, and this decrease is essential for occurrence of the acrosome reaction (Davis, 1980). According to Bearer and Friend (1980), the density of cardiolipin in the plasma membrane over the acrosome of guinea pig spermatozoa increases drastically prior to the acrosome reaction. Fleming and Yanagimachi (1981) have suggested that lysophospholipids (e.g., lysophosphatidylcholine) and acidic phospholipids (e.g., phosphatidylserine) are intricately involved in the preparation of guinea pig sperm membranes for the acrosome reaction.

Extracellular Components Involved in the Acrosome Reaction

The fact that spermatozoa of several mammalian species (e.g., the guinea pig, hamster, dog, and human) can undergo the acrosome reaction in media with simple constituents (Yanagimachi, 1972b; Yanagimachi et al., 1976; Mahi and Yanagimachi, 1978; Mrsny et al., 1979) suggests that extracellular conditions or components necessary for initiation and completion of the acrosome reaction are relatively simple and nonspecific at least in these species. It is difficult and perhaps meaningless to pinpoint which extracellular conditions or components are most important for the acrosome reaction. Perhaps, almost all conditions or components in the medium (including water molecules) are intricately involved in the reaction. The balance among individual conditions or components, rather than a single one, must be important. In the past, numerous papers have been published dealing with the effects of the composition and conditions of the medium and of various reagents on the acrosome reaction of spermatozoa (for reviews, see Meizel, 1978; Rogers, 1978). In most of these studies, spermatozoa were incubated in experimental and control media before the incidence of the acrosome reaction was assessed. For instance, a given component or reagent was added or deleted from the medium from the beginning of sperm incubation and the incidence of acrosome reactions was determined at one time or at various intervals. If the incidence of the acrosome reaction was lower in the medium with a given component than in the medium without it, for instance, it was concluded that the given component inhibited the acrosome reaction. The drawback of this type of approach is obvious. The result does not inform us whether the observed effect is due to inhibition of capacitation or inhibition of the acrosome reaction. The given component might have prevented capacitation rather than the acrosome reaction. As the vast majority of experiments in the past (including my own) have followed this procedure, it is extremely difficult to compile reliable data on the effects of extracellular components or of reagents on the acrosome reaction.

A component in the medium that has unequivocally proven to be essential for the acrosome reaction is Ca^{2+}. At least in the guinea pig, extracellular Ca^{2+} is necessary for initiation of the acrosome reaction, but not for progression and completion of capacitation (Yanagimachi, 1972a; Yanagimachi and Usui, 1974). The necessity of Ca^{2+} for the acrosome reaction has been amply documented (Barros, 1974; Rogers and Yanagimachi, 1975; Roomans, 1975; Yanagimachi, 1975; Summers et al., 1976; Talbot et al., 1976; Green, 1976, 1978a; Rink, 1977; Singh et al., 1978, 1980; Russell et al., 1979b; Garbers and Kopf, 1980). Recently, the presence of calmodulin, a specific Ca^{2+} regulatory protein, was demonstrated in the acrosomal region of guinea pig and rabbit spermatozoa by an immunofluorescence technique (Jones et al., 1980). Other conditions or components of the medium that affect or may affect the acrosome reaction include: *temperature* (Mahi and Yanagimachi, 1973), *pH* (Pavlok, 1968; Bavister, 1969; Mahi and Yanagimachi, 1973; Miyamoto *et al.*, 1974; Hyne and Garbers, 1980), K^+ (Toyoda and Chang, 1974; Mrsny and Meizel, 1980a), Mg^{2+} (Johnson, 1975; Rogers and Yanagimachi, 1976), *energy sources* such as pyruvate and glucose (Pavlok, 1968; Miyamoto and Chang, 1973; Rogers and Yanagimachi, 1975; Hoppe, 1976; Bavister and Yanagimachi, 1977; Niwa and Iritani, 1978; Fraser and Quinn, 1980; Okamoto and Toyoda, 1980), and macromolecules like *albumin* (Yanagimachi, 1969a, 1970a; Miyamoto and Chang, 1973; Hoppe and Whitten, 1974; Johnson, 1975; Blank *et al.*, 1976, Lui and Meizel, 1977; Lui *et al.*, 1977; Davis, 1978; Meizel, 1978) and *complements* (Cabot and Oliphant, 1978). Some of these conditions or components may affect the general physiology of spermatozoa (e.g., physiological integrity of the plasma membrane and energy metabolism) and capacitation rather than the acrosome reaction per se.

Spermatozoa of many species can undergo the acrosome reaction in media without any steroids. However, in the female genital tract steroids may affect capacitation and/or the acrosome reaction (Austin *et al.*, 1973; Rosado *et al.*, 1974). According to Meizel (1978), unphysiologically high concentrations of estrogen and progesterone in the medium prevent hamster spermatozoa from undergoing acrosome reactions. Whether steroids and other types of hormones are involved in capacitation and the acrosome reaction *in vivo* must be studied further.

Spermatozoa of the hamster seem to require certain low-molecular-weight substances ("motility factor") to sustain their motility in a medium (Yanagimachi, 1969a, 1970a; Bavister, 1975; Bavister *et al.*, 1976; Bavister and Yanagimachi, 1977). These substances were identified as neurotransmitter chemicals such as taurine and epinephrine (Cornett and Meizel, 1978; Mrsny *et al.*, 1979). The reason spermatozoa of many other species do not require the presence of the motility factor in the medium could be that these spermatozoa, unlike hamster spermatozoa, strongly retain the factor on their surface or inside (Bavister and Yanagimachi, 1977). At least for the hamster, the motility factor is essential for occurrence of the acrosome reaction, for without it the spermatozoa are simply unable to survive until they initiate the acrosome reaction. Whether survival factors should be included among the factors controlling the acrosome reaction must be a subject of future debate.

Intracellular Components Involved in the Acrosome Reaction

As ATP, ADP, cAMP, cGMP, adenylate cyclase, phosphodiesterase, and protein kinase are known to be intricately involved in the motility, metabolism, and survival of spermatozoa (Bishop, 1961; Mann, 1964; 1967;

Garbers *et al.*, 1971, 1973; Tash and Mann, 1973; Harrison, 1975; Hoskins *et al.*, 1978; Foulkes and MacDonald, 1979; Garbers and Kopf, 1980), it is not surprising that investigators have sought a relationship between these intracellular substances and the acrosome reaction. There are several lines of evidence suggesting that these substances are involved in capacitation and the acrosome reaction (Rogers and Morton, 1973; Mercado *et al.*, 1974; Huacuja *et al.*, 1977; Rogers *et al.*, 1977; Peterson *et al.*, 1978a; Hyne and Garbers, 1979a,b; Rogers and Garcia, 1979; Mrsny and Meizel, 1980b; Santos-Sacchi and Gordon. 1980; Santos-Sacchi *et al.*, 1980). One thing we must bear in mind is that the acrosome reaction is a phenomenon that takes place in the sperm head, not in the midpiece of the tail where the mitochondria are located. According to Fawcett (1975), the sperm plasma membrane is fused with the poreless nuclear envelope at the region of the posterior ring (cf. Figure 1). If this is the case, it would be difficult to conceive of ATP, for instance, being transported from the midpiece to the head unless the poreless nuclear envelope is permeable to such substances or there is a special transport mechanism in the posterior ring region. It will be important to study in the future whether the sperm head possesses enough reserves of energy-carrying substances like ATP for phenomena such as the acrosome reaction to take place, and if not, how these molecules are supplied from the midpiece to the head. A number of investigators have suggested that membrane-bound ATPases are involved in the acrosome reaction (Gordon, 1973, 1977; Yanagimachi and Usui, 1974; Gordon and Dandekar, 1977; Mrsny and Meizel, 1979). Activation of acrosomal proteinase has also been implicated in initiation of the acrosome reaction (Gordon, 1973; Yanagimachi and Usui, 1974; Meizel and Lui, 1976; Lui and Meizel, 1979), but this could be a result rather than the cause of the acrosome reaction (Green, 1978b).

Cytoskeletal systems (microtubules, microfilaments, and actin) present within or around the acrosome (Peterson *et al.*, 1978b; Stambaugh, 1978; Stambaugh and Smith, 1978; Talbot and Kleve, 1978) may participate in the acrosome reaction, but experimental evidence to support this concept has been lacking (Johnson, 1975). In fact, in the hamster, antiactin drugs (cytochalasins B and D, phalloidin) and antimicrotubular drugs (colchicine, podophyllotoxin, vinblastine sulfate, ansamitosin P-3, and *N*-phenylurethane), tested at concentrations of 1 to 100 μM, did not inhibit the acrosome reaction *in vitro* (Yanagimachi and Mohri, unpublished data).

Acrosome Reaction without Prior Capacitation

In vivo, guinea pig spermatozoa seem to require at least 4 hr before they initiate the acrosome reaction (Yanagimachi and Mahi, 1976). Under some *in vitro* conditions, a few guinea pig spermatozoa may initiate the acrosome reaction in 1 hr, but not before (Barros, 1974; Rogers and Yanagimachi,

1975). When the spermatozoa are exposed to media containing a calcium ionophore (A23187), however, the majority undergo the acrosome reaction within 15 min (Green, 1976, 1978a; Talbot *et al.*, 1976). Barros *et al.* (1973a) have demonstrated that guinea pig spermatozoa collected from the epididymis undergo the acrosome reaction within a few minutes when they are compressed between a slide and a coverslip; these spermatozoa are apparently capable of penetrating zona-free hamster eggs *in vitro*. Proper concentrations of various membrane-active reagents can also induce acrosome reactions in a majority of epididymal spermatozoa within 10 to 15 min; these spermatozoa can fertilize zona-intact guinea pig eggs (Yanagimachi, 1975). The "immediate" acrosome reaction described above could be due to acceleration of the removal or modification of sperm surface components, but it is more likely that these conditions or reagents induce the acrosome reaction *directly* by bypassing "capacitation." According to Peterson *et al.* (1978b) and Russell *et al.* (1979a,b), large proportions of boar and human spermatozoa exposed to calcium ionophore for 1 to 3 hr have acrosome reactions. Although we do not know whether spermatozoa of these species can respond to the ionophore within 10–15 min, the acrosome reaction these workers observed could well be identical to the "immediate" acrosome reaction in guinea pig spermatozoa.

Molecular Mechanism of the Acrosome Reaction

We still do not have enough data to present a unified view of the molecular mechanism of the acrosome reaction, but it is hoped that in the near future we can. Investigators who have been engaged in research on the acrosome reaction all have their own working hypotheses. Here, I will introduce five of them as examples. Diagrams based on my interpretation of the descriptions available in the literature are presented here for purposes of clarification.

The hypothesis of Gordon (1973) and Gordon *et al.* (1978) is based largely on observations of ATPase activity in guinea pig, rabbit, and human spermatozoa using cytochemical techniques at the electron microscopic level (Figure 6). A Ca^{2+}-independent ATPase (A) is present on the sperm plasma membrane. This ATPase is activated (B) when a seminal plasma factor (e.g., decapacitation factor) is removed from the sperm surface (C). The activated ATPase transports extracellular Ca^{2+} to the space between the plasma and outer acrosomal membranes. This intracellular Ca^{2+} activates another Ca^{2+}-dependent ATPase (D) on the outer acrosomal membrane, which (E) then transports Ca^{2+} into the acrosome. The Ca^{2+} that has entered the acrosome converts proacrosin (F) to biologically active acrosin (G). Part of the intracellular Ca^{2+} binds to membrane phospholipids (H), and this causes "ballooning" and adhesion of the plasma and outer acrosomal membranes. An increased concentration of Ca^{2+} (I) between the plasma and outer

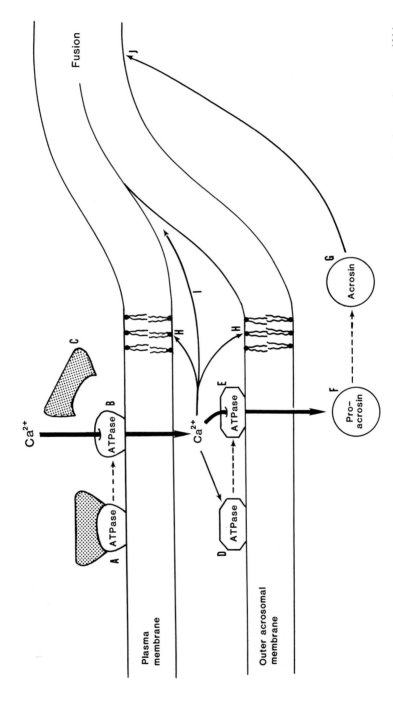

Figure 6. The mechanism of the acrosome reaction proposed by Gordon (1973) and Gordon *et al.* (1978). (For explanation, see the text, p. 101.)

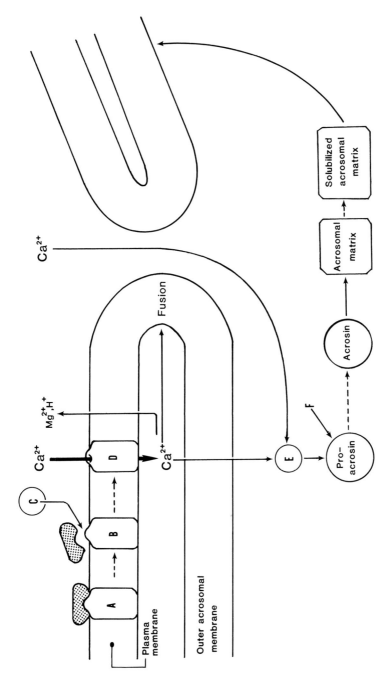

Figure 7. The mechanism of the acrosome reaction proposed by Green (1978c). (For explanation, see the text, p. 104.)

acrosomal membranes promotes their fusion. Activated acrosin (G) then partially digests the fused membranes (J) causing vesiculation and the release of acrosomal enzymes.

The hypothesis of Green (1978c) is based on his work with guinea pig spermatozoa (Figure 7). Green assumes the presence of a receptor (A) (similar to the acetylcholine receptor; Nelson, 1978) in the sperm plasma membrane. This receptor is normally occupied by an antagonist (B) that must first be removed during capacitation before stimulus ligands (C) (follicular cells or zona pellucida?) occupy the receptor. The stimulated receptor (D) allows an influx of extracellular Ca^{2+}, which in turn causes an efflux of Mg^{2+} and protons (e.g., H^+). Either the Ca^{2+} influx or the Mg^{2+} and protein efflux (or both) triggers membrane fusion. Proacrosin within the acrosome is converted to biologically active acrosin by either Ca^{2+}-dependent proteinase (E) or some other factor (F). The acrosin solubilizes the acrosomal matrix with the consequence that the acrosome swells up or "cavitates" due to increased internal colloidal osmotic pressure.

The hypothesis of Meizel (1978) is based on studies of hamster spermatozoa by Meizel and his associates (Figure 8). Through some mechanisms (mediated by catecholamine, ATP, ATPase, adenylate cyclase, cAMP, etc.), Ca^{2+} flows into the space between the plasma and outer acrosomal membranes (A). This leads to increased Ca^{2+} uptake by the acrosome due to stimulation of a Ca^{2+}-dependent ATPase (B), as suggested by Gordon (1973). The Ca^{2+} that has entered the acrosome converts proacrosin (C) to biologically active acrosin (D). Ca^{2+} may activate proacrosin directly, or it may activate proacrosin indirectly by increasing the intraacrosomal pH (by displacing H^+) or by chelating intraacrosomal Zn^{2+}. Acrosin then activates a phospholipase (E) that breaks membrane phospholipid into lysophospholipid and free fatty acid. Fatty acid that may inhibit the phospholipase is absorbed by extracellular albumin (F). Lysophospholipid increases the perturbance of the lipid moieties of the outer acrosomal membrane, which facilitates its fusion with the overlying plasma membrane.

Meizel postulated several different mechanisms for each step of the reaction. Therefore, the above synopsis and the diagram do not represent all that he had in mind.

The hypothesis of Davis (1978) is based on his work with rabbit and rat spermatozoa (Figure 9). When spermatozoa are exposed to seminal plasma, lipid exchange occurs between the sperm membrane and the cholesterol-rich lipoprotein vesicles in the seminal plasma (Davis considers that these vesicles represent the so-called "decapacitation factor"). This results in an increased cholesterol level in the sperm membrane (A to B), which causes stabilization of the membrane. During capacitation, some of the membrane cholesterol is transferred to albumin in the medium (C), resulting in destabilization of the membrane. Ca^{2+} binds to polar heads of membrane phospholipids of both

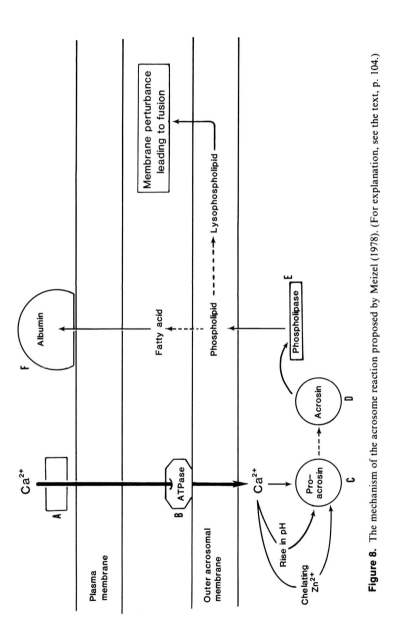

Figure 8. The mechanism of the acrosome reaction proposed by Meizel (1978). (For explanation, see the text, p. 104.)

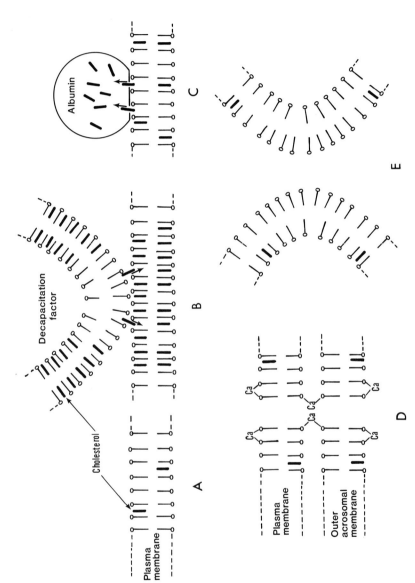

Figure 9. The mechanism of the acrosome reaction proposed by Davis (1978). (For explanation, see the text, p. 104.)

plasma and outer acrosomal membranes, creating aggregation of membrane phospholipids (D) that in turn leads to the fusion between these two membranes (the acrosome reaction).

My own hypothesis for capacitation and the acrosome reaction is outlined in Figure 10. The plasma and acrosomal membranes of mammalian spermatozoa contain numerous protein particles intercalated within the membranes (Koehler, 1972; Friend and Fawcett, 1974; Stackpole and Devorkin, 1974; Fawcett, 1975). Each type of particle must have its own specific function or functions. Some are believed to be for ion transport. For convenience, only one type of protein particle, the Ca^{2+} carrier, is considered here (A). I surmise that this protein particle, like some of the other particles, has a strong affinity for extracellular materials. The particle starts to adsorb the materials while the spermatozoa are within the testis. Other materials are adsorbed onto the particle during transit of spermatozoa through the epididymis and vas deferens as well as while spermatozoa are exposed to the seminal plasma. During capacitation, these adsorbed (coating) materials are removed or modified sequentially by either simple elution or enzymatic action (B). Nonspecific substances like albumin in the surrounding medium may also be involved in the removal or alteration of the coating materials. The coating material that is in direct contact with the protein particle is probably most resistant to removal or alteration. In some species, the removal or alteration of this material may be accomplished by specific substances (C) associated with the cumulus oophorus or egg. The special substances may also stimulate or activate the protein particle. Once the coating material is removed (or altered), or the particle is activated, extracellular Ca^{2+} enters the space between the plasma and outer acrosomal membranes (D). This intracellular Ca^{2+} has at least two functions. It (E) neutralizes the repulsive negative charges of both the plasma and outer acrosomal membranes, facilitating their closer apposition. It also induces both a phase transition (a change from the "fluid" state to the "crystalline" state) and a lateral phase separation (formation of separate domains of lipid species) of the membrane phospholipids. The boundaries between crystalline and noncrystalline (fluid) domains are structurally unstable points of high free energy that offer focal points for mixing of molecules from the two closely apposed membranes (Papahadjopoulos, 1978), i.e., the plasma and outer acrosomal membranes. Ca^{2+} (F) also activates phospholipase (G) in the plasma and outer acrosomal membranes, which then cleaves nearby membrane phospholipids into lysophospholipids and free fatty acids. Part of the free fatty acids (H) are adsorbed by extracellular molecules like albumin or captured by Ca^{2+}. The appearance of lysophospholipids (I) within the membranes induces another type of membrane "perturbance," facilitating membrane fusion (Poole et al., 1970; Lucy, 1975).

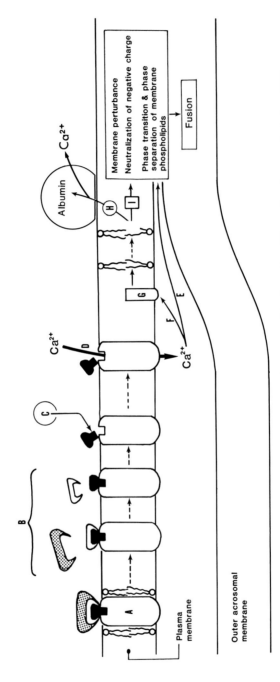

Figure 10. The mechanism of the acrosome reaction proposed by the author. (For explanation, see the text, p. 107.)

Yanagimachi and Usui (1974) have suggested that a Mg^{2+}-dependent ATPase (located on both the inner surface of the plasma membrane and the outer surface of the outer acrosomal membrane) is involved in the acrosome reaction. According to our scheme, Ca^{2+} that has entered the space between the plasma and outer acrosomal membranes inactivates the ATPase, which causes an influx of extracellular water into the acrosome. Swelling of the acrosome brings the plasma and outer acrosomal membranes into close apposition and facilitates their fusion. According to Green (1978a), however, the fusion between the plasma and outer acrosomal membranes begins before the acrosome swells. I have no sound evidence for or against Green's idea. Thus, whether ATPase is directly involved in the acrosome reaction remains to be determined.

Hyperactivation of Spermatozoa

When I incubated hamster spermatozoa in media capable of inducing capacitation and the acrosome reaction (Tyrode's solution with follicular fluid), I noticed that the spermatozoa began to move extremely vigorously shortly before the acrosome reaciton was initiated (Yanagimachi, 1969a,b, 1970a). I tentatively called it *activation* of spermatozoa (Yanagimachi, 1970b). The term activation, however, may be somewhat misleading because some people have already used the same term to refer to the initiation of active movement when motionless epididymal or vas deferens spermatozoa are exposed to seminal plasma or physiological salt solutions. With the consultation of Professor C. R. Austin of Cambridge University, I propose here the revised term *hyperactivation* to refer to the movement in question.

The typical hyperactivated movement of hamster spermatozoa is shown in Figure 11B (Katz and Overstreet, 1980; Katz and Yanagimachi, 1980; Mohri and Yanagimachi, 1980). It is characterized by vigorous whiplashlike beating of the flagellum, with the sperm head tracing erratic figure 8's. Since hyperactivation of spermatozoa was first recognized in the hamster, the same or a similar type of sperm movement has been reported in the guinea pig (Yanagimachi, 1972b; Barros et al., 1973a; Yanagimachi and Usui, 1974; Yanagimachi and Mahi, 1976; Barros and Berrios, 1977; cf. Figure 12), dog (Mahi and Yanagimachi, 1976), mouse (Fraser, 1977b, 1979; Aonuma et al., 1980), and rabbit (Cooper et al., 1979; Overstreet and Cooper, 1979b; Overstreet et al., 1980a).

Hyperactivation *in vitro* is apparently physiological because hamster spermatozoa displaying hyperactivated motility can be seen through the wall of the ampulla about the time of fertilization (Yanagimachi, 1970b; Katz and Yanagimachi, 1980). It is not known whether hyperactivation is limited to certain species or is a general phenomenon throughout the mammals. Human

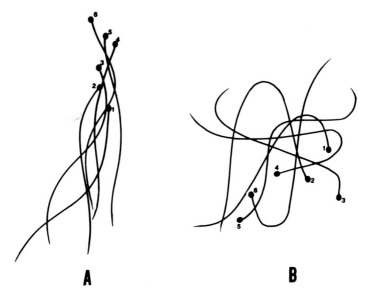

A   **B**

Figure 11. Shapes of typical flagellar beats of fresh epididymal (A) and hyperactivated (B) hamster spermatozoa. Intervals between successive drawings are 0.04 and 0.06 sec, respectively.

spermatozoa in capacitation media usually do not display "typical" activated movement, but the pattern of flagellar motion seems to change (from two dimensional to three dimensional) as capacitation proceeds (Hoshi and Yanagimachi, unpublished observations). Thus, the pattern of hyperactivation may well vary from species to species.

The physiological significance of hyperactivated motility is not clear. In those species in which it has been documented, the great majority of spermatozoa that have been "capacitated" *in vitro* or *in vivo* (in the oviduct) exhibit this type of movement in structureless, low-viscosity fluids. In the rabbit, the resumed ascent of spermatozoa that were quiescent in the lower isthmic region of the oviduct is associated with the onset of hyperactivated motility (Overstreet *et al.*, 1978; Cooper *et al.*, 1979). Whether hyperactivation contributes directly to transoviductal sperm transport or to the initial release from the lower isthmic retention is not clear. When spermatozoa enter the viscous cumulus matrix, they may be physically constrained from expressing the typical pattern of hyperactivated motility. The increased bending ability of the flagellum during hyperactivation may, however, represent a means whereby the spermatozoon can thrust more strongly during cumulus penetration. When hyperactivated spermatozoa of the guinea pig and hamster attach to the zona pellucida, they continue to exhibit large-amplitude, high-curvature flagellar bendings (Katz and Yanagimachi, unpublished observations). With the sperm head anchored against a semisolid zona, such

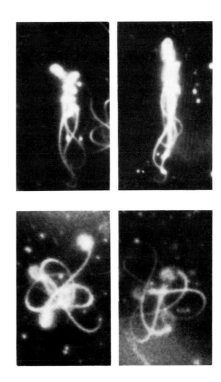

Figure 12. Strobomicrographs of fresh epididymal (upper) and hyperactivated (lower) guinea pig spermatozoa. Eight flashes per second. Micrographed by Dr. Ian Gibbons.

undulations would become an efficient means of generating thrust against the zona (Katz and Overstreet, 1980). Thus, hyperactivated motility would be particularly suited, in a hydrodynamic sense, to facilitate zona penetration.

A clarification is needed for the relationship between capacitation and hyperactivation of spermatozoa. My original article on hyperactivation of hamster spermatozoa (Yanagimachi, 1970b) may lead the reader to infer that capacitated spermatozoa always display hyperactivated motility or conversely that hyperactivated spermatozoa are always capacitated. Under normal conditions, spermatozoa begin hyperactivated movement when capacitation has proceeded to a certain extent. By the time capacitation is completed and the acrosome reaction begins, spermatozoa are already hyperactivated. However, the acrosome reaction and hyperactivation *can* occur independently and should be considered separate phenomena. Hyperactivation without the acrosome reaction (Yanagimachi, 1969a, 1970a, 1975; Mahi and Yanagimachi, 1973; Barros and Berrios, 1977) or the acrosome reaction without hyperactivation (Yanagimachi, 1975) may occur under various experimental conditions. After all, "capacitation" (if we define it strictly as a preparation for the acrosome reaction) and the acrosome reaction are phenomena occurring in the sperm head, whereas hyperactivation is an event in the sperm tail.

We know virtually nothing of the mechanism by which spermatozoa begin hyperactivated motility. Koehler and Gaddum-Rosse (1975) and Friend *et al.* (1977) reported that in the guinea pig the pattern of distribution of intramembranous particles in the plasma membrane of the midpiece changes by the time spermatozoa begin hyperactivation. The significance of this is unknown, but it may indicate an alteration of membrane properties (e.g., membrane permeability to ions and/or to extracellular energy sources) prior to or associated with hyperactivation.

The conditions in the medium surrounding spermatozoa obviously influence the initiation of hyperactivation of spermatozoa. The absence of Ca^{2+} in the medium, for instance, prevents guinea pig and mouse spermatozoa from initiating hyperactivation (Yanagimachi and Usui, 1974; Aonuma *et al.*, 1980). Low temperature (Mahi and Yanagimachi, 1973; Aonuma *et al.*, 1980) and the presence of Zn^{2+} in the medium (Aonuma *et al.*, 1980) also prevent initiation of hyperactivation by hamster and mouse spermatozoa. Mouse spermatozoa seem to require glucose to initiate hyperactivation (Fraser and Quinn, 1980). The addition of caffeine into the medium increases the proportion of hyperactivated mouse spermatozoa (Fraser, 1979). When I treated fresh epididymal spermatozoa of the guinea pig with various membrane-active reagents, both hyperactivation and the acrosome reaction began within several minutes (Yanagimachi, 1975). When I treated the spermatozoa under the same conditions but without exogenous energy sources, they underwent the acrosome reaction without hyperactivation. They were weakly motile. Upon addition of sodium pyruvate (0.3–1 mM), however, they began typical hyperactivated movement. Glucose (1–10 mM) and sodium lactate (1–25 mM) were totally ineffective in inducing hyperactivation (Yanagimachi, unpublished data). These studies suggest that both external and intercellular conditions as well as the metabolism of the spermatozoa are intricately involved in the hyperactivation of spermatozoa. A recent study by Mohri and Yanagimachi (1980) has shown that fresh epididymal and ejaculated hamster spermatozoa demembranated with Triton X-100 initiate hyperactivated motility upon addition of ATP (and cAMP) to a medium containing Mg^{2+}. This and another study (Yanagimachi, 1975) seem to indicate that mature spermatozoa in the epididymis or ejaculate are intrinsically capable of undergoing hyperactivated motility. Spermatozoa with intact membranes must be prevented by some mechanism (intracellular?) from displaying hyperactivated motility until it is needed.

Interaction of Spermatozoa with the Cumulus Oophorus

The Role of Chemotaxis in the Sperm–Cumulus Encounter

The number of spermatozoa present near the eggs at the time of fertilization *in vivo* is amazingly small. According to Zamboni (1972), the number of mouse spermatozoa at the site of fertilization is always lower than the total number of eggs. Only after all the eggs have been penetrated does the number of spermatozoa become equal to or slightly higher than that of the eggs. How do such small numbers of spermatozoa efficiently meet the eggs? Do the eggs or the cumulus oophorus exert some chemotactic attraction toward spermatozoa? Dickmann (1963) transplanted rat eggs into the oviducts of rabbits about the time of ovulation and examined both rabbit and rat eggs 7–11 hr later. He found that far more rabbit spermatozoa were associated with rabbit eggs than with rat eggs. Although this was interpreted by Dickmann as an indication of a chemotactic attraction of rabbit spermatozoa by rabbit eggs, this should more properly be interpreted in terms of the species–specificity of sperm–zona adhesion rather than chemotaxis. Bronson and Hamada (1977) presented experimental evidence that the mouse cumulus oophorus, but not the eggs, secretes a substance that alters the characteristics of the sperm surface. This substance alters the pattern of sperm movement, but not the speed of the movement of individual spermatozoa. The oviduct about the time of fertilization executes a very active adovarian propulsive movement (Blandau, 1978; Battalia and Yanagimachi, 1979), and the ampulla containing the cumulus oophorus displays a vigorous to-and-fro peristaltic movement. Chemotactic attraction of spermatozoa by the cumulus, if any, appears to be of secondary importance for the sperm–cumulus encounter.

Recently, Iqbal et al. (1980) and Vijayasarathy et al. (1980) have claimed that a synthetic peptide (formyl-Met–Leu–Phe) induces chemotaxis of bull spermatozoa. The basis for this is that two to three times as many spermatozoa enter a glass capillary filled with a medium containing this peptide compared to one filled with a control medium (Krebs–Ringer bicarbonate buffer). This method is obviously not suitable for detection of chemotaxis, and the result can be interpreted in terms of extended survival and/or increased motility of the spermatozoa rather than a chemotactic attraction by the peptide. We must be extremely cautious in designing apparatus and in interpreting results obtained when we seek to detect chemotaxis of spermatozoa (Rothschild, 1956; Monroy, 1965; Miller, 1966; Miller and Brokaw, 1970).

State of the Cumulus Oophorus at the Time of Fertilization

The dispersion of the cumulus oophorus from the egg surface was once thought to be an essential preliminary to successful penetration of the spermatozoon into the egg. This concept is no longer valid because in many species (e.g., the mouse, rat, and rabbit) the fertilizing spermatozoa penetrate the eggs long before the cumulus disperses (Lewis and Wright, 1935; Leonard et al., 1947; Austin, 1948; Chang, 1951b; also cf. Figure 13).

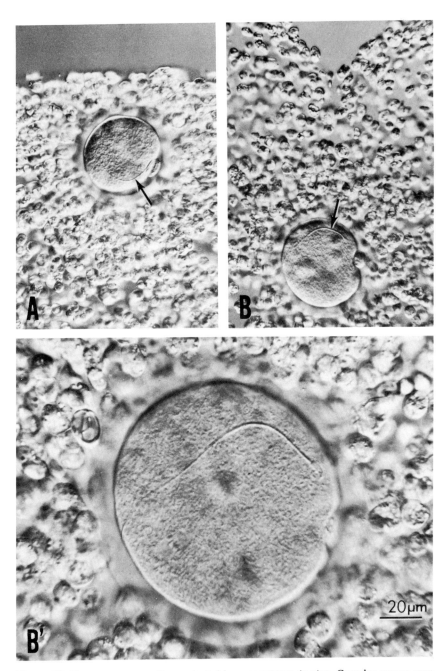

Figure 13. Hamster eggs recently penetrated by spermatozoa *in vivo*. Cumulus masses were collected from oviducts of mated animals and compressed between a slide and a coverslip so that the eggs were clearly visible. Arrows indicate sperm tails in the perivitelline space. (B′) is a high magnification of the same egg photographed in (B).

The condition of the cumulus oophorus obviously changes after ovulation. Immediately or soon after ovulation, the matrix of the cumulus is very viscous and the boundary between the matrix and the surrounding medium can be seen clearly (cf. Figure 74 of Austin, 1961). As time passes, the matrix gradually loosens or disintegrates, resulting in gradual dispersal of the cumulus cells. Thus, the condition of the cumulus matrix at the time of fertilization *in vivo* may well differ depending on when the animals are mated. For instance, when female hamsters are mated soon after the onset of heat (several hours before ovulation), the cumulus matrix is very viscous and the cumulus remains compact during fertilization. When animals are mated toward the end of heat (several hours after ovulation), the cumulus is very loose or may even be absent during fertilization (Yanagimachi, unpublished observations). The "delayed" mating cannot be considered abnormal because the females deliver normal young although the litter size may be greatly reduced. In some species (notably some ungulates), the cumulus oophorus seems to disintegrate very rapidly after ovulation. According to Lorton and First (1979), cow eggs are completely free from follicle cells (both cumulus and corona cells) within 3–4 hr after ovulation. As the fertilizable life of cow eggs is reported to be 18–20 hr (Blandau, 1961), "naked" eggs must be capable of normal fertilization and development. It is, however, important to note that the cow ovulates about 10 hr after the end of behavioral estrus, which lasts 12–22 hr (Asdell, 1964). In other words, under normal circumstances, spermatozoa reside within the female genital tract for at least 10 hr before they meet the eggs. It is therefore most probable that the spermatozoa are capacitated by the time of ovulation and meet the eggs as soon as the eggs are transported from the ovary to the oviduct. The eggs may still be surrounded by the cumulus oophorus (or cumulus matrix) at this time.

According to Braden (1959), the cumulus oophorus surrounding freshly ovulated mouse eggs is too "rigid" to permit penetration by spermatozoa. The cumulus needs "maturation" or "softening" before it will permit penetration by spermatozoa. Circumstantial evidence suggests that the cumulus of naturally ovulated eggs requires a considerably longer time to mature than that of eggs ovulated after exogenous gonadotropin treatments (Braden, 1959). Although the cumulus of rabbit and sheep eggs apparently does not require "maturation" after ovulation (Braden, 1959), it would certainly be worthwhile to carefully investigate whether the cumulus of other species indeed needs to "mature" after ovulation.

Role of the Cumulus Oophorus in Fertilization

The presence of an intact cumulus oophorus around the egg is obviously not an absolute necessity for successful fertilization. Many studies have clearly demonstrated that eggs freed from all the surrounding follicle cells (both cumulus and corona cells) by enzymatic or mechanical means are still capable of fertilization both *in vivo* and *in vitro* (Chang and Bedford, 1962; Cross and Brinster, 1970; Harper, 1970; Chang *et al.*, 1971; Fraser *et al.*, 1971; Fukuda *et al.*, 1972; Miyamoto and Chang, 1972; Moore and Bedford, 1978a) and even develop into normal young (Chang and Bedford, 1962). Without the cumulus oophorus, the fertilization rate may drop, but not always.

As stated previously, the cumulus oophorus is a likely candidate for the induction of the acrosome reaction of spermatozoa *in vivo*. Some investigators maintain that cumulus cells capacitate or participate in capacitating spermatozoa (Gwatkin *et al.*, 1972; Soupart and Morgenstern, 1973; Soupart and Strong, 1974; Gwatkin, 1977). Although these cells may indeed capacitate or assist capacitation or spermatozoa under the *in vitro* conditions these investigators employed, it is not likely that they actually capacitate spermatozoa *in vivo*. *In vivo*, fertilizing spermatozoa very quickly pass through both the cumulus and the zona pellucida (Blandau and Odor, 1952; Austin and Braden, 1956; Zamboni, 1972). The time the fertilizing spermatozoa spend within the cumulus appears to be too short for initiation and completion of capacitation. The notion that the presence of cumulus oophorus around the eggs protects the eggs from polyspermy (Austin, 1961) was contradicted by Bedford and Cooper (1978), who proposed that the condition of the eggs rather than the presence or absence of cumulus cells is important for normal, monospermic fertilization.

Acrosomal Enzymes Implicated in Sperm Penetration through the Cumulus Oophorus

Because the matrix of the cumulus oophorus is made predominantly of hyaluronic acid polymers (Pikó, 1969) and the acrosomes of mammalian spermatozoa are generally rich in hyaluronidase, the involvement of acrosomal hyaluronidase in cumulus penetration by spermatozoa has been inferred for a long time (Austin, 1960, 1961; Pikó, 1969; McRorie and Williams, 1974). The concept that acrosomal hyaluronidase is required for passage of spermatozoa through the cumulus has been supported by the results of immunological studies. Antibodies raised against hyaluronidase effectively block both cumulus dispersion by spermatozoa and fertilization (Metz *et al.*, 1972; Metz, 1973; Dunbar *et al.*, 1976). Synthetic hyaluronidase inhibitors also block fertilization (for references, see Joyce *et al.*, 1979; Reddy *et al.*, 1980). Acrosomal arylsulfatase (Farooqui and Srivastava, 1979a,b) and esterase (Bradford *et al.*, 1976a,b) have also been implicated in the passage of spermatozoa through the cumulus and the dispersion of corona radiata cells. Acidic proteinase (Yanagimachi and Teichman, 1972) and arylsulfatase (Yang and Srivastava, 1974; Farooqui and Srivastava, 1979a,b) of the acrosome may work synergistically with hyaluronidase in depolymerizing the cumulus matrix.

During growth and maturation of eggs in the ovary, the cells of the innermost layer of the cumulus (the corona radiata cells) extend numerous cytoplasmic processes through the intervening zona pellucida to contact the egg. Some of these processes are deeply inserted into the egg cortex (Zamboni and Mastroianni, 1966; Zamboni, 1971; Anderson, 1974). The tight relationship between the processes and the egg is lost during the final phase of preovulatory maturation (Gilula et al., 1978) and the processes begin to retract or degenerate (Zamboni, 1971). In some species (e.g., most laboratory rodents), retraction or degeneration of the processes is completed by the time of ovulation, while in some others (e.g., the rabbit) the processes are still partially inserted in the zona even after ovulation. Although fertilizing spermatozoa of the rabbit seem to penetrate the zona avoiding corona cells and their processes in the zona (cf. Figures 7 and 8 of Bedford, 1972a), some investigators believe that fertilizing spermatozoa release some enzyme to disperse the corona cells. This enzyme is referred to as the corona-penetrating enzyme (Zaneveld and Williams, 1970; McRorie and Williams, 1974) and has been claimed to be an esterase (Bradford et al., 1976a,b). Obviously such enzymes would be unnecessary in species (e.g., most laboratory rodents) whose eggs no longer have a distinct corona radiata at the time of fertilization.

The Role of Acrosomal Enzymes and the Acrosome Reaction in Sperm Penetration through the Cumulus

The mechanism by which acrosomal enzymes are released from fertilizing spermatozoa is generally believed to be by fenestration of the sperm membranes during the acrosome reaction. If acrosomal enzymes are essential for sperm passage through the cumulus, we would expect that all the spermatozoa within the cumulus would have reacting or reacted acrosomes. This is not always the case. For instance, Bedford (1972a) found a few rabbit spermatozoa with apparently intact acrosomes in the close vicinity of the zona pellucida of eggs that were still completely surrounded by cumulus cells, although most spermatozoa in the cumulus were undergoing or had completed the acrosome reaction. How had these acrosome-intact spermatozoa managed to pass through the cumulus? There are at least three possibilities. First, as suggested by Metz et al., (1972), some enzymes (e.g., hyaluronidase) may be bound to the outer surface of the sperm plasma membrane. Although the enzymes released from moribund or dead spermatozoa might be adsorbed onto the surfaces of live spermatozoa before or during ejaculation, it is difficult to believe that the surface hyaluronidase could tolerate elution during capacitation of spermatozoa in vivo. The second possibility is that acrosomal enzymes are released through both acrosomal and plasma membranes that are "intact" morphologically yet altered physiologically (Talbot and Franklin, 1974). Although this possibility cannot be negated, free passage of macromolecules like enzymes through morphologically "intact" membranes is unlikely. Finally, the spermatozoa may pass through the cumulus by purely mechanical means. If this is the case, we should be able to see acrosome-intact spermatozoa within the cumulus rather regularly. Obviously this is not the case, as reported by Bedford (1972a). It is my current belief that acrosome-intact spermatozoa are usually unable to enter or pass through the compact cumulus surrounding freshly ovulated eggs; only spermatozoa that are undergoing the acrosome reaction can readily do so. If the cumulus matrix has been "loosened" either by an autodegradation due to postovulatory aging or by acrosomal enzymes released from preceding spermatozoa, the looser cumulus may permit penetration by acrosome-intact spermatozoa. If the egg had already been penetrated by a spermatozoon, fertilization products (e.g., acids and proteinase known to be released from sea urchin eggs after fertilization: Vacquier *et al.*, 1972; Epel, 1977, 1978; Nishioka and McGwin, 1980) may also loosen the cumulus matrix allowing the mechanical penetration by acrosome-intact spermatozoa.

Function of Acrosomal Hyaluronidase in Bull Spermatozoa

It is very curious that bull spermatozoa, which are very rich in hyaluronidase (Blandau, 1961), fertilize cow eggs, which quickly lose the cumulus oophorus after ovulation. Lorton and First (1979) have surmised that the hyaluronidase of bull spermatozoa is not functional, but an evolutionary relic. As stated earlier (p. 115), cow eggs under normal *in vivo* conditions appear to meet the spermatozoa immediately after they enter the oviduct. At this time, the eggs might still be surrounded by a compact cumulus or at least by the cumulus matrix. According to M. C. Chang (personal communication), the freshly ovulated cow egg is surrounded by a transparent viscous material. This material may originate from follicular fluid or the matrix of the cumulus oophorus. If the material contains polymerized hyaluronic acid complexes, the acrosomal hyaluronidase in bull spermatozoa would have an important function in fertilization. We certainly need more work on the fertilization of cow eggs *in vivo*.

Interaction of Spermatozoa with the Zona Pellucida

Sperm Attachment to Zona Surface

Role of Capacitation and/or the Acrosome Reaction in Sperm Attachment to the Zona. Spermatozoa must firmly attach to the zona

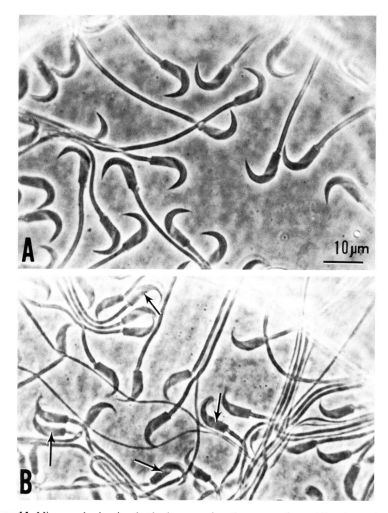

Figure 14. Micrographs showing that both uncapacitated, acrosome-intact (A) and capacitated, acrosome-reacted (B) spermatozoa are able to attach to zona surfaces. Cumulus-free hamster eggs were inseminated *in vitro* and the spermatozoa attached to the zona surfaces were photographed 5–10 min later. Arrows in (B) indicate spermatozoa with swollen (vesiculating?) acrosomal caps.

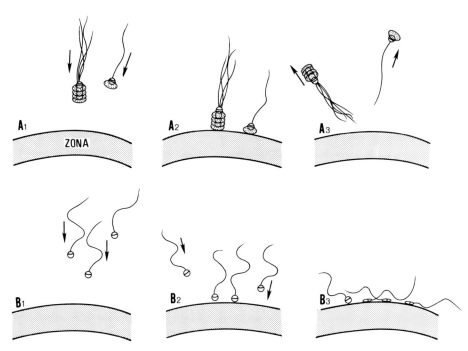

Figure 15. The difference in the behavior of acrosome-intact (A) and acrosome-reacted (B) guinea pig spermatozoa toward zonae pellucidae of guinea pig eggs. Acrosome-intact spermatozoa that hit the zona surface swim away (A_1–A_3); sometimes they may stay on the zona briefly (up to about 30 sec) and then swim away. Acrosome-reacted spermatozoa that hit the zona stay there (B_1–B_3).

pellucida before they penetrate it. According to Bedford (1967a), uncapacitated rabbit spermatozoa mixed with eggs *in vitro* can readily attach to the zona surface. Capacitation may (Bedford, 1967b) or may not (Overstreet and Bedford, 1974b) promote the sperm's ability to attach to the zona. In the hamster, both "uncapacitated" and "capacitated" spermatozoa are able to attach to the zona surface (Hartmann and Hutchison, 1976). Although Phillips and Shalgi (1980a) maintain that only acrosome-intact hamster spermatozoa are able to attach to the external surface of the zona, I have observed that acrosome-intact and acrosome-reacted hamster spermatozoa are equally able to attach to the zona surfaces (Figure 14). According to Saling and Storey (1979) and Saling *et al.* (1979), only acrosome-intact mouse spermatozoa, not acrosome-reacted ones, can stick to the zona. The reverse seems to be true for the guinea pig (Yanagimachi, 1972b; Figure 15). At least in the guinea pig, spermatozoa must undergo the acrosome reaction before they can attach to the zona (Huang *et al.*, 1981).

Mechanism of Sperm Attachment to the Zona Surface. The components with which the spermatozoon attaches to the zona surface must be localized in the sperm head. Saling and Storey (1979) and Saling *et al.* (1979) maintain that the plasma membrane over the intact acrosome of the mouse spermatozoon binds to the zona (Figure 16A). Bedford (personal communication) believes that it is the plasma membrane, after fusing with the underlying outer acrosomal membrane during the acrosome reaction, that binds the zona (Figure 16B). It is conceivable that the "sticky" acrosomal matrix exposed by membrane vesiculation (Figure 16C) binds the acrosome-reacting spermatozoon to the zona as does the "bindin" of sea urchin spermatozoa (Vacquier and Moy, 1977). I (Yanagimachi, 1977) have suggested that in the guinea pig it is the inner acrosomal membrane (Figure 16D) that recognizes and binds to the zona, although the plasma membrane over the equatorial and postacrosomal regions (Figure 16E) may also do so. When I inseminated cumulus-free hamster eggs with acrosome-reacted hamster spermatozoa *in vitro*, many spermatozoa immediately attached to the zona and their tails were seen to beat vigorously (Figure 17). Careful examination of these spermatozoa revealed that the heads tend to pivot about a fixed point (the anterior margin of the equatorial segment), giving the impression that this

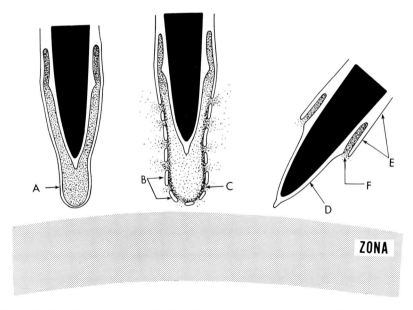

Figure 16. Possible components with which the spermatozoon recognizes and binds to the zona surface. (For explanation, see the text, p. 121.)

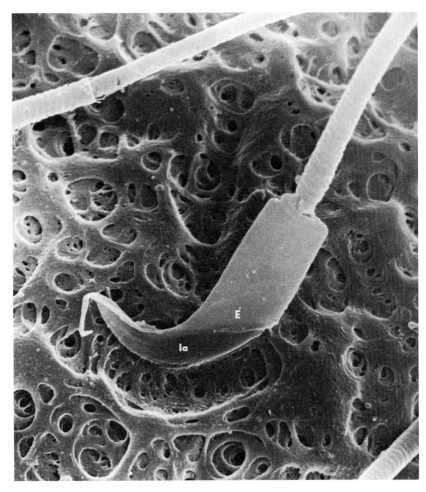

Figure 17. Scanning electron micrograph of an acrosome-reacted hamster spermatozoon attached to the zona surface. Spermatozoa were induced to undergo acrosome reactions *in vitro*, mixed with cumulus-free hamster eggs, and fixed 10 min later. E, equatorial segment of the acrosome; Ia, exposed inner acrosomal membrane of the acrosomal cap region. The specimen was fixed by Yanagimachi and micrographed by Dr. David Phillips.

particular region of the sperm head was very "sticky" to the zona. Some material emanating from the equatorial segment of the acrosome (Figure 16F) could be responsible for this stickiness. Some spermatozoa were also seen sticking to the zona by their inner acrosomal membranes. Thus, in the hamster, both the inner acrosomal and plasma membranes over the equatorial segment (or some substance emanating from this segment of the acrosome) may be structures by which the spermatozoon binds to the zona surface (Yanagimachi, unpublished observations).

According to Hartmann and his associates, sperm attachment to the zona is comprised of a complicated series of events (Hartmann and Hutchison, 1974a–c, 1976, 1977a,b, 1980). According to their scheme, capacitated hamster spermatozoa first loosely associate with the zona (attachment). Two to three minutes after the initial attachment, the spermatozoa become more tightly associated with the zona (binding 1 or B1). This binding is rapidly terminated by a vitelline factor, which probably emanates from the surface of the vitellus or the perivitelline space. Following the termination of B1 binding, the spermatozoa remain attached and are conditioned through the action of the vitelline factor to firmly bind a second time. This second binding (B2) occurs about 30 min after B1 termination. Another factor (S1) acts synergistically with the vitelline factor to terminate B1 binding. The S1 factor is produced by the interaction of spermatozoa with the zona. It would be interesting to learn whether this scheme proposed for the hamster can be applied to other mammalian species. The only comments I would like to make here are that (1) it is not clear at all from the descriptions by Hartmann and his associates whether the spermatozoa they were dealing with were acrosome-reacted or not, and (2) the B2 binding Hartmann and his associates referred to could represent the actual penetration of the sperm head (insertion of the tip of the sperm head) into the zona. If Hartmann and his associates had paid enough attention to the state of the acrosome and the position of the sperm head on and in the zona, the scheme they presented could have been much simplified.

Species Specificity of Sperm Attachment to the Zona. The species specificity of sperm attachment to the zona surface is very distinct in some cases. For instance, human spermatozoa, which readily attach to the human zona, are unable to attach to the zonae of other species (e.g., the baboon, rhesus monkey, squirrel monkey, rabbit, pig, mouse, hamster, and guinea pig: Bedford, 1977; Yanagimachi et al., 1979). The known exception is the zona of the gibbon egg (Bedford, 1977). It permits not only attachment but also penetration by human spermatozoa. Table IV summarizes the results of experiments in which eggs of the guinea pig, hamster, mouse, and rat were

Table IV

Ability of Guinea Pig and Hamster Spermatozoa to Attach to Zonae
of Homologous and Heterologous Species[a,b]

Spermatozoa		Zonae of:			
Species	Acrosome	Guinea pig	Hamster	Mouse	Rat
Guinea pig	Intact	−	−	−	−
	Reacted	+++	−	−	−
Hamster	Intact	++	+++	++	+++
	Reacted	+++	+++	+++	+++

[a] Mature unfertilized eggs were freed from the cumulus oophorus with 0.1–0.2% hyaluronidase and inseminated with spermatozoa. The concentration of spermatozoa in the insemination medium was approximately 5×10^5/ml. The medium used was BWW medium (a modified Krebs-Ringer solution; cf. Biggers *et al.*, 1971). Spermatozoa with intact acrosomes were obtained from the cauda epididymis. Acrosome-reacted spermatozoa were prepared by preincubating epididymal spermatozoa according to the procedures of Yanagimachi (1970a) and Yanagimachi (1972b). The degree of sperm attachement to the zona surface was determined 30 min and 2 hr after insemination. The temperature of the medium was 37–38°C throughout.
[b] +++, Heavy attachment; ++, moderate attachment; −, no attachment at all.

inseminated *in vitro* with spermatozoa of the guinea pig and hamster (Yanagimachi, unpublished data). It can be seen that acrosome-reacted guinea pig spermatozoa specifically attach to the zona of the homologous species, not to the zonae of other species. Hamster spermatozoa, on the other hand, attach to zonae of both homologous and heterologous species regardless of whether or not they are acrosome-reacted.

Conditions or Reagents That Block Sperm Attachment to the Zona. Since the attachment of spermatozoa to the zona is obviously mediated by substances present on the sperm and egg surfaces, it is logical to assume that any conditions or reagents that alter the chemical properties of these substances would either promote or block sperm attachment to the zona. According to Saling *et al.* (1978) and Heffner *et al.* (1980), firm attachment (which they referred to as binding) of mouse spermatozoa to the zona is largely blocked by an absence or deficiency of Ca^{2+} in the medium. Pretreating zonae or spermatozoa with a variety of reagents is also known to inhibit sperm attachment to the zona. For instance, pretreating zonae with antizona antibodies (for reviews, see Shivers and Dudkiewicz, 1974; Shivers, 1979), some plant lectins (Oikawa *et al.*, 1973, 1974), and very low concentrations of trypsin (Hartmann and Gwatkin, 1971; Oikawa *et al.*, 1975) prevent spermatozoa from attaching or firmly adhering to the zona surfaces. These substances must alter or mask "sperm receptor sites" on the zona surface. According to Reyes and Rosado (1975), pretreating rabbit and human spermatozoa with N-4-carboxyl-3-hydroxyl phenylmaleimide (a specific blocking agent for surface SH groups) drastically reduces binding of the spermatozoa to the zona surface. The presence of solubilized zona material

(Gwatkin and Williams, 1977; Bleil and Wasserman, 1980a) and antisperm antibodies (Menge, 1971; Peterson *et al.*, 1979; Tzartos, 1979; Yanagimachi *et al.*, 1981) in the medium also prevents spermatozoa from attaching to the zona surface. These substances must alter or mask the "zona receptor sites" on the sperm surface. As our study (Yanagimachi *et al.*, 1981) demonstrated that autoantibodies to guinea pig spermatozoa blocked binding of acrosome-reacted guinea pig spermatozoa to homologous zona pellucida, it is possible that these "zona receptor sites" are sperm-specific and autoimmunogenic.

To understand the molecular mechanisms of sperm–zona interaction, we must fully understand the chemical characteristics of both the sperm surface and the zona pellucida. Therefore, recent studies on the chemistry of zonae (Menino and Wright, 1979; Bleil and Wasserman, 1980b; Dunbar and Raynor, 1980; Dunbar *et al.*, 1980; Gwatkin *et al.*, 1980) and sperm surface components (Esbenshade and Clegg, 1976; Olson and Hamilton, 1978; O'Rand and Porter, 1979; Vierula and Rajaniemi, 1980) should be appreciated as the "launching pad" for our future exploration of the intermolecular interactions between spermatozoon and zona.

Sperm Penetration through the Zona Pellucida

Manner of Sperm Penetration. In a single observation, I witnessed the entire process of zona penetration by a hamster spermatozoon after eggs were collected from mated females (Yanagimachi, 1966). When this spermatozoon was first observed, it had already undergone the acrosome reaction and was on the zona. At 5 min after the start of the observation, it was still on the zona. Two minutes later, its head was definitely within the zona. The amount of time this spermatozoon spent in crossing the entire thickness of the zona was judged to be 3–4 min. Yang *et al.* (1972) mated 232 hamsters about the time of ovulation and collected 2249 eggs 4–5.5 hr later when fertilization was in progress. Of these, 61 eggs (2.7%) had spermatozoa on the zona or were approached by free spermatozoa during the observations. They reported that when sperm penetration was observed from the beginning of attachment to the zona until the sperm head had completely passed through the zona, the amount of time for penetration averaged 7 min and 3 sec (ranging from 4 min 20 sec to 10 min 53 sec). As Yang and co-workers did not state how long the spermatozoa remained on the zona before they began to penetrate it, the actual time each spermatozoon required to pass through the zona is unknown. If about 4 min is required for the passage of the sperm head through the zona, the spermatozoon must begin to enter the zona almost immediately after its contact with the zona or within at least 7 min after initial contact.

According to Sato and Blandau (1979), who mixed cumulus-free mouse eggs with "preincubated" spermatozoa between a slide and a coverslip, the sperm head spends an average of 20 min (ranging from 15 to 26 min) in crossing the zona. This duration is by no means short, and one wonders if mouse spermatozoa *in vivo* also take this much time to cross the zona.

It has been reported that spermatozoa pass through the zona obliquely in the mouse and rat (Sobbota, 1895, and Sobbota and Burckhard, 1910: cited in Austin, 1961), guinea pig (Austin and Bishop, 1958), hamster (Austin and Bishop, 1958; Yanagimachi, 1966; Yang *et al.*, 1972), pig (Dickmann and Dziuk, 1964; Szollosi and Hunter, 1973), and sheep (Dziuk and Dickmann, 1965). According to Dickmann (1964), 88% of a total of 442 rabbit spermatozoa found within the zona were lying obliquely. Vertical penetration through the zona is certainly possible, but it is probably the exception rather than the rule, at least in the rabbit and hamster (Dickmann, 1964; Yang *et al.*, 1972). In this context, a recent report by Sato and Blandau (1979) deserves special attention. According to them, mouse spermatozoa *in vitro* almost invariably penetrate the zona perpendicularly. Micrographs presented by these authors convincingly demonstrate this. However, one must be aware of the conditions Sato and Blandau employed. They mounted a suspension of eggs and spermatozoa between a slide and a coverslip and compressed the eggs until they were held by the glass surfaces. In other words, the thickness of the suspension under the coverslip was slightly less than the original diameter (about $100 \mu m$?) of the mouse egg. As the mouse spermatozoon is 120–$130 \mu m$ long, the orientations the spermatozoa can assume and still have free, vigorous flagellar motion must be severely limited under such conditions. In other words, the spermatozoa might have been forced to penetrate the zona perpendicularly. The presence or absence of the cumulus oophorus around the eggs may also make a difference in the manner of sperm penetration through the zona. When spermatozoa attach to the surface of cumulus-free eggs, those that attach to the zona surface almost horizontally may not be able to develop enough thrusting power against the zona with the consequence that they are unable to enter the zona. Only spermatozoa that attach to the zona perpendicularly or almost perpendicularly will successfully enter the zona. When the eggs are surrounded by a compact matrix of the cumulus oophorus, the matrix may serve as an anchor to hold each egg in a "fixed" position so that a spermatozoon attached to the zona obliquely (or almost horizontally) can develop enough thrusting power against the zona to successfully penetrate it.

Zona "Maturation" and Sperm Penetration. According to Barros and Munoz (1974), the zonae pellucidae of immature hamster eggs at the germinal vesicle stage are not as readily penetrable by spermatozoa as are the zonae of mature eggs. Mandelbaum *et al.* (1977) and Plachot and Mandelbaum (1978) reported that the zonae of hamster eggs that had been matured *in vitro* were not at all penetrable by spermatozoa. The zonae of eggs that had matured *in vivo*, on the other hand, were readily penetrable by spermatozoa. This led Mandelbaum and her associates to infer that the hamster zona requires "maturation" under the influence of gonadotropin. There are contradictory reports by other investigators. According to Moore and Bedford (1978a), the zonae of immature hamster eggs at the germinal vesicle stage are as penetrable by spermatozoa as are the zonae of mature eggs. In the human, zonae of immature eggs recovered from cadavers (Overstreet and Hembree, 1976) or from ovaries surgically removed from patients (Overstreet *et al.*, 1980b) are readily penetrable by spermatozoa. Similarly, the zonae of immature rabbit and dog eggs are as readily penetrable by spermatozoa as are the zonae of mature eggs (Overstreet and Bedford, 1974c; Mahi and Yanagimachi, 1976).

Species Specificity of Zona Penetration. The zona pellucida is one of the most prominent sites of species specificity (Yanagimachi, 1977). The zona of one species usually does not permit penetration by spermatozoa of other species. This specificity, however, is not absolute. If the zona is challenged by spermatozoa under certain experimental (e.g., *in vitro*) conditions, it may allow penetration by foreign spermatozoa depending on the combination of species. For instance, 0.9–6.3% of the zonae of rat eggs are penetrated by mouse spermatozoa *in vitro* (Hanada and Chang, 1978). A very small proportion (0.3%) of rat zonae are penetrated by hamster spermatozoa *in vitro* (Barros, 1968). As many as 20–21% of the zonae of mouse eggs can be penetrated by dcer mouse spermatozoa *in vitro* (Fukuda *et al.*, 1979). Penetration of the zona by foreign spermatozoa, however, should be considered the exception rather than the rule. If eggs of several different species are inseminated with spermatozoa of a single species in the same dish, one will clearly observe that the eggs of the homologous species are exclusively or at least predominantly penetrated by the spermatozoa (cf. experiments of Yanagimachi, 1977).

Mechanisms of Sperm Penetration through the Zona. Although it is obvious that strong motility of spermatozoa is required for sperm penetration through the zona, the existence of a chemical or enzymatic mechanism by which spermatozoa soften or dissolve the zona material is still expected. This hypothetical zona lytic agent is generally referred to as the zona lysin (Austin and Bishop, 1958; Austin, 1961). As the zona can be dissolved by acrosin (Stambaugh and Buckley, 1968, 1969; Zaneveld *et al.*, 1969; Meizel and Mukerji, 1976) and as acrosin inhibitors prevent both *in vitro* and *in vivo* fertilization (Stambaugh *et al.*, 1969; Zaneveld *et al.*, 1971, 1975; Zaneveld, 1976; Bhattacharyya *et al.*, 1979; Joyce *et al.*, 1979), acrosin has been a popular candidate for the zona lysin. The site of zona lysin is generally believed to be the surface of the inner acrosomal membrane that is exposed directly to the zona material as the spermatozoon passes through the zona (Bedford, 1970a; Brown and Hartree, 1974; Brown et al., 1975).* Koehler (1975), who examined the inner acrosomal membrane using the freeze-fracture technique, inferred that densely packed intramembranous particles could represent the zona lysin. Yanagimachi and Noda (1970a) and Barros et al. (1973b) have proposed that the zona lysin may be located in the equatorial segment; Bedford (1972a, 1974), however, disagrees as he believes the equatorial segment to remain unchanged during sperm passage through the zona. The presence of acrosin on the inner acrosomal membrane has been deduced by sequential extraction of acrosomal enzymes by physical and chemical means (Brown and Hartree, 1974; Brown et al., 1975; Morton, 1976, 1977), but has never been proven unequivocally by cytochemical techniques at the electron microscopic level (see p. 91). If the inner acrosomal membrane indeed carries powerful proteolytic enzymes like acrosin, substrates such as silver proteinate (Yanagimachi and Teichman, 1972) and gelatin (Gaddum-Rosse and Blandau, 1977) exposed directly to the inner acrosomal membrane should be readily digested by the inner acrosomal membrane of acrosome-reacted spermatozoa. This, however, is not the case. It can be argued that these substrates are not readily digested by the acrosin on the inner acrosomal membrane. Bedford and Cross (1978) have questioned whether acrosin is in fact involved in zona penetration by spermatozoa. The basis for this is that rabbit zonae treated with wheat germ agglutinin become very resistant to trypsin and acrosin and yet remain readily penetrable by spermatozoa. A proteinase other than acrosin may be involved in zona penetration by spermatozoa (Srivastava et al., 1979).

The function of acrosomal hyaluronidase is generally believed to be depolymerization of the matrix of the cumulus oophorus. However, it may also serve as a zona lysin (Hartree, 1971; Perreault et al., 1980). Brown (1975) and Morton (1977) maintain that some of the hyaluronidase is bound to the inner acrosomal membrane and functions as a zona lysin. According to Anand et al. (1977), significant proportions of β-N-acetylglucosaminidase, hyaluronidase, and acrosin are tightly bound to spermatozoa. They did not mention the intracellular localization of these enzymes, however, if they are located on the inner acrosomal membrane they may all act as the zona lysin. Recent studies by Farooqui and Srivastava (1980a,b) have shown that rabbit acrosin is much

---

*Austin (1961) stated, "It is possible that the hypothetical zona lysin is active only while attached to the perforatorium." Some investigators use the term *perforatorium* to refer to the apical subacrosomal material, but it should include the overlying inner acrosomal membrane because both structures function as a unit in the functional sense (Yanagimachi and Noda, 1970a,c). Thus, Austin and Bishop (1958) and Austin (1961) should be considered the ones who first suggested the presence of zona lysin on the inner acrosomal membrane.

less effective in dissolving the zona when used alone than when it is combined with β-N-acetylhexosaminidase and arylsulfatase. Thus, the possibility exists that two or more different enzymes work synergistically to function as zona lysins.

The major constituent of the zona pellucida is glycoprotein (Bleil and Wasserman, 1980b; Dunbar *et al.*, 1980). Dissolution of the zona by SS-reducing agents (Braden, 1952; Gould *et al.*, 1971; Nicolson *et al.*, 1975) and high concentrations of urea (Menino and Wright, 1979; Dunbar *et al.*, 1980) suggests that the peptide chains of the zona glycoproteins are held together by SS links and nonconvalent bonds. Therefore, any reagents that can break these links or bonds should be able to dissolve the zona. Thus, Bedford (1974) suggested that the zona lysin could be an enzyme like SS-reductase.

We all tend to think that the zona lysin is an enzyme (or a combination of enzymes), but it could be a nonenzymatic substance. The possibility that the sperm head mechanically cuts through (or into) the zona (Yanagimachi and Noda, 1970a; Bedford, 1974; Noda and Yanagimachi, 1976) should also be considered. Blandau (1961) stated

> The zona pellucida can be softened or disintegrated in buffers with pH values from 3 to 5. Various reducing agents such as glutathione and cysteine cause rapid dissolution of the zona. Oxidizing agents such as the hydrogen peroxide which is produced by sperm are particularly efficacious in removing zona. Several investigators favor the possibility that a specific mucolytic enzyme, zona lysin may be secreted by the sperm as it makes contact with the zona pellucida. It seems likely that the passage of the spermatozoon through the zona pellucida may occur in a variety of ways in different animals. Too few observations have been made to significantly implicate any of the physical, chemical or mechanical mechanisms suggested for sperm penetration of the zona pellucida in the mammalian egg.

This statement is, in essence, still valid today.

Timing of Acrosome Reaction in Relation to Ability of Spermatozoa to Penetrate the Zona. Sea urchin spermatozoa under normal conditions begin their acrosome reactions upon contact with the jelly surrounding the egg or while they are passing through the jelly.* Solubilized jelly material (the so-called "egg water") can also induce the acrosome reaction. The reaction is very fast, being completed within as little as 5 sec (Dan, 1952) or within at most 30 sec (Kinsey *et al.*, 1979). Premature acrosome reaction by spermatozoa

---

*In some species of sea urchins, the acrosome reaction occurs upon contact with the vitelline coat, not within the jelly (Aketa and Ohta, 1977).

(reaction long before contact with the native jelly or with the vitelline coat, which are believed to be analogous to the cumulus matrix and the zona pellucida of a mammalian egg, respectively) is believed to result in the loss of their fertilizing capacity (Monroy, 1965). Takahashi and Sugiyama (1973) have reported that sea urchin spermatozoa remain fully capable of fertilizing eggs for up to 4 min after contact with jelly material, but rapidly lose their fertilizing capacity thereafter. According to Kinsey *et al.* (1979) and Vacquier (1979), the majority of spermatozoa lose their fertilizing capacity by 1 min after the acrosome reaction although they remain motile for some time. The reason the fertilizing capacity of sea urchin spermatozoa is lost so quickly after the acrosome reaction is unknown, but it could be in part the loss of some components on the sperm surface responsible for attachment to the vitelline coat (Vacquier, 1979).

We do not know how long mammalian spermatozoa retain their ability to penetrate the zona after completion of the acrosome reaction. Circumstantial evidence suggests that hamster spermatozoa rapidly lose their fertilizing capacity (the ability to penetrate the zona) after the acrosome reaction (Gwatkin, 1977). Barros *et al.* (1973b) examined the fertilizing capacity of hamster spermatozoa that had been incubated in a sperm-capacitating medium for various periods of time. The medium they used was a gamma-globulin-free human serum fraction which allows for the acrosome reaction of spermatozoa. When spermatozoa were incubated in the medium for 2–3 hr, they were fully capable of penetrating the zona. Spermatozoa incubated for 4 hr or more, on the other hand, were totally incapable of penetrating the zona. Light microscopic examination of both groups of spermatozoa revealed no significant difference in the degree of sperm motility, the incidence of acrosome reaction, or in the ability of spermatozoa to attach to the zona surface. Electron microscopic examination, however, revealed a marked difference in the ultrastructural appearance of the equatorial segment of the acrosome. The majority of spermatozoa incubated 2 hr had either apparently "intact" or slightly vesiculated equatorial segments, whereas in the majority of spermatozoa incubated 5 hr the equatorial segments were extensively vesiculated or completely absent. Although it is not certain whether the loss of the equatorial segment is the only reason the latter spermatozoa fail to penetrate the zona, these observations clearly indicate that acrosome-reacted spermatozoa lose their ability to pass through the zona before they lose their ability to move or attach to the zona surface. As penetration of spermatozoa through the zona requires *vigorous* motility and perhaps zona lysins, the loss of zona-penetrating ability in prematurely acrosome-reacted spermatozoa could be due to a decline in their vigor or degradation of their zona lysins.

In vivo, some spermatozoa may undergo the acrosome reaction away from the oviduct (e.g., in the uterus of the guinea pig; Austin and Bishop, 1958) or several hours before ovulation (in the isthmic region of the rabbit oviduct; Overstreet and Cooper, 1979a). It is unlikely that these precociously acrosome-reacted spermatozoa can retain their fertilizing capacity (the ability to pass through the zona) until they meet the eggs. The site of the acrosome reaction of spermatozoa *in vivo* has not been completely ascertained yet, but it is likely to be the upper region of the oviduct (e.g., the ampulla), in the very vicinity of the eggs, or on/in the egg investments. In any case, achieving the acrosome reaction in the proper site and at the proper time must be of critical importance for successful fertilization *in vivo*.

Sperm–Egg Fusion

Manner of Sperm–Egg Fusion

According to Brackett (1970), a rabbit spermatozoon that has passed through the zona vigorously moves about in the perivitelline space before its head attaches to the vitellus; by 20 min after the attachment, the entire length of the spermatozoon is incorporated into the vitellus. In the hamster, the spermatozoon may occasionally stay free in the perivitelline space for some time (Yang *et al.*, 1972). In most cases, however, the sperm head attaches immediately to the vitellus without wandering about within the perivitelline space (Yanagimachi, 1966; Yang *et al.*, 1972). Austin and Bishop (1957) depicted a diagram of sperm entry into the rat egg, based on their observations of a number of fertilized eggs collected from the oviducts of mated animals. Although almost every step of sperm entry was beautifully illustrated in the diagram, the time intervals between the steps were not presented. Figure 18 diagrams sperm entry into the hamster egg. This was prepared from observations by Yanagimachi (1966) and Yang *et al.* (1972) as well as several observations I have made during the past several years. A spermatozoon passing through the zona beats its tail very vigorously. The sperm head advances through the zona obliquely in almost all cases (Figure 18A). As soon as the entire head has passed through the zona (Figure 18B), the head dashes forward and makes immediate contact with the vitelline surface. The initial point of contact may be the tip of the sperm head (Figure 18C), but the head lies flat almost immediately (Figure 18D). The firm attachment of the sperm head to the vitellus and the vigorous movements of the sperm tail vibrate and rotate the vitellus within the zona until the entire, or almost the entire, length of the sperm tail is within the perivitelline space (Figure 18E–G). Then, rather suddenly the vigor of the tail's movement diminishes; the sperm tail now beats

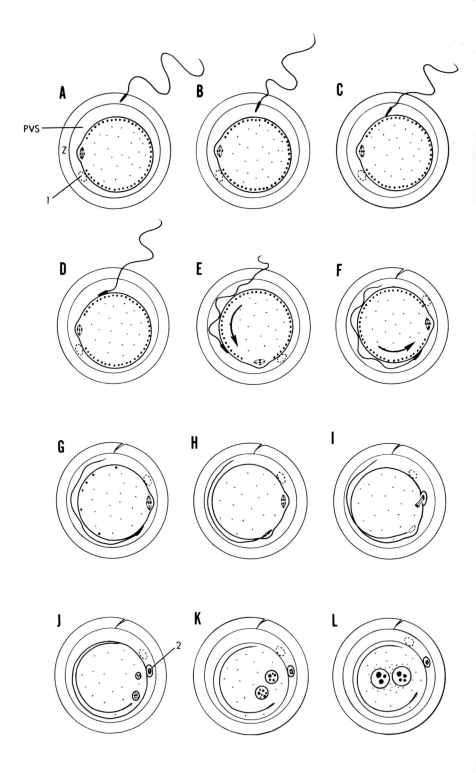

very slowly and intermittently (Figure 18H)*,†. By 30–40 min after the initial contact of the sperm head with the vitellus, decondensation of the sperm head is evident (Figure 18I). The sperm tail is incorporated into the vitellus from the base of the tail toward its tip slowly but steadily (Figure 18H-J). Developing sperm and egg pronuclei are seen in the vitellus 2 hr after sperm entry (Figure 18K).

According to Shalgi and Phillips (1980b), hamster spermatozoa mixed with zona-intact or zona-free hamster eggs *in vitro* commonly penetrate the egg vitelli perpendicularly. I have also witnessed this form of penetration in the hamster when eggs with or without zonae pellucidae were inseminated *in vitro*. In these cases, a large part of the sperm tail often remained outside of the vitellus even after the sperm nuclei had been transformed into pronuclei. *In vivo*, spermatozoa are invariably incorporated into the egg horizontally, and the entire length of the sperm tail enters the vitellus. The perpendicular penetration by the sperm head and the incomplete incorporation of its tail into the egg vitellus must be due to abnormal or subnormal conditions of the gametes and their environment.

One of the most dramatic events during fertilization is the sudden loss of vigor by the sperm tail soon after the sperm head contacts with the vitellus (Yanagimachi, 1966; Yang *et al.*, 1972; Sato and Blandau, 1979). This also can be seen when zona-free eggs are inseminated *in vitro* (Figure 3 of Yanagimachi, 1978a). The cause is unknown. Since uncapacitated, acrosome-intact spermatozoa that have attached to (are trapped by) the vitelline surface of zona-free eggs continue their vigorous tail movement (Yanagimachi, unpublished data), sperm–egg contact per se cannot be considered as the cause. It is most likely

---

*Professor R. J. Blandau of the University of Washington kindly showed me unpublished cinematographs (taken with Dr. K. Sato) of mouse spermatozoa fertilizing mouse eggs *in vitro*. The manner of sperm contact with the vitellus in the mouse was almost the same as that in the hamster, although the spermatozoa penetrated the zona perpendicularly and hit the vitellus with their tips. The next moment, however, the heads were laid flat on the vitellus. Within the next 10 sec or so, the entire sperm tail was incorporated into the perivitelline space and the vigor of the sperm tail diminished in about 15 sec.

†According to Brackett (1970), the tail of the rabbit spermatozoon retains its vigorous motility during the entire course of sperm penetration into the vitellus. Wolf and Armstrong (1978), who inseminated zona-free mouse eggs *in vitro*, state, "Although attached sperm underwent a marked reduction in flagellar activity prior to incorporation, active motility continued at least in short bursts throughout the incorporation sequence." Thus, the tail of the mouse spermatozoon seems to display intermittent motility during its incorporation into the vitellus.

← _____

Figure 18. Diagrams of successive stages of fertilization in the hamster. PVS, perivitelline space; Z, zona pellucida; 1, first polar body; 2, second polar body. Time intervals between: B and D, a few seconds or less than 1 sec; D and G, 10–15 sec; G and I, about 45 min; I and K, about 2 hr. (For explanation, see the text, p. 131.)

that sperm–egg fusion causes drastic changes in the physiological properties (e.g., depolarization?) of the entire area of the sperm plasma membrane.

Acrosome Reaction as a Necessary Preliminary to Sperm–Egg Fusion

As stated already, spermatozoa undergo the acrosome reaction before they begin to penetrate the zona pellucida. Therefore, under normal conditions, spermatozoa that have passed through the zona and are about to fuse with the egg plasma membrane have already undergone the acrosome reaction. Must the spermatozoa be acrosome-reacted to fuse with the egg? To answer this question, Yanagimachi and Noda (1970b) removed the zonae from unfertilized hamster eggs and inseminated the "naked" eggs *in vitro* with either fresh epididymal spermatozoa with intact acrosomes or spermatozoa incubated *in vitro* until they had acrosome-reacted. The results clearly demonstrated that only acrosome-reacted spermatozoa were capable of fusing with the eggs. Acrosome-intact spermatozoa may be trapped by the egg microvilli, but they never fuse with the egg. Toyoda and Chang (1968) inseminated rat eggs (surrounded by both cumulus cells and zonae pellucidae) with epididymal spermatozoa in the presence of chymotrypsin. When they examined the eggs 4–8 hr later, the zonae had disappeared and some of the eggs contained swelling sperm heads or sperm pronuclei. This led them to conclude that capacitation is not necessary for sperm entry into the egg. The same conclusion was reached by Pavlok and McLaren (1972) after observing the penetration of zona-free mouse eggs by epididymal spermatozoa. We must be aware that these workers did not actually examine the state of the acrosomes at the time the spermatozoa entered the eggs. It is highly probable that the spermatozoa underwent some membrane modifications (Chang and Hunter, 1977) and acrosome reaction sometime during incubation with the eggs. In fact, Wolf *et al.* (1976) demonstrated that capacitation and acrosome reaction are necessary for the fusion of mouse spermatozoa with zona-free eggs.

Yanagimachi and Noda (1970b) originally stated that capacitation is necessary for sperm–egg fusion. This statement is somewhat misleading because we now know that capacitation and the acrosome reaction are separate phenomena (Bedford, 1970a; Yanagimachi and Usui, 1974). It is the acrosome reaction that is required for fusion, not capacitation per se (Yanagimachi, 1977). To clarify this point, I performed two series of experiments using hamster gametes (Yanagimachi, unpublished). In the first series, I mixed fresh epididymal spermatozoa with zona-free eggs in a medium capable of inducing the acrosome reaction, and incubated them for various periods. In the second series, I preincubated spermatozoa in the medium until their acrosomes just began to react, then mixed the spermatozoa with zona-free eggs and continued incubation for various periods. These procedures should have given the zona-free eggs opportunity to meet spermatozoa at various stages of capacitation and acrosome reaction. If capacitation per se is the condition necessary for sperm–egg fusion, some acrosome-intact (yet capacitated) spermatozoa should have been seen fusing with eggs. In no instance did I find such spermatozoa at either the light or the electron microscopic level. All the spermatozoa fusing with eggs had already undergone the acrosome reaction. Thus, we may conclude that the acrosome reaction, not capacitation per se, is the necessary preliminary to sperm–egg fusion. The notion that capacitation is needed for sperm–egg fusion (Yanagimachi and Noda, 1970b; Niwa and Chang, 1975a; Wolf et al., 1976) is not incorrect in a sense because capacitation precedes the acrosome reaction. However, I would like to stress here again that capacitation per se is not enough to render the spermatozoa capable of fusing with the eggs. Moore (1972), who microsurgically injected sheep spermatozoa into the perivitelline space of unfertilized sheep eggs, found that neither freshly ejaculated spermatozoa nor uterine spermatozoa could penetrate the eggs. It is most likely that neither type of spermatozoa Moore (1972) used had undergone the acrosome reaction even though the uterine spermatozoa may have been capacitated. According to Soupart and Strong (1975), human spermatozoa can fuse with zona-free eggs regardless of whether or not the spermatozoa are acrosome-reacted. The micrographic evidence presented by these workers, however, is not convincing enough to substantiate their statement.

The mechanisms by which the acrosome reaction renders the spermatozoon capable of fusing with the egg plasma membrane are unknown. What seems to be certain is that the plasma membrane of either the equatorial segment or the postacrosomal region (or both) of the spermatozoon changes radically as a result of (or concurrent with) the acrosome reaction. According to Friend et al. (1977) and Friend (1980), particle-free patches emerge within the plasma membrane over both the equatorial segment and the postacrosomal region of the guinea pig spermatozoon following the acrosome reaction. Development of these particle-free areas may make the sperm membrane capable of fusing with the egg plasma membrane. I suspect that the outer acrosomal membrane of the equatorial segment has unique properties and its exposure to external medium upon the acrosome reaction somehow triggers changes in the plasma membrane of the equatorial segment or the postacrosomal region (or both).

Sites of Initiation of Sperm–Egg Fusion

In many invertebrates (Colwin and Colwin, 1967), domestic fowl (Okamura and Nishiyama, 1978), and perhaps marsupials (Rodger and Bedford, 1980), sperm–egg fusion is initiated between the egg plasma

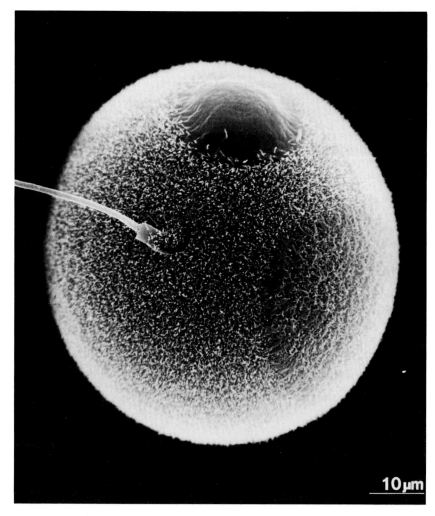

Figure 19. Scanning electron micrograph of a hamster spermatozoon fusing with the vitellus. Zona-free hamster eggs were inseminated *in vitro* with acrosome-reacted spermatozoa and fixed about 10 min later. The specimen was fixed by Yanagimachi and micrographed by Dr. David Phillips. Note the elevated microvilli-free area of the egg at the top of the micrograph; the metaphase II chromosomes are located under this area.

membrane and the inner acrosomal membrane of the spermatozoon. In eutherian mammals, it is the sperm plasma membrane, not the inner acrosomal membrane, that initially fuses with the egg plasma membrane (Pikó and Tyler, 1964; Barros and Franklin, 1968; Yanagimachi and Noda, 1970d; Bedford and Cooper, 1978; Yanagimachi, 1978a).

The surface of the mammalian egg has numerous microvilli except for the area over the metaphase spindle of the second meiotic division. In the mouse, this microvilli-free area occupies almost one fifth of the entire surface of the egg (Eager *et al.*, 1976; Phillips and Shalgi, 1980b). Sperm–egg fusion does not occur or seldom occurs in this "bald" area (Johnson *et al.*, 1975). In the hamster, the microvilli-free (or microvilli-poor) area over the second meiotic spindle is much smaller than in the mouse (Yanagimachi and Noda, 1970d; Shalgi and Phillips, 1980b), but again we seldom encounter spermatozoa fusing in this area (Figure 19). The importance of microvilli as a means of facilitating the fusion of somatic cells has been stressed by Poste (1970, 1972). Participation of egg microvilli in sperm–egg fusion is obvious at least in the hamster (Yanagimachi and Noda, 1970d; Shalgi and Phillips, 1980a,b), but Bedford and Cooper (1978) have raised a question about the role of microvilli in the fusion process. They have suggested that the intervillous regions rather than the microvilli themselves fuse with the sperm plasma membrane. The bases for this suggestion are that (1) immature rabbit eggs at the germinal vesicle stage have sparsely distributed microvilli and yet can readily fuse with spermatozoa (Berrios and Bedford, 1979) and (2) the plasma membrane of egg microvilli may lack "fluidity" as does that of intestinal microvilli. An argument against this suggestion can be made, however. First, even though immature rabbit eggs may have relatively few microvilli, the distance between two adjacent microvilli is probably far less than the length of the sperm head. When the sperm head hits or moves over the egg surface, it will come in contact with many microvilli. Second, at least in the hamster, mouse, and rat, the microvilli are so dense on the egg surface(Jackowski and Dumont, 1979; Horiuchi *et al.*, 1980; Shalgi and Phillips, 1980a) that it would be impossible for the sperm head to avoid contact with microvilli when it hits or moves over the egg surface. On some occasions, the spermatozoon may land on the microvilli-free (or -poor) area over the meiotic spindle, but this is the area where spermatozoa in fact seldom fuse. Finally, egg microvilli are probably not entirely comparable to intestinal microvilli. Intestinal microvilli are very stationary structures reinforced by distinct bundles of microfilaments. Egg microvilli are rather dynamic structures and can disappear and reappear, suggesting high "fluidity" of their membranes.

The structure with which the spermatozoon first fuses with the egg plasma membrane is believed to be the plasma membrane of the postacrosomal region (Pikó and Tyler, 1964; Pikó, 1967, 1969; Stefanini *et al.*, 1969;

Yanagimachi and Noda, 1970d) or of the equatorial segment (Bedford, 1972a; Bedford and Cooper, 1978; Bedford *et al.*, 1979). According to Bedford and his associates, a spermatozoon that has passed through the zona has an "intact" equatorial segment and the plasma membrane over the equatorial segment fuses specifically with the egg plasma membrane. Yanagimachi and Noda's (1970d) belief that the sperm plasma membrane in the postacrosomal region fuses with the egg membrane is based on their observations of spermatozoa fusing with zona-free eggs *in vitro*. Although the manner of sperm entry into the egg under these conditions may not be entirely normal (Shalgi and Phillips, 1980b), some of the micrographs we presented (e.g., Figures 10 and 11 of Yanagimachi and Noda, 1970d) clearly indicate that the plasma membrane of the postacrosomal region *can* fuse with egg microvilli. Under certain *in vitro* conditions, spermatozoa of the hamster (Barros *et al.*, 1973b), guinea pig (Barros and Herrera, 1977), and human (Soupart and Strong, 1974; McMaster *et al.*, 1978) completely lose their equatorial segments (together with the overlying plasma membrane) either in the medium or within the zona, yet these spermatozoa still seem to be able to fuse with eggs if they are brought directly to the egg surfaces (Barros et al., 1973b;

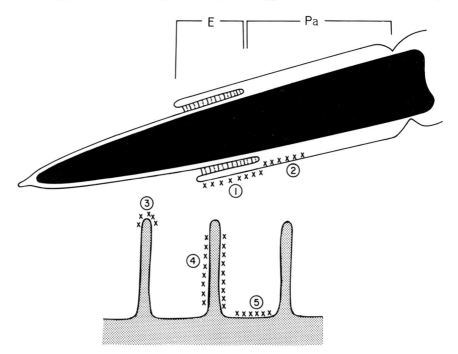

Figure 20. Diagram showing the probable sites of initiation of sperm–egg membrane fusion. E, equatorial segment of the acrosome; Pa, postacrosomal region. (For explanation, see the text, p. 137.)

Barros and Herrera, 1977). Barros (1977) is of the opinion that the plasma membranes of both the equatorial segment and the postacrosomal region are capable of fusing with the egg plasma membrane. Chacon and Talbot (1980), who examined zona-free hamster eggs fusing with human spermatozoa *in vitro*, found that the plasma membranes of both the equatorial segment and the anterior third of the postacrosomal region of the spermatozoon fuse with the egg plasma membrane. Figure 20 illustrates the proposed or probable sites of initiation of membrane fusion between spermatozoon and egg.

Recently, Jones *et al.* (1980) demonstrated the presence of high concentrations of calmodulin in the postacrosomal region of guinea pig and rabbit spermatozoa. The significance of this finding remains to be determined.

Intermixing of Sperm and Egg Plasma Membranes during Fertilization

Obviously, the sperm plasma membrane intermingles with the egg plasma membrane during their fusion (Figure 21). Yanagimachi *et al.* (1973) demonstrated this by labeling hamster eggs and spermatozoa with positively charged colloidal iron particles, which bind to the egg plasma membrane but not to the plasma membrane over the sperm head. In a more sophisticated method, O'Rand (1977b) prepared a specific antibody against rabbit spermatozoa. This antibody in the presence of guinea pig complement caused 90% of the fertilized rabbit eggs, but none of the unfertilized eggs, to cytolyse. This clearly indicates that the sperm membrane becomes part of the egg plasma membrane during fertilization. Some sperm surface components seem to remain on the egg surface even long after fertilization. Gabel *et al.* (1979) labeled mouse epididymal spermatozoa with tetramethylrhodamine isothiocyanate and deposited them in the uteri of ovulating mice. Subsequent examination of eggs with fluorescence microscopy revealed that the surfaces of recently fertilized eggs and even those in four- to eight-cell stages had fluorescent patches.

Species Specificity of Sperm–Egg Fusion

Sperm–egg fusion appears to be less species specific than sperm–zona interaction (Yanagimachi, 1977). For instance, mouse spermatozoa, which seldom penetrate the zonae of rat eggs, can readily enter (fuse with) zona-free rat eggs (Hanada and Chang, 1972; Pavlok, 1979). Similarly, human spermatozoa, which cannot penetrate hamster zonae, can enter (fuse with) zona-free hamster eggs (Yanagimachi *et al.*, 1976). These facts, however, should not be taken as implying that the egg plasma membranes are totally lacking in species specificity. The plasma membrane of the mouse egg, for

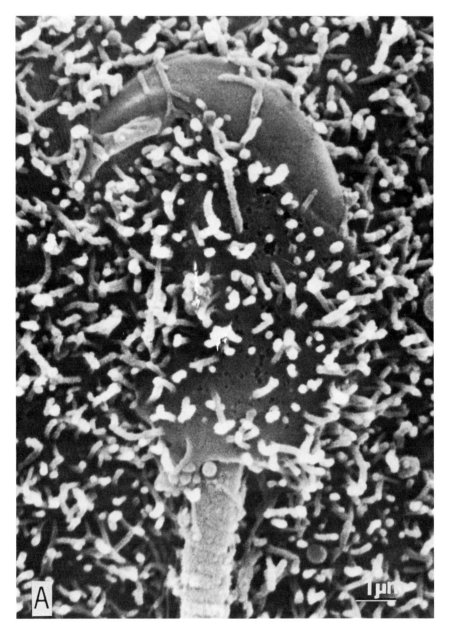

Figure 21. Scanning electron micrographs of hamster spermatozoa fusing with eggs. Zona-free hamster eggs were inseminated *in vitro* with acrosome-reacted spermatozoa and fixed between 15

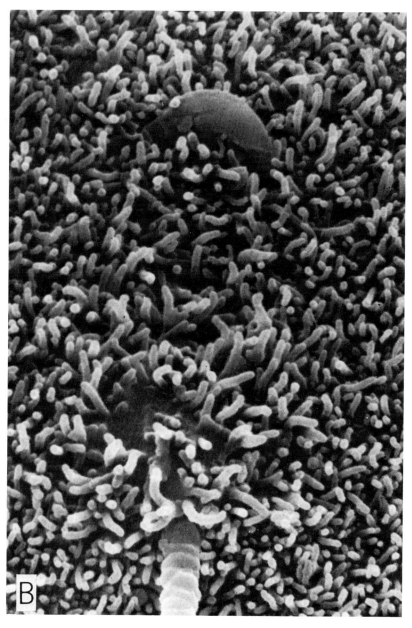

and 30 min later. The specimens were fixed by Yanagimachi and micrographed by Dr. David
Phillips.

Table V

Penetration of Zona-Free Eggs by Spermatozoa of Homologous
and Heterologous Species[a]

Spermatozoa of:	Zona-free eggs of:				
	Hamster	Mouse	Rat	Guinea pig	Rabbit
Hamster	Yes[1]	No[4,14]	No[4,14]	Yes[14]	No[7]
Mouse	Yes[2-4]	Yes[4,5]	Yes[2,4,16]		Yes[3]
Rat	Yes[2-4]	No[4]	Yes[4]		Yes[3]
Guinea pig	Yes[6]	No[7]	No[7]	Yes[8]	No[7]
Deer mouse	Yes[7]	No[7]	No[7,16]		
(*P. maniculatus*)					
Rabbit	Yes[7]				Yes[9]
Pig	Yes[10]				
Bull	Yes[11]				
Dolphin	Yes[12]				
Human	Yes[13]	No[14,15]	No[14,15]		
Goat	Yes[17]				

[a] References: (1) Yanagimachi and Noda (1970b,d); (2) Hanada and Chang (1972); (3) Hanada and Chang (1976); (4) Pavlok (1979); (5) Wolf *et al.* (1976); (6) Yanagimachi (1972c); (7) Hanada and Chang (1978); (8) Yanagimachi (1972b); (9) Brackett *et al.* (1971); Gordon and Dandekar (1976); (10) Imai *et al.* (1979, 1980); (11) Lorton and First (1979); (12) Fleming *et al.* (1981); (13) Yanagimachi *et al.* (1976); Barros *et al.* (1978, 1979); Hall *et al.* (1979); Kanwar *et al.* (1979); Menge and Black (1979); Rogers *et al.* (1979); Binor *et al.* (1980); Hall *et al.* (1980); (14) Yanagimachi (unpublished data); (15) Quinn (1979); (16) Thadani (1980); (17) Kim *et al.* (1980).

example, manifests strong species specificity and permits the fusion of only mouse spermatozoa (Table V). Although the hamster egg plasma membrane allows fusion of a variety of foreign spermatozoa (Table V), it does show some degree of specificity. For instance, when zona-free hamster eggs are inseminated in a dish containing approximately equal numbers of acrosome-reacted hamster, guinea pig, and human spermatozoa, a greater number of hamster spermatozoa will later be found within each egg than guinea pig or human spermatozoa; the numbers of spermatozoa in each hamster egg will be hamster $>$ guinea pig $\gg$ human (Yanagimachi, unpublished data). Obviously, the hamster egg plasma membrane has the greatest affinity for the spermatozoa of its own species. It is important to emphasize here that the acrosome reaction is a sine qua non condition even for cross-fertilization of zona-free eggs (Yanagimachi, 1972c, 1978a; Yanagimachi *et al.*, 1976).

Role of Sperm Motility in Sperm–Egg Fusion

The spermatozoon that has passed through the zona and is about to contact the egg plasma membrane is very vigorously motile. This does not imply that the motility of the spermatozoon is essential for the initiation of sperm–egg fusion. I have often observed that hamster spermatozoa that have undergone the acrosome reaction *in vitro* several hours earlier are very weakly motile and unable to penetrate the zona, yet readily fuse with zona-free eggs (Yanagimachi, unpublished data). When actively motile, acrosome-reacted hamster spermatozoa were treated with 0.03% formaldehyde in Tyrode's solution for 5 min, the vast majority became completely motionless only about 3% of them being feebly motile. When these spermatozoa were washed and mixed with zona-free eggs *in vitro* (with occasional agitation to increase the chance of sperm–egg collision), no active movement of the spermatozoa was seen in the medium or on the egg surfaces, yet 50–100% of the eggs were penetrated by spermatozoa within 1 hr after insemination. When the spermatozoa were killed by treating them with higher concentrations ($>0.7\%$) of formaldehyde, however, none of them penetrated the eggs (Yanagimachi, unpublished data). It appears, therefore, that as long as the plasma membrane is "alive," the spermatozoon is able to fuse with the egg plasma membrane regardless of the vigor or quality of flagellar movement.

Egg Maturation and Sperm–Egg Fusion

When immature ovarian eggs at the germinal vesicle stage (for the mouse, rat, hamster, and rabbit) are inseminated either *in vitro* or *in vivo* and examined several hours later by light microscopy, spermatozoa are commonly found in the perivitelline space. However, swollen (decondensing) sperm heads are seldom seen within the egg cytoplasm. This has led investigators to conclude that immature eggs are not penetrable or are barely penetrable by spermatozoa (Iwamatsu and Chang, 1972; Barros and Munoz, 1973, 1974; Overstreet and Bedford, 1974c; Niwa and Chang, 1975b). Electron microscopic studies, however, have revealed that immature hamster eggs at the germinal vesicle stage are fully capable of fusing with spermatozoa. The membrane fusion between egg and spermatozoon occurs normally, but decondensation of sperm nuclei fails to occur (Usui and Yanagimachi, 1976; Moore and Bedford, 1978b; Berrios and Bedford, 1979). In the dog, spermatozoa are not only able to penetrate immature eggs at the germinal vesicle stage, but also their heads decondense in the egg cytoplasm (Mahi and Yanagimachi, 1976). Thus, the plasma membrane of the eggs of the hamster, dog, and perhaps all other mammalian species seems to have full capacity to fuse with the sperm membrane even before the egg begins its nuclear maturation. How early in oogenesis the egg plasma membrane gains the ability to fuse with spermatozoa must be the subject of future studies.

Effects of Ionic Composition and Temperature of Medium on Sperm–Egg Fusion

The presence of Ca^{2+} in the medium is essential for sperm–egg fusion (Yanagimachi, 1978b). In Ca^{2+}-free or Ca^{2+}-deficient medium, acrosome-reacted spermatozoa may attach to the egg plasma membranes, but are unable to fuse with them. Mg^{2+}, Ba^{2+}, and Sr^{2+} can replace Ca^{2+}, but they are less effective. Excess Ca^{2+} (10 mM) or Mg^{2+} (100 mM) in the medium does not seem to disturb sperm–egg fusion in the hamster (Yanagimachi, unpublished data). The pH of the medium is critical (Yanagimachi *et al.*, 1980). The rate of sperm–egg fusion (in the hamster) in media with pH values above 7.1 is 100%; it declines sharply below 7.1 and is 0 at pH 6.1. At pH 6.1 or below, acrosome-reacted spermatozoa may attach to the egg plasma membranes, but are unable to fuse with them. The block of sperm–egg fusion at low pH or under Ca^{2+}-free conditions is reversible, as the eggs that are not penetrated by spermatozoa at low pH or in Ca^{2+}-free medium are penetrated when they are transferred to more alkaline or Ca^{2+}-containing media (Yanagimachi, 1978b; Yanagimachi *et al.*, 1980). Sperm–egg fusion is also temperature dependent, and cannot occur at temperatures below 10° C (Hirao and Yanagimachi, 1978a).

Effects of Enzymes on Egg Plasma Membrane

Hirao and Yanagimachi (1978b) treated zona-free hamster eggs with a variety of enzymes to determine whether enzyme treatments would render the eggs incapable of fusing with acrosome-reacted spermatozoa. Unexpectedly, of the 29 different enzymes tested, only phospholipase C markedly reduced the ability of the egg plasma membrane to fuse with spermatozoa. Eggs treated with trypsin, chymotrypsin, Pronase, and several other proteinases remained fully capable of fusing with spermatozoa. Unlike hamster eggs, mouse eggs seem to be rather sensitive to proteinases. According to Wolf *et al.* (1976), treating zona-free eggs with trypsin and chymotrypsin greatly reduces the ability of the eggs to fuse with spermatozoa. In the mouse, the egg plasma membrane quickly becomes incapable of fusing with spermatozoa after the first fertilizing spermatozoon penetrates the egg (Wolf, 1978; Sato, 1979). A proteinase (a trypsinlike enzyme?) released from the cortical granules at the time of fertilization (Wolf and Hamada, 1977) may alter the properties of surface components of the egg plasma membrane. In the hamster, the egg plasma membrane remains fusible with spermatozoa for many hours after fertilization (Usui and Yanagimachi, 1976). A trypsinlike enzyme in the cortical granules of the hamster egg may alter characteristics of the zona (Gwatkin *et al.*, 1973), but not those of the surface components of the egg plasma membrane.

Effects of Miscellaneous Reagents on Sperm–Egg Fusion

According to Carroll and Levitan (1978a,b), micromolar concentrations of erythrosin B and structurally related anionic, lipophilic dyes (e.g., rose bengal and eosin) block fertilization in a variety of invertebrates as well as frogs and fish. The mechanism by which these dyes block fertilization is unknown. Caroll and Levitan (1978a) postulated that the dyes are adsorbed by or integrated into the gametes' membranes, altering the electrostatic properties of the membranes and thereby inhibiting membrane fusion of the gametes. High concentrations of erythrosin B (0.5–1 mM) block the fusion of zona-free mouse eggs with spermatozoa (Carroll and Wolf, 1979), but I could not confirm this with the hamster (Yanagimachi, unpublished data). When I separately treated acrosome-reacted spermatozoa and zona-free eggs for 10 min with media containing 0.1–1 mM erythrosin B and then mixed them in the presence of erythrosin B at the same concentrations, 100% of the eggs were penetrated by spermatozoa within 1 hr (as evidenced by the presence of swollen sperm heads within the egg cytoplasm). A higher concentration of erythrosin (3 mM) reduced the incidence of sperm penetration, but the dye at this concentration obviously had cytotoxic effects on the spermatozoa.

Hirao and Yanagimachi (1978b) treated zona-free hamster eggs with various enzymes and examined the ability of the treated eggs to fuse with acrosome-reacted spermatozoa. Of the 29 enzymes tested (9 protein-hydrolyzing, 8 carbohydrate-hydrolyzing, 4 lipid-hydrolyzing, and 8 others), only phospholipase C rendered the egg plasma membrane incapable of fusing with spermatozoa. Excessive treatment of eggs with this enzyme inevitably resulted in their cytolysis probably due to disintegration of the egg plasma membranes. A brief treatment of eggs with low concentrations of the enzyme caused neither cytolysis nor visible changes in the eggs, yet rendered the eggs completely incapable of fusing with spermatozoa. Phospholipase C must prevent sperm–egg fusion by drastically altering the molecular configuration of the lipid moiety of the egg plasma membrane. That alteration of the lipid composition of the egg and sperm plasma membranes would change the ability of the membranes to fuse is expected. Fleming and Yanagimachi (1981) found that acrosome-reacted guinea pig spermatozoa were unable to fuse with the egg plasma membrane in the presence of exogenous phosphatidylserine or lysophosphatidylserine. Integration of excess phosphatidylserine and lysophosphatidylserine into the egg and sperm plasma membranes may prevent a proper phase separation of membrane phospholipids (Papahadjopoulos *et al.*, 1979), which might be necessary for sperm–egg fusion (cf. Fleming and Yanagimachi, 1981, for discussion).

Cytochalasin B (an antiactin agent) at concentrations of 1–50 μg/ml (= 2×10^{-6}–1×10^{-4} M) blocks sperm–egg fusion in the sea urchin, but not in the mouse (Longo, 1978a). Cytochalasin D (1.7×10^{-4} M) drastically changes the surface characteristics (e.g., viscosity of egg cortex and morphology of microvilli) of the hamster egg, but does not prevent sperm–egg fusion (Yanagimachi and Mohri, unpublished data).

Proteinase inhibitors (e.g., ovomucoid, soybean and lima bean inhibitors, and p-aminobenzamidine) inhibit sperm–egg fusion in the mouse (Wolf, 1977), but not in the hamster (Yanagimachi *et al.*, 1980). I suspect that proteinase inhibitors block sperm–egg fusion in the mouse by preventing the acrosome reaction rather than sperm–egg fusion per se. Conway and Metz (1976) suggested the possible involvement of phospholipase in sperm–egg fusion in the sea urchin. Mepacrine (a phospholipase inhibitor), however, did not prevent sperm–egg fusion in the hamster at nontoxic levels (< 0.1 mM) (Yanagimachi, unpublished data).

Unexpectedly, zona-free hamster and rabbit eggs treated with plant lectins (e.g., concanavalin A, wheat germ agglutinin, and *Ricinus communis* agglutinin) are still able to fuse with spermatozoa (Nicolson *et al.*, 1975; Gordon and Dandekar, 1976). When these lectins bind to plasma membranes, they may induce extensive aggregations of intramembranous glycoprotein particles, thus creating numerous particle-free areas within the egg membrane. These conditions may promote sperm–egg fusion rather than prevent it.

Tsunoda and Sugie (1979) prepared rabbit antiserum against a homogenate of zona-free mouse eggs. When tested *in vitro*, this antiserum did not at all prevent fusion of mouse spermatozoa with zona-free eggs. The antiserum Tsunoda and Sugie prepared may have contained antibodies against intracellular components of the egg, but probably not anti-egg plasma membrane antibodies. Antibodies raised against spermatozoa may block fertilization by interfering with sperm passage through the egg investments (Russo and Metz, 1974a,b; Tsunoda and Chang, 1976), but there is convincing evidence that the antibodies can also block sperm–egg fusion. Oikawa and Suzuki (1979) prepared antibodies against saline extracts of hamster epididymis (epididymal tissue plus spermatozoa). When female hamsters were injected with the antibodies and mated, spermatozoa were seen to have penetrated the zonae, but not the vitelli. The antibodies seem to bind to the sperm plasma membrane, particularly the membrane of the postacrosomal region. Tzartos (1979) prepared Fab fragments of antibodies against hamster epididymal spermatozoa. When acrosome-reacted hamster spermatozoa were exposed to the antibodies and mixed with zona-free eggs *in vitro*, the spermatozoa remained highly motile but none of them penetrated the eggs. We isolated IgG antibodies from antisperm autoantiserum of the guinea pig. The antibodies neither agglutinated nor slowed down the movement of the acrosome-reacted guinea pig spermatozoa, but prevented the spermatozoa from attaching to and penetrating zona-free eggs (Yanagimachi *et al.*, 1981). To our surprise, Fab antibodies were not as effective as IgG antibodies in preventing sperm penetration into the eggs. According the Menge and Black (1979), Fab antibodies prepared from antisera against human spermatozoa or testis completely or largely blocked the entry of human spermatozoa into zona-free hamster eggs. However, it is not clear from their report whether the antibodies blocked the acrosome reaction or sperm–egg fusion.

Decondensation of the Sperm Nucleus and Development of Sperm and Egg Pronuclei

When a spermatozoon enters the egg cytoplasm, the nuclear envelope surrounding the sperm nucleus disappears and decondensation of the nucleus begins. A new nuclear envelope then appears around the decondensed chromatin. Under normal conditions, the new envelope appears after decondensation of the sperm chromatin is completed (Bedford, 1970b, 1972a). Under some experimental conditions, however, the new envelope may begin to appear before the completion of chromatin decondensation (Yanagimachi and Noda, 1970d). Complete loss of basic (arginine-rich) proteins from the sperm nucleus is concomitant with decondensation of the chromatin (Kopecny and Pavlok, 1975). DNA synthesis in both sperm and egg nuclei is more or less synchronous with the development of pronuclei (Szollosi, 1966; Luthardt and Donahue, 1973; Krishna and Generoso, 1977). Fully developed sperm and egg pronuclei come into close proximity in the center of the egg, their nuclear envelopes disappear, and the chromosomes of both sperm and egg pronuclei mingle for the first mitotic division (Longo and Anderson, 1969; Gondos *et al*., 1972; Zamboni, 1972; Longo, 1973; Anderson *et al*., 1975).

In almost all mammals, the inner acrosomal membrane, perinuclear materials, basal body, connecting piece, centrioles, mitochondria, and other tail components are incorporated into the egg cytoplasm during sperm–egg fusion. According to Szollosi (1965, 1976), all of these sperm components disintegrate sooner or later and do not seem to directly participate in the development of the zygote. However, it is not known at the present time whether the degenerated (digested?) products of these elements are utilized or eliminated by the zygote. Possible involvement of the sperm mitochondrial DNA in the development of the embryo is conceivable, but this has not been proven or disproven unequivocally. According to Iwamatsu *et al*. (1976), flagellar microtubules isolated from sea urchin and oyster spermatozoa induce normal cleavages of *Oryzias* (a teleost) eggs when injected microsurgically. The flagellar microtubules may serve as a "seed" for polymerization of ooplasmic tubulins and the formation of the mitotic spindle. Thus, part of the microtubules in the mammalian sperm flagellum that are incorporated into the egg cytoplasm during fertilization may well function as a cleavage-inducing or cleavage-promoting factor.

Egg Cytoplasmic Factors Controlling Decondensation
of the Sperm Nucleus

Sperm nuclei incorporated into the cytoplasm of mature eggs soon begin to decondense. There must be some specific chemicals or factors in the egg cytoplasm that induce nuclear decondensation. Thibault and his associates (Thibault and Gerard, 1970; Thibault, 1973b; Thibault et al., 1975) were the first to suggest the presence of such factors in the egg cytoplasm. When they isolated immature oocytes from ovaries of the rabbit and cow and cultured them in vitro, the oocytes matured in vitro were able to incorporate spermatozoa. Sperm nuclei, however, invariably failed to decondense to the full extent. Obviously, the in vitro-matured oocytes lacked some factor necessary for decondensation of the sperm nucleus. This factor has been referred to as the male pronucleus growth factor. Yanagimachi and Usui (1972) and Usui and Yanagimachi (1976) reported a similar but somewhat different factor in the egg cytoplasm. We found that hamster sperm nuclei incorporated into the cytoplasm of immature eggs at the germinal vesicle stage were unable to decondense despite the fact that the nuclear envelope surrounding the nucleus disappeared soon after sperm entry. Sperm nuclei incorporated into the cytoplasm of eggs matured in vivo, on the other hand, rapidly decondensed. It is obvious that the cytoplasm of the immature hamster egg lacks some factor necessary for decondensation of the sperm nucleus. This factor was called sperm nucleus-decondensing factor (SNDF). By comparing the speed of sperm nuclear decondensation after sperm entry into eggs at various stages of maturation, Usui and Yanagimachi (1976) inferred that SNDF begins to appear in the egg cytoplasm after breakdown of the germinal vesicle, increases in amount as egg maturation advances, and reaches a maximum level shortly before or after ovulation. Interestingly, SNDF quickly disappears after fertilization and reappears shortly before the first mitosis (cleavage) begins. The lack of SNDF in immature rat eggs at the germinal vesicle stage has also been demonstrated by Thadani (1979), who microsurgically injected rat spermatozoa into eggs and did not observe decondensed sperm nuclei.

The SNDF seems to be abundant in the egg matured in vivo. Hirao and Yanagimachi (1979) observed as many as 56 decondensing sperm nuclei in the cytoplasm of a hamster egg. In the pig, more than 80 spermatozoa may enter the egg, but when more than 20 have entered, their nuclei decondense only to a limited degree, suggesting that the amount of SNDF accessible for decondensation of sperm nuclei is limited (Hunter, 1976).

The SNDF does not appear to be highly species specific because the nuclei of spermatozoa that enter the cytoplasm of foreign eggs are able to decondense (e.g., Hanada and Chang, 1972, 1976, 1978; Yanagimachi, 1972b,

1977; Uehara and Yanagimachi, 1976; Yanagimachi *et al.*, 1976; Barros *et al.*, 1979; Thandani, 1980). The SNDF is resistant to light (Hirao and Yanagimachi, 1978c) and seems to retain its activity even after extensive "aging" of the egg cytoplasm under some experimental conditions (Barros and Leal, 1980).

We originally thought that SNDF becomes biologically active only after the egg is activated by a spermatozoon or parthenogenetic agent (Uehara and Yanagimachi, 1976; Yanagimachi, 1977). This notion, however, must be revised as we subsequently found the hamster sperm nuclei injected microsurgically into a mature egg decondense even if the egg shows no sign of activation (Uehara and Yanagimachi, 1977). Our criteria for egg activation were the exocytosis of cortical granules and the resumption of meiosis. As these are merely the visible indications of egg activation and many invisible, physiological and biochemical events must be involved also, the "unactivated" eggs containing decondensing sperm nuclei may have been "partially" activated. It would be hasty to conclude that activation of the egg cytoplasm is unnecessary for SNDF, but we may at least say that full activation of the egg cytoplasm is not required for SNDF to achieve its function.

The origin of SNDF is unknown. Usui and Yanagimachi (1976) speculated that SNDF is synthesized in the egg cytoplasm, transported to and accumulated in the germinal vesicle, and then released into the egg cytoplasm at the time of germinal vesicle breakdown. The amount of free SNDF in the cytoplasm of the hamster egg at the germinal vesicle stage may never reach a level high enough to induce decondensation of sperm nuclei. This does not seem to be the case of the dog because the cytoplasm of immature dog eggs with intact germinal vesicles can readily induce decondensation of sperm nuclei (Mahi and Yanagimachi, 1976). In this context, it is interesting to note the results of experiments performed by Iwamatsu and Ohta (1980) using *Oryzias* eggs. They centrifuged eggs at the germinal vesicle stage to displace the germinal vesicle from the cytoplasm into the yolk mass. When the egg was cultured *in vitro*, the germinal vesicle remained intact. When eggs matured in this way were inseminated, the sperm nuclei decondenses and developed into pronuclei just like those that penetrated normally matured eggs. Thus, at least in this fish, SNDF seems to appear in the cytoplasm independently of the germinal vesicle material. We do not know whether this is true also for mammals. It is conceivable that in most mammals, SNDF is gradually accumulated in the cytoplasm during the growth of the oocyte and is "activated" by germinal vesicle material during the final stage of maturation.

The chemical nature of SNDF is unknown. Eng and Metz (1980) have recently isolated a macromolecule from sea urchin eggs that is capable of decondensing sperm nuclei. This molecule has a molecular weight of about 100,000, is heat labile, and requires Ca^{2+} to manifest its activity. No similar substance has even been isolated from mammalian eggs. As the isolation and identification of SNDF from mammalian eggs are difficult due to the limited numbers of eggs available, inferences regarding its nature have been based on artificial decondensation of sperm nuclei *in vitro*. There are numerous reagents capable of decondensing sperm nuclei (cf. Delgado *et al.*, 1980, and Kvist, 1980, for references). As the sperm nuclei of eutherian mammals are very rich in S–S cross-linkings, and the S–S-reducing agents can induce decondensation of the nuclei (Calvin and Bedford, 1971), Bedford (1972b) postulated that the egg possesses the ability to cleave S–S bonds within the sperm chromatin. Mahi and Yanagimachi (1975) suggested that reduced glutathione and/ or some specific SH-dependent enzymes may be involved in decondensation of sperm chromatin. The reagents most commonly used for inducing decondensation of sperm nuclei are S–S-reducing agents (like dithiothreitol) combined with detergents (like sodium dodecyl sulfate). Although the native SNDF within the egg cytoplasm is unlikely to contain such harsh substances, both SNDF and these reagents must have some common characteristics. An acrosinlike proteinase intrinsic to sperm chromatin has been implicated in decondensation of the chromatin (Marushige and Marushige, 1975, 1978; Gall and Ohsumi, 1976; Zirkin and Chang, 1977; Chang and Zirkin, 1978; Zirkin *et al.*, 1980), although some doubt has been cast about this (Young, 1979). However, it is certainly possible that proteinase within the egg cytoplasm constitutes part of the SNDF or assists the action of the SNDF.

Factors Controlling Development of the Pronuclei

Little is known about the mechanisms by which sperm and egg pronuclei develop. When excessively large numbers of spermatozoa enter an egg, the sperm nuclei decondense but fail to develop into pronuclei, whereas the egg chromosomes develop into a pronucleus with distinct nucleoli (Hirao and Yanagimachi, 1979; cf. Figure 22). This may suggest that the egg cytoplasmic factor responsible for development of the egg pronucleus is not the same as that which controls the development of the sperm pronucleus.

The factor controlling the development of the sperm pronucleus (*sperm pronucleus development factor*, SPDF) is not strictly species specific because sperm nuclei incorporated into the cytoplasm of foreign eggs (e.g., human sperm nuclei in hamster eggs) can develop into apparently normal pronuclei (e.g., Imai *et al.*, 1977; Yanagimachi, 1977; Barros *et al.*, 1979; Thadani, 1980).

When Uehara and Yanagimachi (1977) microsurgically injected hamster sperm nuclei into unfertilized eggs, decondensation of the sperm nuclei occurred regardless of whether the eggs were activated or not. The nuclei decondensed even if the eggs were not activated at all or were activated only

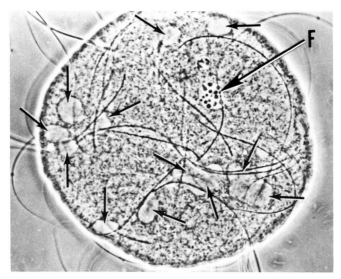

Figure 22. A heavily polyspermic zona-free hamster egg. The swollen sperm heads (arrows) failed to develop into pronuclei, but the egg chromosomes did develop into a pronucleus (F). Photographed 3 hr after the egg was inseminated *in vitro* with acrosome-reacted spermatozoa.

partially. Well-developed sperm pronuclei, however, formed only when the eggs were fully activated. Thus, SPDF seems to be able to function only when the egg cytoplasm is fully activated.

The amount of SPDF present in the egg cytoplasm seems to be limited. When excessively large numbers of spermatozoa enter an egg, the sperm nuclei apparently "compete" for SPDF; in the hamster, five spermatozoa per egg appears to be the limit for all the sperm nuclei to develop into pronuclei (Hirao and Yanagimachi, 1979).

Perinuclear materials (subacrosomal material and postacrosomal dense lamina; cf. Fawcett, 1975) in the spermatozoa of some species contain distinct microtubular structure (Blom and Birch-Andersen, 1965; Plattner, 1971; Wooding and O'Donnell, 1971; Koehler, 1978; Peterson *et al.*, 1978b) and actin (Clarke and Yanagimachi, 1978; Tamblyn, 1980). As these perinuclear materials are definitely incorporated into the egg during sperm–egg fusion, microtubules and actin of sperm origin may join the actin (Amsterdam *et al.*, 1977) and microtubules of the egg and participate in the migration of the sperm and egg pronuclei to the center of the egg. According to Longo (1978b), puromycin inhibits the migration of pronuclei to the center of the rabbit egg, and actinomycin D blocks the breakdown of nuclear envelopes. Thus, the migration of pronuclei and subsequent breakdown of their nuclear envelopes seem to require postfertilization synthesis of proteins and RNA within egg cytoplasm. Activation and rearrangement of cytoskeletal systems within the egg cytoplasm may also be involved in migration of the sperm and egg pronuclei to the center of the egg as demonstrated in the sea urchin (Schatten and Schatten, 1979).

Conclusions

Figure 23 depicts the possible relationships among the major events that occur before and during fertilization. The diagram is of course tentative and should be revised as we accumulate more solid information.

1. As far as we are aware, spermatozoa of all eutherian mammals must undergo both maturation (A) and capacitation (B) before they are capable of undergoing the acrosome reaction. Although some important intracellular changes may occur during capacitation, removal or modification of substances adsorbed on the plasma membrane prior to or during ejaculation seems to constitute the major part of capacitation.

2. When a fully capacitated spermatozoon nears the site of fertilization or comes into contact with the cumulus oophorus surrounding the egg, the acrosome reaction (C) is initiated. Although some substances emanating from the cumulus could be the "native" factors that induce the acrosome reaction *in vivo*, the acrosome reaction can be induced under a variety of experimental conditions without any contribution from the cumulus or cumulus factors. As long as the spermatozoon is fully capacitated, any conditions that cause "perturbation" or increase "excitability" of the membrane seem to be able to trigger the acrosome reaction.

3. Although Ca^{2+} in the medium is known to be essential for the acrosome reaction, a proper overall balance of extra- and intracellular conditions or components, rather than a single condition or component, must be important for initiation and completion of the reaction.

Under certain experimental conditions, spermatozoa may undergo an "immediate" acrosome reaction without capacitation.

4. The site where the spermatozoon initiates its acrosome reaction may not be strictly fixed under either *in vivo* or *in vitro* conditions. Under ordinary *in vivo* conditions, the fertilizing spermatozoon probably initiates its acrosome reaction when it comes into close approximation with the cumulus, on contact with the cumulus, or while it is passing through the cumulus. If the cumulus has been "softened" or dispersed (e.g., due to postovulatory aging prior to fertilization) or if the cumulus has been artificially removed, acrosome-intact spermatozoa may undergo acrosome reactions on the surface of the zona.

The proper timing of the acrosome reaction seems to be important. If the spermatozoon undergoes the acrosome reaction too long before meeting the egg, its ability to penetrate the zona may be lost before it ceases moving.

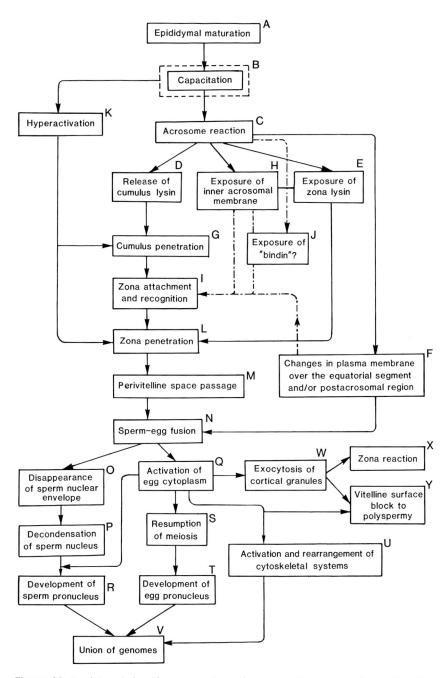

Figure 23. Possible relationships among the major events that occur before and during fertilization in mammals. (For explanation, see the text, pp. 152–155.)

5. The acrosome reaction has at least two biological functions. It provides for the release or exposure of "lysins" (D and E) with which the spermatozoon makes its way through the egg investments. It also renders, by some unknown mechanism, the plasma membrane over the equatorial segment and/or postacrosomal region capable of fusing with the egg plasma membrane (F).

6. The most probable candidates for the cumulus and zona lysins are hyaluronidase and acrosin. However, it is certainly possible that other enzymes or nonenzymatic substances are functional lysins that work independently or synergistically with hyaluronidase and acrosin.

7. The structure with which the spermatozoon attaches (binds) to or recognizes the zona could be the plasma membrane of the acrosomal and/or the postacrosomal region. At least in the guinea pig, the inner acrosomal membrane exposed after the acrosome reaction (H) appears to be one of the structures with which the spermatozoon recognizes the zona (I). A substance like the "bindin" of sea urchins could be involved in firm attachment of the spermatozoon to the zona surface (J).

8. In some species, the spermatozoon begins extremely vigorous flagellar movement shortly before the acrosome reaction. This movement, which has been referred to as activation, is renamed *hyperactivation* (K). The biological significance of hyperactivation is unknown, but it could provide strong thrusting power to the spermatozoon for passing through the cumulus and zona (G and L). Although hyperactivation and the acrosome reaction may occur almost simultaneously, they are separate phenomena. After all, hyperactivation is a phenomenon that occurs in the sperm flagellum, and the acrosome reaction is an event that occurs in the sperm head. Whether the term *capacitation* should be confined to changes in the spermatozoon that render it capable of undergoing the acrosome reaction or whether it should include changes that render the sperm tail capable of manifesting hyperactivated motility must be the subject of future debate.

9. Sperm penetration through the zona (L) seems to be achieved by both mechanical and chemical means. Although it is generally believed that acrosin bound on the inner acrosomal membrane serves as the zona lysin, unequivocal evidence is needed to substantiate this belief.

10. The spermatozoon that has passed through the perivitelline space (M) fuses with egg plasma membrane (N). Fusion is initiated between the egg plasma membrane (most probably the microvilli) and the sperm plasma membrane of the equatorial and/or postacrosomal regions.

11. As soon as the sperm nucleus enters the egg cytoplasm, the nuclear envelope surrounding the nucleus starts to break down (O) and the nucleus begins to decondense (P). Activation of the egg cytoplasm (Q) by the fertilizing spermatozoon may not be necessary for decondensation of the

sperm nucleus, but it does seem necessary for transformation of the decondensed nucleus into the sperm pronucleus (R). The cytoplasmic factor controlling the resumption of meiosis (S) and the development of the egg pronucleus (T) may not be identical with that regulating the development of the sperm pronucleus. Activation and rearrangement of cytoskeletal systems (U) will bring the developing sperm and egg pronuclei to the center of the egg, and the union of sperm and egg genomes (V) ensues.

12. Activation of the egg by the fertilizing spermatozoon causes exocytosis of cortical granules (W), which in turn induces the zona reaction (X) and vitelline surface changes (Y) to prevent polyspermy. The block to polyspermy at the vitelline surface may occur independently from cortical granule exocytosis, however (cf. Wolf, Chapter 6, this volume).

ACKNOWLEDGMENTS

I wish to express my sincere thanks to Mrs. Cherrie A. Mahi-Brown, Dr. James M. Cummins, Dr. Kenneth S. K. Tung, and Dr. David F. Katz for their invaluable advice and suggestions. I am also indebted to Dr. Luigi Mastroianni and Mrs. Michele Ikeda for their assistance in the preparation of the manuscript. The studies by my associates and me were supported by grants from the National Institute of Child Health and Human Development (HD-03402), the Population Council, the Ford Foundation, the International Planned Parenthood Federation, the Morris Animal Foundation, and the University of Hawaii Research Administration.

References

Adams, C. E., and Chang, M. C., 1962, Capacitation of rabbit spermatozoa in the fallopian tube and in the uterus, *J. Exp. Zool.* **151**:159–165.

Aketa, K., and Ohta, T., 1977, When do sperm of sea urchin, *Pseudocentrotus depressus*, undergo the acrosome reaction at fertilization?, *Dev. Biol.* **61**:366–372.

Allison, A. C., and Hartree, E. F., 1970, Lysosomal enzymes in the acrosome and their possible role in fertilization, *J. Reprod. Fertil.* **21**:501–515.

Amsterdam, A., Lindner, H. R., and Groeschel-Stewart, U., 1977, Localization of actin and myosin in the rat oocyte and follicular wall by immunofluorescence, *Anat. Rec.* **187**:311–328.

Anand, S. R., Kaur, S. P., and Chaudhry, P. S., 1977, Distribution of β-N-acetylglucosaminidase, hyaluronoglucosaminidase and acrosin in buffalo and goat spermatozoa, *Hoppe-Seyler's Z. Physiol. Chem.* **358**:685–688.

Anderson, E., 1974, Comparative aspects of the ultrastructure of the female gamete, *Int. Rev. Cytol. Suppl.* **4**:1–70.

Anderson, E., Hoppe, P. C., Whitten, W. K., and Lee, G. S., 1975, *In vitro* fertilization and early embryogenesis: A cytological analysis, *J. Ultrastruct. Res.* **50**:231–252.

Aonuma, S., Mayumi, T., Suzuki, T., Noguchi, T., Iwai, M., and Okabe, M., 1973, Studies on sperm capacitation. I. The relationship between a guinea pig sperm-coating antigen and a sperm capacitation phenomenon, *J. Reprod. Fertil.* **35**:425–432.

Aonuma, S., Okabe, M., Kawaguchi, M., and Kishi, Y., 1980, Studies on sperm capacitation. IX. Movement characteristics of spermatozoa in relation to capacitation, *Chem. Pharm. Bull. Jpn.* **28**:1497-1502.

Asdell, S. A., 1964, *Pattern of Mammalian Reproduction*, 2nd ed., Cornell University Press, Ithaca, N.Y.

Austin, C. R., 1948, Function of hyaluronidase in fertilization, *Nature (London)* **162**:63.

Austin, C. R., 1951, Observations on the penetration of the sperm into the mammalian egg, *Aust. J. Sci. Res. Ser. B* **4**:581-596.

Austin, C. R., 1952, The "capacitation" of the mammalian sperm, *Nature* (London) **170**:326.

Austin, C. R., 1960, Capacitation and the release of hyaluronidase from spermatozoa, *J. Reprod. Fertil.* **1**:310-311.

Austin, C. R., 1961, *The Mammalian Egg*, Thomas, Springfield, Ill.

Austin, C. R., 1968, *Ultrastructure of Fertilization*, Holt. Rinehart & Winston, New York.

Austin, C. R., and Bishop, M. W. H., 1957, Fertilization in mammals, *Biol. Rev.* **32**:296-349.

Austin, C. R., and Bishop, M. W. H., 1958, Role of the rodent acrosome and perforatorium in fertilization, *Proc. R. Soc. London Ser. B* **149**:241-248.

Austin, C. R., and Braden, A. W. H., 1956, Early reactions of the rodent egg to spermatozoon penetration, *J. Exp. Biol.* **33**:358-365.

Austin, C. R., and Walton, A., 1960, Fertilization, in: *Marshall's Physiology of Reproduction*, Volume 1, Part 2 (A. S. Parkes, ed.), Longmans, Green, London, pp. 310-416.

Austin, C. R., Bavister. B. D., and Edwards, R. G., 1973, Components of capacitation, in: *The Regulation of Mammalian Reproduction* (S. J. Segal, R. Crozier, P. A. Corfman, and P. Condliffe, eds.), Thomas, Springfield, Ill., pp. 247-254.

Babcock, D. F., Singh, J. P., and Lardy, H. A., 1979, Alteration of membrane permeability to calcium ions during maturation of bovine spermatozoa, *Dev. Biol.* **69**:85-93.

Back, D. J., Shenton, J. C., and Glover, T. D., 1974, The composition of epididymal plasma from the cauda epididymis of the rat, *J. Reprod. Fertil.* **40**:211-214.

Baker, L. D. S., and Amann, R. P., 1970, Epididymal physiology. I. Specificity of antisera against bull spermatozoa and reproductive fluids, *J. Reprod. Fertil.* **22**:441-452.

Baker, L. D. S., and Amann, R. P., 1971, Epididymal physiology. II. Immunofluorescent analyses of epithelial secretion and absorption, and of bovine sperm maturation, *J. Reprod. Fertil.* **26**:319-332.

Barros, C., 1968, *In vitro* capacitation of golden hamster spermatozoa with fallopian tube fluid of the mouse and rat, *J. Reprod. Fertil.* **17**:203-206.

Barros, C., 1974, Capacitation of mammalian spermatozoa, in: *Physiology and Genetics of Reproduction*, Part B (E. M. Coutinho and F. Fuchs, eds.), Plenum Press, New York, pp. 3-24.

Barros, C., 1977, The fertile mammalian spermatozoon, *Microsc. Electronica (Santiago, Chile)* **4**:107-113.

Barros, C., and Berrios, M., 1977, Is the activated spermatozoa really capacitated?, *J. Exp. Zool.* **201**:65-72.

Barros, C., and Franklin, L. E., 1968, Behavior of the gamete membranes during sperm entry into the mammalian egg, *J. Cell Biol.* **37**:C13-C18.

Barros, C., and Herrera, E., 1977, Ultrastructural observation of the incorporation of guinea-pig spermatozoa into zona-free hamster oocytes, *J. Reprod. Fertil.* **49**:47-50.

Barros, C., and Leal, J., 1980, *In vitro* fertilization technique and application to study gamete interactions, *Arch. Androl.* **5**:61-62.

Barros, C., and Munoz, G., 1973, Sperm–egg interaction in immature hamster oocytes, *J. Exp. Zool.* **186**:73-78.

Barros, C., and Munoz, G., 1974, Sperm penetration through the zona pellucida of immature hamster oocytes, *Acta Physiol. Lat. Am.* **24**:612-615.

Barros, C., Bedford, J. M., Franklin, L. E., and Austin, C. R., 1967, Membrane vesiculation as a feature of the mammalian acrosome reaction, *J. Cell Biol.* **34**:C1–C5.

Barros, C., Berrios, M., and Herrera, E., 1973a, Capacitation *in vitro* of guinea-pig spermatozoa in a saline solution, *J. Reprod. Fertil.* **34**:547–549.

Barros, C., Fujimoto, M., and Yanagimachi, R., 1973b, Failure of zona penetration of hamster spermatozoa after prolonged preincubation in a blood serum fraction, *J. Reprod. Fertil.* **35**:89–95.

Barros, C., Gonzalez, J., Herrera, E., and Bustos-Obregon, E., 1978, Fertilizing capacity of human spermatozoa evaluated by actual penetration of foreign eggs, *Contraception* **17**:87–93.

Barros, C., Gonzalez, J., Herrera, E., and Bustos-Obregon, E., 1979, Human sperm penetration into zona-free hamster oocytes as a test to evaluate the sperm fertilizing ability, *Andrologia* **11**:197–210.

Battalia, D. B., and Yanagimachi, R., 1979, Enhanced and co-ordinated movement of the hamster oviduct during the periovulatory period, *J. Reprod. Fertil.* **56**:515–520.

Bavister, B. D., 1969, Environmental factors important for *in vitro* fertilization in the hamster, *J. Reprod. Fertil.* **18**:544–545.

Bavister, B. D., 1973, Capacitation of golden hamster spermatozoa during incubation in culture medium, *J. Reprod. Fertil.* **35**:161–163.

Bavister, B. D., 1975, Properties of the sperm motility-stimulating component derived from human serum, *J. Reprod. Fertil.* **43**: 363–366.

Bavister, B. D., and Yanagimachi, R., 1977, The effects of sperm extracts and energy sources on the motility and acrosome reaction of hamster spermatozoa *in vitro*, *Biol. Reprod.* **16**:228–237.

Bavister, B. D., Yanagimachi, R., and Teichman, R. J., 1976, Capacitation of hamster spermatozoa with adrenal gland extracts, *Biol. Reprod.* **14**:219–221.

Bearer, E. L., and Friend, D. S., 1980, Modifications of anionic phospholipid distribution preceding membrane fusion, *J. Cell Biol.* **87**:199a (ME [534).

Bedford, J. M., 1963, Changes in the electrophoretic properties of rabbit spermatozoa during passage through the epididymis, *Nature (London)* **200**:1178–1180.

Bedford, J. M., 1964, Fine structure of sperm head in ejaculate and uterine spermatozoa of the rabbit, *J. Reprod. Fertil.* **7**:221–228.

Bedford, J. M., 1965, Effect of environment on phagocytosis of rabbit spermatozoa, *J. Reprod. Fertil.* **9**: 249–256.

Bedford, J. M., 1966, Development of the fertilizing ability of spermatozoa in the epididymis of the rabbit, *J. Exp. Zool.* **163**:319–329.

Bedford, J. M., 1967a, Experimental requirement for capacitation and observations on ultrastructural changes in the rabbit spermatozoa during fertilization, *J. Reprod. Fertil. Suppl.* **2**:35–48.

Bedford, J. M., 1967b, The importance of capacitation for establishing contact between eggs and sperm in the rabbit, *J. Reprod. Fertil.* **13**:365–367.

Bedford, J. M., 1968, Ultrastructural changes in the sperm head during fertilization in the rabbit, *Am. J. Anat.* **123**:329–358.

Bedford, J. M., 1969a, Limitation of the uterus in the development of the fertilizing ability (capacitation) of spermatozoa, *J. Reprod. Fertil. Suppl.* **8**:19–26.

Bedford, J. M., 1969b, Morphological aspects of sperm capacitation in mammals, in: *Advances in Biosciences*, Volume 4 (G. Raspe, ed.), Pergamon Press, Oxford, pp. 35–50.

Bedford, J. M., 1970a, Sperm capacitation and fertilization in mammals, *Biol. Reprod. Suppl.* **2**:128–158.

Bedford, J. M., 1970b, The saga of mammalian sperm from ejaculation to syngamy, in:

Mammalian Reproduction (H. Gibian and E. J. Plotz, eds.), Springer-Verlag, Berlin, pp. 124–182.

Bedford, J. M., 1972a, An electron microscopic study of sperm penetration into the rabbit egg after natural mating, *Am. J. Anat.* **133**:213–254.

Bedford, J. M., 1972b, Sperm transport, capacitation and fertilization, in: *Reproductive Biology* (H. Balin and S. Glasser, eds.), Excerpta Medica, Amsterdam, pp. 338–392.

Bedford, J. M., 1974, Mechanisms involved in penetration of spermatozoa through the vestments of the mammalian egg, in: *Physiology and Genetics of Reproduction*, Part B (E. M. Coutinho and F. Fuchs, eds.), Plenum Press, New York, pp. 55–68.

Bedford, J. M., 1975, Maturation, transport, and fate of spermatozoa in the epididymis, in: *Handbook of Physiology*, Section 7, Volume 5 (R. O. Greep, ed.), American Physiological Society, Washington, D.C., pp. 303–317.

Bedford, J. M., 1977, Sperm/egg interaction: The specificity of human spermatozoa, *Anat. Rec.* **188**:477–488.

Bedford, J. M., 1979, Evolution of the sperm maturation and sperm storage function of the epididymis, in: *The Spermatozoa* (D. W. Fawcett and J. M. Bedford, eds.), Urban & Schwarzenberg, Munich, pp. 7–21.

Bedford, J. M., and Cooper, G. W., 1978, Membrane fusion events in the fertilization of vertebrate eggs, in: *Cell Surface Reviews*, Volume 5 (G. Poste and G. L. Nicolson, eds.), North-Holland, Amsterdam, pp. 65–125.

Bedford, J. M., and Cross, N. L., 1978, Normal penetration of rabbit spermatozoa through a trypsin- and acrosin-resistant zona pellucida, *J. Reprod. Fertil.* **54**:385–392.

Bedford, J. M., Calvin, H., and Cooper, G. W., 1973, The maturation of spermatozoa in the human epididymis, *J. Reprod. Fertil. Suppl.* **18**:199–213.

Bedford, J. M., Moore, H. D. M., and Franklin, L. E., 1979, Significance of the equatorial segment of the acrosome of the spermatozoon in eutherian mammals, *Exp. Cell Res.* **119**:119–126.

Bedirian, K. N., Shea, B. F., and Baker, R. D., 1975, Fertilization of bovine follicular oocytes in bovine and porcine oviducts, *Can. J. Anim. Sci.* **55**:251–256.

Berrios, M., and Bedford, J. M., 1979, Oocyte maturation: Aberrant post-fusion responses of the rabbit primary oocyte to penetrating spermatozoa, *J. Cell Sci.* **39**:1–12.

Bhattacharyya, A. K., Goodpasteuer, J. C., and Zaneveld, L. J. D., 1979, Acrosin of mouse spermatozoa, *Am. J. Physiol.* **237**:E40–E44.

Biggers, J. D., Whitten, W. K., and Whittingham, D. G., 1971, The culture of mouse embryos *in vitro*, in: *Methods in Mammalian Embryology* (J. C. Daniel, ed.), Freeman, San Francisco, pp. 86–116 (cf. Table 6-5 for the composition of BWW medium).

Binor, Z., Sokoloski, J. E., and Wolf, D. P., 1980, Penetration of the zona-free hamster egg by human sperm, *Fertil. Steril.* **33**:321–327.

Bishop, D. W., 1961, Biology of spermatozoa, in: *Sex and Internal Secretions*, Volume 2 (W. C. Young, ed.), Williams & Wilkins, Baltimore, pp. 707–796.

Bishop, D. W., 1969, Sperm physiology in relation to the oviduct, in: *The Mammalian Oviduct* (E. S. E. Hafez and R. J. Blandau, eds.), University of Chicago Press, Chicago, pp. 231–290.

Blandau, R. J., 1961, Biology of eggs and implantation, in: *Sex and Internal Secretions*, Volume 2 (W. C. Young, ed.), Williams & Wilkins, Baltimore, pp. 797–882.

Blandau, R. J., 1969, Gamete transport—Comparative aspects, in: *The Mammalian Oviduct* (E. S. E. Hafez and R. J. Blandau, eds.), University of Chicago Press, Chicago, pp. 129–162.

Blandau, R. J., 1978, Gamete transport in oviduct of rats, *Anat. Rec.* **190**:593a.

Blandau, R. J., and Gaddum-Rosse, P., 1974, Mechanisms of sperm transport in pig oviducts, *Fertil. Steril.* **25**:61–67.

Blandau, R. J., and Odor, D. L., 1952, Observations on sperm penetration into the ooplasm and changes in the cytoplasmic components of the fertilizing spermatozoon in rat ova, *Fertil. Steril.* **3**:13-26.

Blandau, R. J., and Rumery, R. E., 1964, The relationship of swimming movement of epididymal spermatozoa to their fertilizing capacity, *Fertil. Steril.* **15**:571-579.

Blank, M., Soo, L., and Britten, J. S., 1974, The properties of rabbit sperm membranes in contact with electrode surfaces, *J. Membr. Biol.* **18**:351-364.

Blank, M., Soo, L., and Britten, J. S., 1976, Absorption of albumin in rabbit sperm membranes, *J. Membr. Biol.* **29**:401-409.

Bleil, J. D., and Wasserman, P. M., 1980a, Mammalian sperm–egg interaction: Identification of a glycoprotein in mouse egg zonae pellucidae possessing receptor activity for sperm, *Cell* **20**:873-882.

Bleil, J. D., and Wasserman, P. M., 1980b, Structure and function of the zona pellucida: Identification and characterization of the proteins of the mouse oocyte's zona pellucida, *Dev. Biol.* **76**:185-203.

Blom, E., and Birch-Andersen, A., 1965, The ultrastructure of the bull sperm, *Nord. Veterinaermed.* **17**:193-212.

Boettcher, B., 1968, Correlation between human ABO blood group antigens in seminal plasma and on seminal spermatozoa, *J. Reprod. Fertil.* **16**:49-54.

Brackett, B. G., 1970, *In vitro* fertilization of rabbit ova: Time sequence of events, *Fertil. Steril.* **21**:169-176.

Brackett, B. G., and Oliphant, G., 1975, Capacitation of rabbit spermatozoa *in vitro*, Biol. Reprod. **12**:260-274.

Brackett, B. G., Killen, D. K., and Peace, M. D., 1971, Cleavage of rabbit ova inseminated *in vitro* after removal of follicular cells and zonae pellucidae, *Fertil. Steril.* **22**:816-828.

Braden, A. W. H., 1952, Properties of the membranes of rat and rabbit eggs, *Aust. J. Sci. Res.* **5**:460-471.

Braden, A. W. H., 1958, Variations between strains of mice in phenomena associated with sperm penetration and fertilization, *J. Genet.* **56**:37-47.

Braden, A. W. H., 1959, Sperm penetration and fertilization in the mouse, *Proc. Int. Symp. Exp. Biol.* Pavia, Italy, May 2-7, *Symp. Genet. Biol. Ital.* **9**:1-8.

Bradford, M. M., McRorie, R. A., and Williams, W. L., 1976a, A role for esterases in the fertilization process, *J. Exp. Zool.* **197**:297-301.

Bradford, M. M., McRorie, R. A., and Williams, W. L., 1976b, Involvement of esterases in sperm penetration of the corona radiata of the ovum, *Biol. Reprod.* **15**:102-106.

Bronson, R., and Hamada, Y., 1977, Gamete interactions *in vitro*, *Fertil. Steril.* **28**:570-576.

Brooks, D. E., 1979, Carnitine, acetylcarnitine and activity of carnitine acyltransferase in seminal plasma and spermatozoa of men, rams and rats, *J. Reprod. Fertil.* **56**:667-673.

Brooks, D. E., Hamilton, D. W., and Mallek, A. H., 1974, Carnitine and glycerylphosphoryl-choline in the reproductive tract of the male rat, *J. Reprod. Fertil.* **36**:141-160.

Brown, C. R., 1975, Distribution of hyaluronidase in the ram spermatozoa, *J. Reprod. Fertil.* **45**:537-539.

Brown, C. R., and Hartree, E. F., 1974, Distribution of trypsin-like proteinase in the ram spermatozoa, *J. Reprod. Fertil.* **36**:195-198.

Brown, C. R., Andani, Z., and Hartree, E. F., 1975, Studies on ram acrosin: Isolation from spermatozoa, activation by cations and organic solvents, and influence of cations on its reaction with inhibitors, *Biochem. J.* **149**:133-146.

Bryant, J. H. D., 1974, Capacitation in the mouse: The response of murine acrosomes to the environment of the female reproductive tract, *Biol. Reprod.* **10**:414-421.

Bryant, J. H. D., and Unnithan, R. R., 1973, Cytochemical localization of non-specific esterase and acid phosphatase in spermatozoa of the mouse (*Mus musculus*), *Histochemie* **33**:169-180.

Byrd, E. W., Goodeaux, L. L., Pool, S. H., and Godke, R. A., 1979, Effect of bovine serum albumin and Ca^{++} on capacitation of bovine spermatozoa, *Theriogenology* **11**:93.

Cabot, C. L., and Oliphant, G., 1978, The possible role of immunological complement in induction of rabbit sperm acrosome reaction, *Biol. Reprod.* **19**:666–672.

Calvin, H. I., and Bedford, J. M., 1971, Formation of disulphide bonds in the nucleus and accessory structures of mammalian spermatozoa during maturation in the epididymis, *J. Reprod. Fertil. Suppl.* **13**:65–75.

Carroll, E. J., and Levitan, H., 1978a, Fertilization in the sea urchin, *Strongylocentrotus purpuratus*, is blocked by fluorescein dyes, *Dev. Biol.* **63**:432–440.

Carroll, E. J., and Levitan, H., 1978b, Fertilization is inhibited in five diverse animal phyla by erythrosin B, *Dev. Biol.* **64**:329–331.

Carroll, E. J., and Wolf, D. P., 1979, Mouse egg penetration is inhibited by erythrosin B, *Gamete Res.* **1**:293–298.

Casillas, E. R., and Chaipayungpan, S., 1979, The distribution of carnitine and acetylcarnitine in the rabbit epididymis and the carnitine content of rabbit spermatozoa during maturation, *J. Reprod. Fertil.* **56**:439–444.

Chacon, R. S., and Talbot, P., 1980, Early stages in mammalian sperm–oocyte plasma membrane fusion, *J. Cell Biol.* **87**:131a (FE 1004).

Chang, M. C., 1951a, Fertilizing capacity of spermatozoa deposited into fallopian tubes, *Nature (London)* **168**:697–698.

Chang, M. C., 1951b, Fertility and sterility as revealed in the study of fertilization and development of rabbit eggs, *Fertil. Steril.* **2**:205–222.

Chang, M. C., 1958, Capacitation of rabbit spermatozoa in the uterus with special reference to the reproductive phase of the female, *Endocrinology* **63**:619–623.

Chang, M. C., 1969, Hormonal regulation of sperm capacitation, in: *Advances in Biosciences*, Volume 4 (G. Raspe, ed.), Pergamon Press, Oxford, pp. 13–33.

Chang, M. C., and Bedford, J. M., 1962, Fertilizability of rabbit ova after removal of the corona radiata, *Fertil. Steril.* **13**:421–425.

Chang, M. C., and Hunter, R. H. F., 1977, Capacitation of mammalian sperm: Biological and experimental aspects, in: *Handbook of Physiology*, Section 7, Volume 5 (R. O. Greep, ed.), American Physiological Society, Washington, D.C., pp. 339–351.

Chang, M. C., Hanada, A., and Hunt, D. M., 1971, Fertilization of denuded rabbit eggs *in vitro* by sperm recovered from the uterus or vagina, *Nature (London)* **232**:343–344.

Chang, T. S. K., and Zirkin, B. R., 1978, Proteolytic degradation of protamine during thiol-induced nuclear decondensation in rabbit spermatozoa, *J. Exp. Zool.* **204**:283–289.

Chulavantnatol, M., and Yindipit, S., 1976, Changes in surface ATPase of rat spermatozoa in transit from the caput to the cauda epididymis, *J. Reprod. Fertil.* **48**:91–97.

Clarke, G. N., and Yanagimachi, R., 1978, Actin in mammalian sperm heads, *J. Exp. Zool.* **205**:125–132.

Clegg, E. D., and Foote, R. H., 1973, Phospholipid composition of bovine sperm fractions, seminal plasma and cytoplasmic droplet, *J. Reprod. Fertil.* **34**:379–383.

Clegg, E. D., Morre, D. J., and Lunstra, D. D., 1975, Porcine sperm membrane: *In vivo* phospholipid changes, isolation and electron microscopy, in: *The Biology of Male Gametes* (J. G. Duckett and P. A. Racey, eds.), Academic Press, London, pp. 321–335.

Colwin, L. H., and Colwin, A. L., 1967, Membrane fusion in relation to sperm–egg association, in: *Fertilization*, Volume 1 (C. B. Metz and A. Monroy, eds.), Academic Press, New York, pp. 295–367.

Conway, A. F., and Metz, C. B., 1976, Phospholipase activity of sea urchin sperm: Its possible involvement in membrane fusion, *J. Exp. Zool.* **198**:39–48.

Cooper, G. W., and Bedford, J. M., 1971, Acquisition of surface charge by the plasma membrane of mammalian spermatozoa during epididymal maturation, *Anat. Rec.* **169**:300–301.

Cooper, G. W., Overstreet, J. W., and Katz, D. F., 1979, The motility of rabbit spermatozoa recovered from the female reproductive tract, *Gamete Res.* **2**:35–42.

Cornett, L. E., and Meizel, S., 1978, Stimulation of *in vitro* activation and the acrosome reaction of hamster spermatozoa by catecholamines, *Proc. Natl. Acad. Sci. USA* **75**:4954–4958.

Courtens, J. L., and Fournier-Delpech, S., 1979, Modifications in the plasma membranes of epididymal ram spermatozoa during maturation and incubation *in utero*, *J. Ultrastruct. Res.* **68**:136–148.

Crabo, B., Gustafsson, B., Bane, A., Meschks, P., and Ringmar, J. E., 1967, The concentration of sodium, potassium, calcium, inorganic phosphate, protein and glycerylphosphorylcholine in the epididymal plasma of bull calves, *J. Reprod. Fertil.* **13**:589–591.

Cross, P. C., and Brinster, R. L., 1970, *In vitro* development of mouse oocytes, *Biol. Reprod.* **3**:298–307.

Cummins, J. M., and Orgebin-Crist, M. C., 1971, Investigations into the fertility of epididymal spermatozoa, *Biol. Reprod.* **5**:13–19.

Cummins, J. M., and Teichman, R. J., 1974, The accumulation of malachite green stainable phospholipid in rabbit spermatozoa during maturation in epididymis, and its possible role in capacitation, *Biol. Reprod.* **10**:555–564.

Cummins, J. M., Bernstein, M. H., and Teichman, R. J., 1974, Light and electron microscopic studies of lipid stained by malachite green in the male reproductive tract of the rabbit, hamster and mongoose, *J. Reprod. Fertil.* **41**:75–83.

Dan, J. C., 1952, Studies on the acrosome. I. Reaction to egg-water and other stimuli, *Biol. Bull.* **103**:54–66.

Dan, J. C., 1956, The acrosome reaction, *Int. Rev. Cytol.* **5**:365–393.

Dan, J. C., 1967, Acrosome reaction and lysins, in: *Fertilization*, Volume 1 (C. B. Metz and A. Monroy, eds.), Academic Press, New York, pp. 237–293.

Darin-Benett, A., White, I. G., and Hoskins, D. D., 1977, Phospholipids and phospholipid-bound fatty acids and aldehydes of spermatozoa and seminal plasma of rhesus monkey, *J. Reprod. Fertil.* **49**:119–122.

Davis, B. K., 1976, Inhibitory effect of synthetic phospholipid vesicles containing cholesterol on the fertilizing capacity of rabbit spermatozoa, *Proc. Soc. Biol. Med.* **152**:257–261.

Davis, B. K., 1978, Inhibition of fertilizing capacity in mammalian spermatozoa by natural and synthetic vesicles, in: *Symposium on the Pharmacological Effects of Lipids*, AOCS Monogr. No. 5, pp. 145–158.

Davis, B. K., 1980, Interaction of lipids with the plasma membrane of sperm cells. I. The antifertilization action of cholesterol, *Arch. Androl.* **5**:249–254.

Davis, B. K., Byrne, R., and Hungund, B., 1979, Studies on the mechanism of capacitation. II. Evidence for lipid transfer between plasma membrane of rat sperm and serum albumin during capacitation *in vitro*, *Biochim. Biophys. Acta* **558**:257–266.

Davis, B. K., Byrne, R., and Bedigian, K., 1980, Studies on the mechanism of capacitation: Albumin-mediated changes in the plasma membrane lipids during *in vitro* incubation of rat sperm cells, *Proc. Natl. Acad. Sci. USA* **77**:1546–1550.

Dawson, R. M. C., and Scott, T. W., 1964, Phospholipid composition of epididymal spermatozoa prepared by density gradient centrifugation, *Nature (London)* **202**:292–293.

Decker, G. L., Joseph, D. B., and Lennarz, W. J., 1976, A study of factors involved in induction of the acrosome reaction in sperm of the sea urchin, *Arbacia punctulata*, *Dev. Biol.* **53**:115–125.

Delgado, N. M., Huacuja, L., Pancardo, R. M., and Rosado, A., 1976a, Modification of human sperm metabolism by induced release of intracellular zinc, *Life Sci.* **16**:1483–1488.

Delgado, N. M., Haucuja, L., Pancardo, R. M., Merchant, H., and Rosado, A., 1976b, Changes in the protein conformation of human spermatozoal membranes after treatment with cyclic adenosine 3′:5′-monophosphate and human follicular fluid, *Fertil. Steril.* **27**:413–420.

Delgado, N. M., Huacuja, L., Merchant, H., Reyes, R., and Rosado, A., 1980, Species specific decondensation of human spermatozoa nuclei by heparin, *Arch. Androl.* **4:**305–313.

DeMayo, F. J., Mizoguchi, H., and Dukelow, W. R., 1980, Fertilization of squirrel monkey and hamster ova in the rabbit oviduct, *Science* **208:**1468–1469.

Dickmann, Z., 1963, Chemotaxis of rabbit spermatozoa, *J. Exp. Biol.* **40:**1–5.

Dickmann, Z., 1964, The passage of spermatozoa through and into the zona pellucida of the rabbit egg, *J. Exp. Biol.* **41:**177–182.

Dickmann, Z., and Dziuk, P. J., 1964, Sperm penetration of the zona pellucida of the pig egg, *J. Exp. Biol.* **41:**603–608.

Dunbar, B. S., and Raynor, B. D., 1980, Characterization of porcine zona pellucida antigens, *Biol. Reprod.* **22:**941–954.

Dunbar, B. S., Munoz, C. G., Cordle, C. T., and Metz, C. B., 1976, Inhibition of fertilization *in vitro* by treatment of rabbit spermatozoa with univalent isoantibodies to rabbit sperm hyaluronidase, *J. Reprod. Fertil.* **47:**381–384.

Dunbar, B. S., Wardrip, N. I., and Hedrick, J. L., 1980, Isolation, physicochemical properties, and macromolecular composition of zona pellucida from porcine oocytes, *Biochemistry* **19:**356–365.

Dziuk, P. J., 1965, Double mating of rabbit to determine capacitation time, *J. Reprod. Fertil.* **10:**389–395.

Dziuk, P. J., and Dickmann, Z., 1965, Sperm penetration through the zona pellucida of the sheep egg, *J. Exp. Zool.* **158:**237–240.

Eager, D. D., Johnson, M. H., and Thurley, K. W., 1976, Ultrastructural studies on the surface membrane of the mouse egg, *J. Cell Sci.* **22:**345–353.

Edwards, R. G., Ferguson, L. C., and Coombs, R. R. A., 1964, Blood group antigens on human spermatozoa, *J. Reprod. Fertil.* **7:**153–161.

Eng, L. A., and Metz, C. B., 1980, Sperm head decondensation by a high molecular weight fraction of sea urchin egg homogenates, *J. Exp. Zool.* **212:**159–167.

Eng, L. A., and Oliphant, G., 1978, Rabbit sperm reversibl. decapacitation by membrane stabilization with a highly purified glycoprotein from seminal plasma, *Biol. Reprod.* **19:**1083–1094.

Epel, D., 1977, The egg surface in relation to metabolic activation at fertilization, in: *Immunobiology of Gametes* (M. Edidin and M. H. Johnson, eds.), Cambridge University Press, London, pp. 235–254.

Epel, D., 1978, Mechanisms of activation of sperm and egg during fertilization of sea urchin gametes, in: *Current Topics in Developmental Biology*, Volume 12 (A. Moscona and A. Monroy, eds.), Academic Press, New York, pp. 185–246.

Ericsson, R. J., 1967, Technology, physiology and morphology of sperm capacitation, *J. Reprod. Fertil. Suppl.* **2:**65–74.

Ericsson, R. J., 1969, Capacitation *in vitro* of rabbit sperm with mule eosinophils, *Nature* (*London*) **221:**568–569.

Ericsson, R. J., 1970, Leucocytes and sperm capacitation, *J. Reprod. Fertil. Suppl.* **10:**147–151.

Esbenshade, K. E., and Clegg, E. D., 1976, Electrophoretic characterization of proteins in the plasma membrane of porcine spermatozoa, *J. Reprod. Fertil.* **47:**333–337.

Esbenshade, K. L., and Clegg, E. D., 1977, Surface proteins of porcine spermatozoa: Identification and influence of incubation in the uterus, *Proc. 10th Annu. Meet. Soc. Study Reprod.*, abstract No. 82.

Evans, R. W., and Setchell, B. P., 1979, Lipid changes in boar spermatozoa during epididymal maturation with some observation on the flow and composition of boar rete testis fluid, *J. Reprod. Fertil.* **57:**189–196.

Farooqui, A. A., and Srivastava, P. N., 1979a, Role of rabbit testicular arylsulfatase in fertilization, *Fed. Proc.* **38:**1125a.

Farooqui, A. A., and Srivastava, P. N., 1979b, Isolation, characterization and the role of rabbit testicular arylsulfatase A in fertilization, *Biochem. J.* **181**:331–337.

Farooqui, A. A., and Srivastava, P. N.. 1980a, Concanavalin A immobilization induced changes in the kinetic parameters of the rabbit plasma β-N-acetylhexosaminidase, *Fed. Proc.* **39**:3198a.

Farooqui, A. A., and Srivastava, P. N., 1980b, Isolation of β-N-acetyl-hexosaminidase from the rabbit semen and its role in fertilization, *Biochem. J.* **191**:827–834

Fawcett, D. W., 1975, The mammalian spermatozoa, *Dev. Biol.* **44**:394–436.

Fléchon, J. E., 1975, Ultrastructural and cytochemical modifications of rabbit spermatozoa during epididymal transport, in: *The Biology of Spermatozoa* (E. S. E. Hafez and C. Thibault, eds.), Karger, Basel, pp. 36–45.

Fléchon, J. E., and Dubois, M. P., 1975, Localisation immunocytochemique de la hyaluronidase dans les spermatozoides de mamifères domestiques, *C. R. Acad. Sci.* **280**:877–880.

Fléchon, J. E., and Morstin, J., 1975, Localisation des glycoprotéines et des charges négatives et positives dans le rêvetement de surface des spermatozoides éjaculés de lapin et de taureau, *Ann. Histochem.* **20**:291–300.

Fleming, A. D., and Yanagimachi, R., 1981, Effects of various lipids on the acrosome reaction and fertilizing capacity of guinea pig spermatozoa with special reference to the possible involvement of lysophospholipids in the acrosome reaction, *Gamete Res.* **4**, in press.

Fleming, A. D., Yanagimachi, R., and Yanagimachi, H., 1981, Spermatozoa of the Atlantic bottlenose dolphin, *Tursiops truncatus, J. Reprod. Fertil.*, in press.

Foulkes, J. A., and MacDonald, B. J., 1979, The relationship between ATP content and motility of bovine spermatozoa, *Theriogenology* **11**:313–319.

Fraser, L. E., 1977a, Differing requirements for capacitation *in vitro* of mouse spermatozoa from two strains, *J. Reprod. Fertil.* **49**:83–87.

Fraser, L. E., 1977b, Motility pattern in mouse spermatozoa before and after capacitation, *J. Exp. Zool.* **202**:439–444.

Fraser, L. E., 1979, Accelerated mouse sperm penetration *in vitro* in the presence of caffeine, *J. Reprod. Fertil.* **57**:377–384.

Fraser, L. E., and Drury, L. M., 1976, Mouse sperm genotype and the rate of egg penetration *in vitro, J. Exp. Zool.* **197**:13–20.

Fraser, L. E., and Quinn, P. J., 1981, A glycolytic product is obligatory for initiation of the sperm acrosome reaction and whiplash motility required for the fertilization in the mouse, *J. Reprod. Fertil.*, **61**:25–35.

Fraser, L. E., Dandekar, P. V., and Vaidya, R. A., 1971, *In vitro* fertilization of tubal rabbit ova partially or totally denuded of follicle cells, *Biol. Reprod.* **4**:229–233.

Friend, D. S., 1977, The organization of the sperm membrane, in: *Immunobiology of Gametes* (M. Edidin and M. H. Johnson, eds.), Cambridge University Press, London, pp. 5–30.

Friend, D. S., 1980, Freeze-fracture alterations in guinea pig sperm membranes preceding gamete fusion, in: *Membrane–Membrane Interactions* (N. B. Gilula, ed.), Raven Press, New York, pp. 153–165.

Friend, D. S., and Fawcett, D. W., 1974, Membrane differentiations in freeze-fractured mammalian sperm, *J. Cell Biol.* **63**:641–664.

Friend, D. S., Orci, L., Perrelet, A., and Yanagimachi, R., 1977, Membrane particle changes attending the acrosome reaction in guinea pig spermatozoa, *J. Cell Biol.* **74**:561–577.

Fritz, H., Schleuning, D., Schiessler, H., Schill, W. B., Wendt, V., and Winkler, G., 1975, Boar, bull and human sperm acrosin: Isolation properties and biological aspects, in: *Proteases and Biological Control* (E. Reich, D. B. Rifkin, and E. Shaw, eds.), Cold Spring Harbor Laboratory, Cold Spring Harbor, N.Y., pp. 715–735.

Fukuda, Y., Okada, O., and Toyoda, Y., 1972, Studies on the fertilization of mouse eggs *in vitro*. IV. Fertilization of denuded eggs by capacitated spermatozoa, *Jpn. J. Anim. Reprod.* **18**:73–77.

Fukuda, Y. Maddock, M. B., and Chang, M. C., 1979, *In vitro* fertilization of two species of deer mouse eggs by homologous or heterologous sperm and penetration of laboratory mouse eggs by deer mouse sperm, *J. Exp. Zool.* **207**:481–490.

Gabel, C. A., Eddy, E. M., and Shapiro, B. M., 1979, After fertilization, sperm surface components remain as a patch in sea urchin and mouse embryos, *Cell* **18**:207–215.

Gaddum-Rosse, P., and Blandau, R. J., 1977, Proteolytic activity of guinea pig spermatozoa after induction of the acrosome reaction *in vitro*, *Am. J. Anat.* **149**:423–430.

Gall, W. E., and Ohsumi, Y., 1976, Decondensation of sperm nuclei *in vitro*, *Exp. Cell Res.* **102**:349–358.

Garbers, D. L., and Kopf, G. S., 1980, The regulation of spermatozoa by calcium and cyclic nucleotides, in: *Advances in Cyclic Nucleotide Research*, Volume 13 (P. Greengard and A. Robinson, eds.), Raven Press, New York, pp. 251–306.

Garbers, D. L., Lust, W. D., First, N. L., and Lardy, H. A., 1971, Effects of phosphodiesterase inhibitors and cyclic nucleotides on sperm respiration and motility, *Biochemistry* **10**:1825–1831.

Garbers, D. L., First, N. L., and Lardy, H. A., 1973, The stimulation of bovine epididymal sperm metabolism by cyclic nucleotide phosphodiesterase inhibitors, *Biol. Reprod.* **8**:589–598.

Gilula, N. B., Epstein, M. L., and Beers, W. H., 1978, Cell-to-cell communication and ovulation: A study of the cumulus–oocyte complex, *J. Cell Biol.* **78**:58–75.

Gondos, B., Bhiraleus, P., and Conner, L. A., 1972, Pronuclear membrane alterations during approximation of pronuclei and initiation of cleavage in the rabbit, *J. Cell Sci.* **10**:61–78.

Gordon, M., 1973, Localization of phosphatase activity on the membrane of the mammalian sperm head, *J. Exp. Zool.* **185**:111–120.

Gordon, M., 1977, Cytochemical analysis of the membranes of the mammalian sperm head, in: *Male Reproductive System* (R. D. Yates and M. Gordon, eds.), Masson, New York, pp. 15–33.

Gordon, M., and Dandekar, P. V., 1976, Electron microscope assessment of fertilization of rabbit ova treated with concanavalin A and wheat germ agglutinin, *J. Exp. Zool.* **198**:437–442.

Gordon, M., and Dandekar, P. V., 1977, Fine-structural localization of phosphatase activity on the plasma membrane of the rabbit sperm head, *J. Reprod. Fertil.* **49**:155–156.

Gordon, M., Dandekar, P. V., and Bartoszwicz, W., 1974, Ultrastructural localization of surface receptors for concanavalin A on rabbit spermatozoa, *J. Reprod. Fertil.* **36**:211–214.

Gordon, M., Dandekar, P. V., and Bartoszwicz, W., 1975, The surface coat of epididymal, ejaculated and capacitated sperm, *J. Ultrastruct. Res.* **50**:199–207.

Gordon, M., Dandekar, P. V., and Eager, P. R., 1978, Identification of phosphatases on the membranes of guinea pig sperm, *Anat. Rec.* **191**:123–134.

Gould, K., Zaneveld, L. J. D., Srivastava, P. N., and Williams, W. L., 1971, Biochemical changes in the zona pellucida of rabbit ova induced by fertilization and sperm enzymes, *Proc. Soc. Exp. Biol. Med.* **136**:6–10.

Gould, S. F., and Bernstein, M. H., 1975, Localization of bovine sperm hyaluronidase, *Differentiation* **3**:123–132.

Green, D. P. L., 1976, Induction of the acrosome reaction in guinea-pig spermatozoa *in vitro* by Ca ionophore A23187, *J. Physiol.* **260**:18P–19P.

Green, D. P. L., 1978a, The induction of the acrosome reaction in guinea pig spermatozoa by the divalent metal cation ionophore A23187, *J. Cell Sci.* **32**:137–151.

Green, D. P. L., 1978b, The activation of proteolysis in acrosome reaction of guinea-pig spermatozoa, *J. Cell Sci.* **32**:153–164.

Green, D. P. L., 1978c, The mechanism of the acrosome reaction, in: *Development in Mammals*, Volume 3 (M. H. Johnson, ed.), North-Holland, Amsterdam, pp. 65–81.

Green, D. P. L., and Hockaday, A. R., 1978, The histochemical localization of acrosin in guinea-pig sperm after the acrosome reaction, *J. Cell Sci.* **32**:177–184.

Grogan, D. E., Mayer, D. T., and Sikes, J. D., 1966, Quantitative differences in phospholipids of ejaculated spermatozoa and spermatozoa from three levels of the epididymis of the boar, *J. Reprod. Fertil.* **12**:431–436.

Grotjan, H. E., Day, B. N., and Mayer, D. T., 1974, Porcine spermatozoan respiration in the presence of porcine follicular fluid, *J. Anim. Sci.* **38**:1235–1238.

Gwatkin, R. B. L., 1976, Fertilization, in: *Cell Surface Reviews*, Volume 1 (G. Poste and G. L. Nicolson, eds), Elsevier/North-Holland, Amsterdam, pp. 1–54.

Gwatkin, R. B. L., 1977, *Fertilization Mechanisms in Man and Mammals*, Plenum Press, New York.

Gwatkin, R. B. L., and Williams, D. T., 1977, Receptor activitiy of hamster and mouse solubilized zona pellucida before and after the zona reaction, *J. Reprod. Fertil.* **49**:55–59.

Gwatkin, R. B. L., Andersen, O. F., and Hutchison, C. F., 1972, Capacitation of hamster spermatozoa *in vitro:* The role of cumulus components, *J. Reprod. Fertil.* **30**:389–394.

Gwatkin, R. B. L., Williams, D. T., Hartmann, J. F., and Kniazuk, M., 1973, The zona reaction of hamster and mouse eggs: Production *in vitro* by a trypsin-like protease from cortical granules, *J. Reprod. Fertil.* **32**:259–265.

Gwatkin, R. B. L., Andersen, O. F., and Williams, D. T., 1980, Large scale isolation of bovine and pig zonae pellucidae: Chemical, immunological, and receptor properties, *Gamete Res.* **3**:217–231.

Hafez, E. S. E., and Thibault, C. G., (eds.), 1975, *The Biology of Spermatozoa*, Karger, Basel.

Hall, J. L., Sloan, C. S., and Willis, W. D., 1979, Evaluation of freeze preserved human sperm fertilization potential using zona-free animal ova, *Biol. Reprod.* **20**:96a.

Hall, J. L., Sloan, M. G., and Hammond, M. G., 1980, Correlation of heterologous *in vitro* fertilization using human sperm and hamster ova with clinical evaluation of male fertility, *Fertil. Steril.* **33**:238a.

Hamilton, D. W., 1977, The epididymis, in: *Frontiers in Reproduction and Fertility Control* (R. O. Greep, ed.), MIT Press, Cambridge, Mass., pp. 411–426.

Hamilton, D. W., and Fawcett, D. W., 1970, *In vitro* synthesis of cholesterol and testosterone from acetate by rat epididymis and vas deferens, *Proc. Soc. Exp. Biol. Med.* **133**:693–695.

Hamilton, D. W., and Gould, R. P., 1980, Galactosyltransferase activity associated with rat epididymal spermatozoan maturation, *Anat. Rec.* **196**:71a.

Hammerstedt, R. H., Keith, A. D., Hay, S., Deluca, N., and Amann, R. P., 1979, Changes in ram sperm membrane during epididymal maturation, *Arch. Biochem. Biophys.* **196**:7–12.

Hamner, C. E., and Sojka, N. J., 1967, Capacitation of rabbit spermatozoa: Species and organ specificity, *Proc. Soc. Exp. Biol. Med.* **124**:689–691.

Hamner, C. E., and Williams, W. L., 1963, Effect of the female reproductive tract on sperm metabolism in the rabbit and fowl, *J. Reprod. Fertil.* **5**:143–150.

Hanada, A., and Chang, M. C., 1972, Penetration of zona-free eggs by spermatozoa of different species, *Biol Reprod.* **6**:300–309.

Hanada, A., and Chang, M. C., 1976, Penetration of hamster and rabbit zona-free eggs by rat and mouse spermatozoa with special reference to sperm capacitation, *J. Reprod. Fertil.* **46**:239–241.

Hanada, A., and Chang, M. C., 1978, Penetration of the zona-free or intact eggs by foreign spermatozoa and the fertilization of deer mouse eggs *in vitro, J. Exp. Zool.* **203**:277–286.

Harding, H. R., Carrick, F. N., and Shorey, C. D., 1976, Acrosome development during spermatogenesis in some Australian marsupials: An ultrastructural study, *Theriogenology* **6**:657.

Harper, M. J. K., 1970, Factors influencing sperm penetration of rabbit eggs *in vivo, J. Exp. Zool.* **173**:47–62.

Harper, M. J. K., 1973, Relationship between sperm transport and penetration of eggs in the rabbit oviduct, *Biol. Reprod.* **8**:441–450.

Harrison, R. A. P., 1975, Aspects of the enzymology of mammalian spermatozoa, in: *Biology of Male Gametes* (J. D. Dukelow and P. A. Racey, eds.), Academic Press, London, pp. 301–316.

Hartmann, J. F., and Gwatkin, R. B. L., 1971, Alteration of sites on the mammalian sperm surface following capacitation, *Nature (London)* **234:**479–481.

Hartmann, J. F., and Hutchison, C. F., 1974a, Nature of the pre-penetration contact interactions between hamster gametes *in vitro, J. Reprod. Fertil.* **36:**49–57.

Hartmann, J. F., and Hutchison, C. F., 1974b, Mammalian fertilization *in vitro:* Sperm-induced preparation of the zona pellucida of golden hamster ova for final binding, *J. Reprod. Fertil.* **37:**443–445.

Hartmann, J. F., and Hutchison, C. F., 1974c, Contact between hamster spermatozoa and the zona pellucida releases a factor which influences early binding stages, *J. Reprod. Fertil.* **37:**61–66.

Hartmann, J. F., and Hutchison, C. F., 1976, Surface interactions between mammalian sperm and egg: Variation of spermatozoa concentration as a probe for the study of binding *in vitro, J. Cell Physiol.* **88:**219–226.

Hartmann, J. F., and Hutchison, C. F., 1977a, Release of a factor during early stages of contact between hamster sperm and eggs *in vitro, J. Cell Physiol.* **93:**41–48.

Hartmann, J. F., and Hutchinson, C. F., 1977b, Involvement of two carbohydrate-containing components in the binding of uncapacitated spermatozoa to eggs of the golden hamster *in vitro, J. Exp. Zool.* **201:**383–380.

Hartmann, J. F., and Hutchison, C. F., 1980, Nature and fate of the factors released during early contact interactions between hamster sperm and egg prior to fertilization *in vitro, Dev. Biol.* **78:**380–393.

Hartree, E. F., 1971, Lysosomes and fertilization, in: *Of Microbes and Life* (J. Monod and E. Borek, eds.), Columbia University Press, New York, pp. 271–303.

Hartree, E. F., 1975, The acrosome–lysosome relatinship, *J. Reprod. Fertil.* **44:**125–126.

Hartree, E. F., and Mann, T., 1960, Phospholipids in mammalian semen, *J. Reprod. Fertil.* **1:**23–29.

Heffner, L. J., Saling, P. M., and Storey, B. T., 1980, Separation of calcium effects on motility and zona binding ability of mouse spermatozoa, *J. Exp. Zool.* **212:**53–60.

Hekman, A., and Ruemke, P., 1969, The antigens of human seminal plasma, with special reference to lactoferrin as a spermatozoa-coating antigen, *Fertil. Steril.* **20:**312–323.

Herrmann, W. P., and Uhlenbruck, G., 1972, Studies on glycoproteins of the human seminal plasma, *Z. Klin. Chem. Klin. Biochem.* **10:**363–366.

Hicks, J. J., Martinez-Manautou, J., Pedron, N., and Rosado, A., 1972a, Metabolic changes in human spermatozoa related to capacitation, *Fertil. Steril.* **23:**172–179.

Hicks, J. J., Pedron, N., and Rosado, A., 1972b, Modification of human spermatozoa glycolysis by cyclic adenosine monophosphate (cAMP), estrogen, and follicular fluid, *Fertil. Steril.* **23:**886–893.

Hirao, Y., and Yanagimachi, R., 1978a, Temperature dependence of sperm–egg fusion and post-fusion events in hamster fertilization, *J. Exp. Zool.* **205:**433–438.

Hirao, Y., and Yanagimachi, R., Effects of various enzymes on the ability of hamster egg plasma membrane to fuse with spermatozoa, *Gamete Res.* **1:**3–12.

Hirao, Y., and Yanagimachi, R., 1978c, Detrimental effect of visible light on meiosis of mammalian eggs *in vitro, J. Exp. Zool.* **206:**365–370.

Hirao, Y., and Yanagimachi, R., 1979, Development of pronuclei in polyspermic eggs of the golden hamster: Is there any limit to the number of sperm heads that are capable of developing into male pronuclei? *Zool. Mag. (Tokyo)* **88:**24–33.

Holt, W. V., 1980, Surface-bound sialic acid on ram and bull spermatozoa: Deposition during epididymal transit and stability during washing, *Biol. Reprod.* **23:**847–857.

Hoppe, P. C., 1976, Glucose requirement for mouse sperm capacitation *in vitro, Biol. Reprod.* **15**:39–45.

Hoppe, P. C., 1980, Genetic influences on mouse sperm capacitation *in vivo* and *in vitro, Gamete Res.* **3**:343–349.

Hoppe, P. C., and Whitten, W. K., 1974, An albumin requirement for fertilization of mouse egg *in vitro, J. Reprod. Fertil.* **39**:433–436.

Horiuchi, T., Takahashi, J., Sugawara, S., and Masaki, J., 1980, Scanning electron microscopical observations on the rat sperm head trapped by ovum microvilli during penetration into ovum *in vivo, Jpn. J. Anim. Reprod.* **26**:98–99.

Hoskins, D. D., and Casillas, E. R., 1975, Hormones, second messengers and the mammalian spermatozoa, in: *Molecular Mechanisms of Gonadal Hormone Action*, Volume 1 (J. A. Thomas and R. L. Sinhal, eds.), University Park Press, Baltimore, pp. 293–324.

Hoskins, D. D., Brandt, H., and Acott, T. S., 1978, Initiation of sperm motility in the mammalian epididymis, *Fed. Proc.* **37**:2534–2542.

Huacuja, L., Sosa, A., Delgado, N. M., and Rosado, A., 1973, A kinetic study of the participation of zinc in human spermatozoa metabolism, *Life Sci.* **13**:1383–1394.

Huacuja, L., Delgado, N. M., Merchant, H., Pancardo, R. M., and Rosado, A., 1977, Cyclic AMP induced incorporation of ^{33}P into human spermatozoa membrane components, *Biol. Reprod.* **17**:89–96.

Huang. T. T. F., Fleming, A. D., and Yanagimachi, R., 1981, Only acrosome-reacted spermatozoa can bind to and penetrate zona pellucida: A study using the guinea pig, *J. Exp. Zool.*, in press.

Hunter, A. G., and Hafs, H. D., 1964, Antigenicity and cross-reactions of bovine spermatozoa, *J. Reprod. Fertil.* **7**:357–365.

Hunter, A. G., and Nornes, H. O., 1969, Characterization and isolation of a sperm-coating antigen from rabbit seminal plasma with capacity to block fertilization, *J. Reprod. Fertil.* **20**:419–427.

Hunter, R. H. F., 1968, Capacitation in the golden hamster, with special reference to the influence of the uterine environment, *J. Reprod. Fertil.* **20**:223–237.

Hunter, R. H. F., 1975, Transport, migration and survival of spermatozoa in the female genital tract: Species with intra-uterine deposition of semen, in: *Biology of Spermatozoa* (E. S. E. Hafez and C. Thibault, eds.), Karger, Basel, pp. 145–155.

Hunter, R. H. F., 1976, Sperm–egg interactions in the pig: Monospermy, extensive polyspermy, and the formation of chromatin aggregates, *J. Anat.* **122**:43–59.

Hunter, R. H. F., 1980, *Physiology and Technology of Reproduction in Female Domestic Animals*, Academic Press, London/New York.

Hunter, R. H. F., and Hall, J. P., 1974, Capacitation of boar spermatozoa: The influence of post-coital separation of the uterus and fallopian tubes, *Anat. Rec.* **180**:597–604.

Hyne, R. V., and Garbers, D. L., 1979a, Calcium-dependent increase in adenosine 3′,5′-monophosphate and induction of the acrosome reaction in guinea pig spermatozoa, *Proc. Natl. Acad. Sci. USA* **76**:5699–5703.

Hyne, R. V., and Garbers, D. L., 1979b, Regulation of guinea pig sperm adenylate cyclase by calcium, *Biol. Reprod.* **21**:1135–1142.

Hyne, R. V., and Garbers, D. L., 1980, Induction of an *in vitro* acrosome reaction of guinea pig spermatozoa by biological factors at pH 7.4, *Biol. Reprod.* **22**(Suppl. 1):9a.

Imai, H., Niwa, K., and Iritani, A., 1977, Penetration *in vitro* of zona-free hamster eggs by ejaculated boar spermatozoa, *J. Reprod. Fertil.* **51**:495–497.

Imai, H., Niwa, K., and Iritani, A., 1979, Time requirement for capacitation of boar spermatozoa assessed by their ability to penetrate zona-free hamster egg, *J. Reprod. Fertil.* **56**:489–492.

Imai, H., Niwa, K., and Iritani, A., 1980, Ultrastructural observations of boar spermatozoa penetrating zona-free hamster eggs, *Biol. Reprod.* **23**:481–486.

Iqbal, M., Shivaji, S., Vijayasarathy, S., and Balaram, P., 1980, Synthetic peptides as chemoattractants for bull spermatozoa: Structures–activity correlations, *Biochem. Biophys. Res. Commun.* **96:**235–242.

Iritani, A., Gomes, W., and Van Demark, N. L., 1969, The effect of whole, dialysed and heated female genital tract fluids on respiration of rabbit and rat spermatozoa, *Biol. Reprod.* **1:**77–82.

Iritani, A., Tsunoda, Y., Miyake, M., and Nishikawa, M., 1975, Enhanced respiration and reduction of tetracycline binding of boar and bull spermatozoa following incubation in the female genital tract, *Jpn. J. Zootech. Sci.* **46:**531–537.

Iwamatsu, T., and Chang, M. C., 1972, Sperm penetration *in vitro* of mouse oocytes at various times after maturation, *J. Reprod. Fertil.* **31:**237–247.

Iwamatsu, T., and Ohta, T., 1980, The changes in sperm nuclei after penetrating fish oocytes matured without germinal vesicle material in their cytoplasm, *Gamete Res.* **3:**121–132.

Iwamatsu, T., Miki-Nomura, T., and Ohta, T., 1976, Cleavage initiation activities of microtubules and *in vitro* reassembled tubulins of sperm flagella, *J. Exp. Zoo.* **195:**97–106.

Jackowski, S., and Dumont, J. N., 1979, Surface alterations of the mouse zona pellucida and ovum following *in vivo* fertilization: Correlation with the cell cycle, *Biol. Reprod.* **20:**150–161.

Jain, Y. C., and Anand, S. R., 1976, The lipids of buffalo spermatozoa and seminal plasma, *J. Reprod. Fertil.* **47:**255–260.

Johnson, M. H., 1975, The macromolecular organization of membranes and its bearing on events leading up to fertilization, *J. Reprod. Fertil.* **44:**167–184.

Johnson, M. H., Eager, D., and Muggleton-Harris, A., 1975, Mosaicism in organization of concanavalin A receptors on surface membrane of mouse egg, *Nature (London)* **257:** 321–322.

Johnson, O., and Eliasson, R., 1978, Destabilization of human sperm membranes by albumin, *Int. J. Androl.* **1:**485–488.

Johnson, W. L., and Hunter, A. G., 1972, Seminal antigens: Their alteration in the genital tract of female rabbits and during partial *in vitro* capacitation with beta-amylase and beta-glucuronidase, *Biol Reprod.* **7:**332–340.

Jones, H. P., Lenz, R. W., Palevitz, B. A., and Cormier, M. J., 1980, Calmodulin localization in mammalian spermatozoa, *Proc. Natl. Acad. Sci. USA* **77:**2772–2776.

Joyce, C., Freund, M., and Peterson, R. N., 1979, Contraceptive effects of intravaginal application of acrosin and hyaluronidase inhibitors in rabbit, *Contraception* **19:**95–106.

Kanwar, K. C., Yanagimachi, R., and Lopata, A., 1979, Effects of human seminal plasma on the fertilizing capacity of human spermatozoa, *Fertil. Steril.* **31:**321–327.

Katz, D. F., and Overstreet, J. W., 1980, Mammalian sperm movement in the secretions of the male and female genital tracts, in: *Testicular Development, Structure, and Function* (A. Steinberger and E. Steinberger, eds.), Raven Press, New York, pp. 481–489.

Katz, D. F., and Yanagimachi, R., 1980, Movement characteristics of hamster spermatozoa within the oviduct, *Biol. Reprod.* **22:**759–764.

Kerek, G., Biberfeld, P., and Afzelius, B. A., 1973, Demonstration of HL-A antigens, "species", and "semen"-specific antigens on human spermatozoa, *Int. J. Fertil.* **18:**145–155.

Killian, G. J., and Amann, R. P., 1973, Immunoelectrophoretic characterization of fluid and sperm entering and leaving the bovine epididymis, *Biol. Reprod.* **9:**489–499.

Kim, C. I., Niwa, K., Imai, H., and Iritani, A., 1980, Penetration of zona-free hamster eggs *in vitro* by goat spermatozoa preincubated in the reproductive tract isolated from a maturing gilt, *J. Exp. Zool.* **213:**181–183.

Kinsey, W. H., and Koehler, J. K., 1978, Cell surface changes associated with *in vitro* Capacitation of hamster sperm, *J. Ultrastruct. Res.* **64:**1–13.

Kinsey, W. H., SeGall, G. K., and Lennarz, W. J., 1979, The effect of the acrosome reaction on the respiratory activity and fertilizing capacity of echinoid sperm, *Dev. Biol.* **71:**49–59.

Kirton, K. T., and Hafs, H. D., 1965, Sperm capacitation by uterine fluid or by beta-amylase *in vitro, Science* **150:**618–619.

Koehler, J. K., 1972, Human sperm head ultrastructure: A freeze-etching study, *J. Ultrastruct. Res.* **39:**520–539.

Koehler, J. K., 1975, Periodicities in the acrosome or acrosomal membrane: Some observations on mammalian spermatozoa, in: *Biology of the Male Gamete* (J. G. Duckett and P. A. Racey, eds.), Linnean Society of London/Academic Press, London, pp. 337–342.

Koehler, J. K., 1976, Changes in antigenic site distribution on rabbit spermatozoa after incubation in "capacitating" media, *Biol. Reprod.* **15:**444–456.

Koehler, J. K., 1978, Observations on the fine structure of vole spermatozoa with particular reference to cytoskeletal elements in the mature sperm head, *Gamete Res.* **1:**247–259.

Koehler, J. K., and Gaddum-Rosse, P., 1975, Media induced alterations of the membrane associated particles of the guinea pig sperm tail, *J. Ultrastruct. Res.* **51:**106–118.

Koehler, J. K., Nudelman, E. D., and Hakomori, S., 1980, A collagen-binding protein on the surface of ejaculated guinea pig spermatozoa, *J. Cell Biol.* **86:**529–536.

Kohane, A. C., Cameo, M. S., Pineiro, L., Garberi, J. C., and Blaquier, J. A., 1980a, Distribution and site of production of specific proteins in the rat epididymis, *Biol. Reprod.* **23:**181–187.

Kohane, A. C., Gomzalez-Echeverria, F. M. C., Pineiro, L., and Blaquier, J. A., 1980b, Interaction of proteins of epididymal origin with spermatozoa, *Biol. Reprod.* **23:**737–742.

Kopecny, V., and Pavlok, A., 1975, Autoradiographic study of mouse spermatozoan arginine-rich nuclear protein in fertilization, *J. Exp. Zool.* **191:**85–96.

Kopf, G. S., and Garbers, D. L., 1980, Calcium and a fucose-sulfate-rich polymer regulate sperm cyclic nucleotide metabolism and the acrosome reaction, *Biol. Reprod.* **22:**1118–1126.

Krishna, M., and Generoso, W. M., 1977, Timing of sperm penetration, pronuclear formation, pronuclear DNA synthesis, and first cleavage in naturally ovulated mouse eggs, *J. Exp. Zool.* **202:**245–252.

Kunze, H., and Bohn, E., 1978, Phospholipase A_2 and prostaglandins in human seminal plasma, in: *Advances in Prostaglandin and Thromboxane Research*, Volume 3 (C. Galli, G. Galli, and G. Porcellati, eds.), Raven Press, New York, pp. 159–165.

Kvist, U., 1980, Sperm nuclear chromatin decondensation ability, *Acta Physiol. Scand. Suppl.* **486:**1–24.

Langlais, J., Bleau, G., Hoel, H., Chapdelaine, A., and Roberts, K. K., 1980, Localization of sterol sulfatases on the plasma membrane of spermatozoa: A proposed mechanism for their role in membrane stabilization, *Biol. Reprod.* **22:**(Suppl. 1):11a.

Lavon, U., Volcani, R., and Danon, D., 1970, The lipid content of bovine spermatozoa during maturation and ageing, *J. Reprod. Fertil.* **23:**215–222.

Lavon, U., Volcani, R., and Danon, D., 1971, The proteins of bovine spermatozoa from the caput and cauda epididymis, *J. Reprod. Fertil.* **24:**219–232.

Lea, O. A., Petrusz, P., and French, F. S., 1978, Purification and localization of acidic epididymal glycoprotein (AEG): A sperm coating protein secreted by the rat epididymis, *Int. J. Androl. Suppl.* **2:**592–607.

Leblond, C. P., and Clermont, Y., 1952, Spermatogenesis of rat, mouse, hamster and guinea pig as revealed by the periodic acid–fuchsin sulfurous acid technique, *Am. J. Anat.* **90:**167–215.

Legault, Y., Van den Heuvel, W. J. A., Arison, B. H., Bleau, G., Chapdelaine, A., and Roberts, K. D., 1978, 5 alpha-cholesta-7,24-dien-3 beta-ol as a major sterol of the hamster reproductive tract, *Steroids* **32:**649–658.

Legault, Y., Bleau, G., Chapdelaine, A., and Roberts, K. K., 1979a, The binding of sterol sulfates to hamster spermatozoa, *Steroids* **34:**89–99.

Legault, Y., Bouthiller, M., Bleau, G., Chapdelaine, A., and Roberts, K. D., 1979b, The sterol and sterol sulfate content of the male hamster reproductive tract, *Biol. Reprod.* **20:**1213–1219.

Leonard, S. L., Perlman, P. L., and Kurzrok, R., 1947, Relation between time of fertilization and follicle cell dispersion in rat ova, *Proc. Soc. Exp. Biol. Med.* **66**:517-518.

Lewin, L. M., Weissenberg, R., Sobel, J. S., Marcus, Z., and Nebel, L., 1979, Differences in concanavalin A-FITC binding to rat spermatozoa during epididymal maturation and capacitation, *Arch. Androl.* **2**:279-281.

Lewis, W. H., and Wright, E. S., 1935, On the early development of the mouse, *Contrib. Embryol. Carnegie Inst.* **25**:113-146.

Longo, F. J., 1973, Fertilization: A comparative ultrastructural review, *Biol. Reprod.* **9**:149-215.

Longo, F. J., 1978a, Effects of cytochalasin B on sperm–egg interactions, *Dev. Biol.* **67**:249-265.

Longo, F. J., 1978b, Effects of puromycin and actinomycin D on fertilized rabbit eggs cultured *in vitro*, *J. Exp. Zool.* **203**:223-250.

Longo, F. J., and Anderson, E., 1969, Cytological events leading to the formation of two-cell stage in the rabbit: Association of the maternally and paternally derived genomes, *J. Ultrastruct. Res.* **29**:86-118.

Lorton, S. F., and First, N. L., 1979, Hyaluronidase does not disperse the cumulus oophorus surrounding bovine ova, *Biol. Reprod.* **21**:301-308.

Lucy, J. A., 1975, The fusion of cell membrane, in: *Cell Membranes* (G. Weismann and R. C. Clairborn, ed.), HP Pub., New York, pp. 75-83.

Lui, C. W., and Meizel, S., 1977, Biochemical studies of the *in vitro* acrosome reaction inducing ability of bovine serum albumin, *Differentiation* **9**:59-66.

Lui, C. W., and Meizel, S., 1979, Further evidence in support of a role for hamster sperm hydrolytic enzymes in the acrosome reaction, *J. Exp. Zool.* **207**:173-186.

Lui, C. W., Cornett, L. E., and Meizel, S., 1977, Identification of the bovine follicular fluid protein involved in the *in vitro* induction of the hamster sperm acrosome reaction, *Biol. Reprod.* **17**:34-41.

Luthardt, F. W., and Donahue, R. P., 1973, Pronuclear DNA synthesis in mouse eggs, *Exp. Cell Res.* **82**:143-151.

McMaster, R., Yanagimachi, R., and Lopata, A., 1978, Penetration of human eggs by human spermatozoa *in vitro*, *Biol. Reprod.* **19**:212-216.

McRorie, R. A., and Williams, W. L., 1974, Biochemistry of mammalian fertilization, *Annu. Rev. Biochem.* **43**:777-803.

Mahi, C. A., and Yanagimachi, R., 1973, The effect of temperature, osmolality and hydrogen ion concentration on the activation and acrosome reaction of golden hamster spermatozoa, *J. Reprod. Fertil.* **35**:55-66.

Mahi, C. A., and Yanagimachi, R., 1975, Induction of nuclear decondensation of mammalian spermatozoa *in vitro*, *J. Reprod. Fertil.* **44**:293-296.

Mahi, C. A., and Yanagimachi, R., 1976, Maturation and sperm penetration of canine ovarian oocytes *in vitro*, *J. Exp. Zool.* **196**:189-196.

Mahi, C. A., and Yanagimachi, R., 1978, Capacitation, acrosome reaction and egg penetration by canine and spermatozoa in a simple defined medium, *Gamete Res.* **1**:101-109.

Mancini. R. E., Alonso, A., Barquet, J., and Nemirovski, B., 1964, Histo-immunological localization of hyaluronidase in bull testis, *J. Reprod. Fertil.* **8**:325-330.

Mandelbaum, J., Plachot, M., and Thibault, C., 1977, Role of the follicle in zona pellucida maturation of hamster oocyte, *Ann. Biol. Anim. Biochim. Biophys.* **17**:389-391.

Mann, T., 1964, *The Biochemistry of Semen and the Male Reproductive Tract*, Methuen, London.

Mann, T., 1967, Sperm metabolism, in: *Fertilization*, Volume 1 (C. B. Metz and A. Monroy, eds.), Academic Press, New York, pp. 99-116.

Martan, J., and Risley, P. L., 1963, Holocrine secretory cells of the rat epididymis, *Anat. Rec.* **146**:173-190.

Martan, J., Risley, P. L., and Hruban, Z., 1964, Holocrine cells of the hamster epididymis, *Fertil. Steril.* **15**:180–187.

Marushige, Y., and Marushige, K., 1975, Enzymatic unpacking of the bull sperm chromatin, *Biochim. Biophys. Acta* **403**:180–191.

Marushige, Y., and Marushige, K., 1978, Dispersion of mammalian sperm chromatin during fertilization: An *in vitro* study, *Biochim. Biophys. Acta* **519**:1–22.

Meizel, S., 1978, The mammalian sperm acrosome reaction: A biochemical approach, in: *Development in Mammals*, Volume 3 (M. H. Johnson, Ed.), North-Holland, Amsterdam, pp. 1–62.

Meizel, S., and Lui, C. W., 1976, Evidence for a role of a trypsin-like enzyme in the hamster sperm acrosome reaction, *J. Exp. Zool.* **195**:137–144.

Meizel, S., and Mukerji, S. K., 1975, Proacrosin from rabbit epididymal spermatozoa: Partial purification and initial biochemical characterization, *Biol. Reprod.* **13**:83–93.

Meizel, S., and Mukerji, S. K., 1976, Biochemical studies of proacrosin and acrosin from hamster cauda epididymal spermatozoa, *Biol. Reprod.* **14**:444–450.

Menge, A. C., 1971, Antiserum inhibition of rabbit spermatozoal adherence to ova, *Proc. Soc. Exp. Biol. Med.* **138**:98–102.

Menge, A. C., and Black, C. B., 1979, Effects of antisera on human sperm penetration of zona-free hamster ova, *Fertil. Steril.* **32**:214–218.

Menino, A. R., and Wright, W., 1979, Characterization of porcine oocyte zona pellucida by polyacrylamide gel electrophoresis, *Proc. Soc. Exp. Biol. Med.* **160**:449–452.

Mercado, E., Hicks, J. J., Drago, C., and Rosado, A., 1974, A study of the interaction of human spermatozoa membrane with ATP and cyclic-AMP, *Biochem. Biophys. Res. Commun.* **56**:185–192.

Metz, C. B., 1973, Role of specific sperm antigens in fertilization, *Fed. Proc.* **32**:2057–2064.

Metz, C. B., Seiguer, A. C., and Castro, A. E., 1972, Inhibition of the cumulus dispersing and hyaluronidase activities of sperm by heterologous and isologous antisperm antibodies, *Proc. Soc. Exp. Biol. Med.* **140**:766–781.

Miller, R. L., 1966, Chemotaxis during fertilization in the hydroid, *Campanularia*, *J. Exp. Zool.* **161**:23–44.

Miller, R. L., and Brokaw, C. J., 1970, Chemotactic turning behavior in *Tubularia* spermatozoa, *J. Exp. Biol.* **52**:699–706.

Millette, C. F., and Bellve, A. R., 1977, Temporal expression of membrane antigens during mouse spermatogenesis, *J. Cell Biol.* **74**:86–97.

Miyamoto, H., and Chang, M. C., 1972, Fertilization *in vitro* of mouse and hamster eggs after the removal of follicle cells, *J. Reprod. Fertil.* **30**:309–312.

Miyamoto, H., and Chang, M. C., 1973, The importance of serum albumin and metabolic intermediates for capacitation of spermatozoa and fertilization of mouse eggs *in vitro*, *J. Reprod. Fertil.* **32**:193–205.

Miyamoto, H., Toyoda, Y., and Chang, M. C., 1974, Effect of hydrogen ion concentration on *in vitro* fertilization of mouse, golden hamster, and rat eggs, *Biol. Reprod.* **10**:487–493.

Mohri, H., and Yanagimachi, R., 1980, Characteristics of motor apparatus in testicular, epididymal and ejaculated spermatozoa: A study using demembranated sperm model, *Exp. Cell Res.* **129**:191–196.

Monroy, A., 1965, *Chemistry and Physiology of Fertilization*, Holt, Rinehart & Winston, New York.

Moore, H. D. M., 1979, The net surface charge of mammalian spermatozoa as determined by isoelectric focusing: Changes following sperm maturation, ejaculation, incubation in the female tract, and after enzyme treatment, *Int. J. Androl.* **2**:449–462.

Moore, H. D. M., 1980, Localization of specific glycoproteins secreted by the rabbit and hamster epididymis, *Biol. Reprod.* **22**:705–718.

Moore, H. D. M., and Bedford, J. M., 1978a, An *in vitro* analysis of factors influencing the fertilization of hamster eggs, *Biol. Reprod.* **19**:879–885.

Moore, H. D. M., and Bedford, J. M., 1978b, Ultrastructure of the equatorial segment of hamster spermatozoa during penetration of oocytes, *J. Ultrastruct. Res.* **62**:110–117.

Moore, H. D. M., and Hibbitt, K. G., 1975, Isoelectric focusing of boar spermatozoa *J. Reprod. Fertil.* **44**:329–332.

Moore, N. W., 1972, Fertilization of sheep ova following mechanical penetration of the zona pellucida, *Aust. J. Biol. Sci.* **25**:443–436.

Morton, D. B., 1975, Acrosomal enzymes: Immunological localization of acrosin and hyaluronidase in ram spermatozoa, *J. Reprod. Fertil.* **45**:375–378.

Morton, D. B., 1976, Lysosomal enzymes in mammalian spermatozoa, in: *Lysosomes in Biology and Pathology*, Volume 5 (J. D. Dingle and R. T. Dean, eds.), Elsevier/North-Holland, Amsterdam, pp. 203–255.

Morton, D. B., 1977, Lysosomal enzymes in mammalian spermatozoa, in: *Immunobiology of Gametes* (M. Edidin and M. H. Johnson, eds.), Cambridge University Press, London, pp. 115–155.

Mounib, M. S., and Chang, M. C., 1974, Effect of *in utero* incubation on the metabolism of rabbit spermatozoa, *Nature (London)* **201**:943–944.

Mrsny, R. J., and Meizel, S., 1979, Inhibition of hamster sperm acrosome reaction by inhibitors of $(Na^+ + K^+)$-ATPase, *J. Cell Biol.* **83**:602a.

Mrsny, R. J., and Meizel, S., 1980a, K^+ influx is required for the hamster sperm acrosome reaction, *J. Cell Biol.* **87**:103a (FE 1003).

Mrsny, R. J., and Meizel, S., 1980b, Evidence suggesting a role for cyclic nucleotides in acrosome reactions of hamster sperm *in vitro*, *J. Exp. Zool.* **211**:153–158.

Mrsny, R. J., Waxman, L., and Meizel, S., 1979, Taurine maintains and stimulates motility of hamster sperm during capacitation *in vitro*, *J. Exp. Zool.* **210**:123–128.

Multamaki, S., and Suominen, J., 1976, Distribution and removal of the acrosin of bull spermatozoa, *Int. J. Fertil.* **21**:69–81.

Murdoch, R. N., and White, I. G., 1967, The metabolism of labelled glucose by rabbit spermatozoa after incubation *in utero*, *J. Reprod. Fertil.* **14**:213–223.

Nelson, L., 1978, Chemistry and neurochemistry of sperm motility control, *Fed. Proc.* **37**:2543–2547.

Nicolson, G. L., and Yanagimachi, R., 1972, Terminal saccharides on sperm plasma membranes: Identification by specific agglutinins, *Science* **177**:276–279.

Nicolson, G. L., and Yanagimachi, R., 1979, Cell surface changes associated with the epididymal maturation of mammalian spermatozoa, in: *The Spermatozoa* (D. W. Fawcett and J. M. Bedford, eds.), Urban & Schwarzenberg, Munich, pp. 187–194.

Nicolson, G. L., Yanagimachi, R., and Yanagimachi, H., 1975, Ultrastructural localization of lectin-binding sites on the zonae pellucidae and plasma membranes of mammalian eggs, *J. Cell. Biol.* **66**:263–274.

Nicolson, G. L., Usui, N., Yanagimachi, R., Yanagimachi, H., and Smith, J. R., 1977, Lectin-binding sites on the plasma membrane of rabbit spermatozoa: Changes in surface receptors during epididymal maturation and after ejaculation, *J. Cell Biol.* **74**:950–962.

Nicolson, G. L., Bronginski, A. B., Beattie, G., and Yanagimachi, R., 1979, Cell surface changes in the protein of rabbit spermatozoa during epididymal maturation, *Gamete Res.* **2**:153–162.

Nishikawa, Y., and Waide, Y., 1952, Studies on the maturation of spermatozoa. I. Mechanism and speed of transition of spermatozoa in the epididymis and their functional changes, *Bull. Jpn. Natl. Inst. Agric. Sci. Ser. G* **3**:68–78.

Nishioka, D., and McGwin, N. E., 1980, Relationships between the release of acid, the cortical reaction, and the increase of protein synthesis in sea urchin eggs, *J. Exp. Zool.* **212**:215–223.

Niwa, K., and Chang, M. C., 1974, Optimal sperm concentration and minimum number of spermatozoa for fertilization *in vitro* of rat eggs, *J. Reprod. Fertil.* **40**:471–474.

Niwa, K., and Chang, M. C., 1975a, Requirement of capacitation for sperm penetration of zona-free rat eggs, *J. Reprod. Fertil.* **44:**305–308.

Niwa, K., and Chang, M. C., 1975b, Fertilization of rat eggs *in vitro* at various times before and after ovulation with special reference to fertilization of ovarian oocytes matured *in vitro*, *J. Reprod. Fertil.* **43:**435–451.

Niwa, K., and Iritani, A., 1978, Effect of various hexoses on sperm capacitation and penetration of rat eggs *in vitro*, *J. Reprod. Fertil.* **53:**267–271.

Niwa, D., Arai, M., and Iritani, A., 1980, Fertilization *in vitro* of eggs and first cleavage of embryos in different strains of mice, *Biol. Reprod.* **22:**1155–1159.

Noda, Y. D., and Yanagimachi, R., 1976, Electron microscopic observations of guinea pig spermatozoa penetrating eggs *in vitro*, *Dev. Growth Differ.* **18:**15–23.

Noyes, R. W., Walton, A., and Adams, C. E., 1958, Capacitation of rabbit spermatozoa, *J. Endocrinol.* **17:**374–380.

Oikawa, T., and Suzuki, T., 1979, Demonstration of male reproductive tissue specific antigen and induction of the failure of fusion between gametes in golden hamster, *Biol. Reprod.* **20:**(Suppl.1):41a.

Oikawa, T., Yanagimachi, R., and Nicolson, G. L., 1973, Wheat germ agglutinin blocks mammalian fertilization, *Nature (London)* **241:**256–259.

Oikawa, T., Nicolson, G. L., and Yanagimachi, R., 1974, Inhibition of hamster fertilization by phytoagglutinins, *Exp. Cell Res.* **83:**239–246.

Oikawa, T., Nicolson, G. L., and Yanagimachi, R., 1975, Trypsin-mediated modification of the zona pellucida glycopeptide structure of the hamster egg, *J. Reprod. Fertil.* **43:**133–136.

Okamoto, M., and Toyoda, Y., 1980, Effects of glucose and pyruvate on the sperm penetration and fertilization of mouse eggs *in vitro*, *Jpn. J. Zootech, Sci.* **51:**171–180.

Okamura, F., and Nishiyama, H., 1978, Penetration of spermatozoa into ovum and transformation of the sperm nucleus into the male pronucleus in the domestic fowl, *Gallus gallus*, *Cell Tissue Res.* **190:**89–98.

Oliphant, G., 1976, Removal of sperm-bound seminal plasma components as a prerequisite to induction of the rabbit acrosome reaction, *Fertil. Steril* **27:**28–38.

Oliphant, G., and Brackett, B. G., 1973, Immunological assessment of surface changes of rabbit sperm undergoing capacitation, *Biol. Reprod.* **9:**404–414.

Oliphant, G., and Singhas, C. A., 1979, Iodination of rabbit sperm plasma membrane: Relationship of specific surface proteins to epididymal function and sperm capacitation, *Biol. Reprod.* **21:**937–944.

Olson, G. E., 1980, Changes in intramembranous particle distribution in the plasma membranes of *Didelphis virginiana* spermatozoa during maturation in the epididymis, *Anat. Rec.* **197:**471–488.

Olson, G. E., and Hamilton, D. W., 1978, Characterization of the surface glycoproteins of rat spermatozoa, *Biol. Reprod.* **19:**26–35.

Onuma, H., and Nishikawa, Y., 1963, Studies on the acrosomic system of spermatozoa of domestic animals. I. Cytochemical nature of the PSA positive materials in the acrosomic system of boar spermatozoa, *Bull. Jpn. Natl. Inst. Anim. Ind. Chiba* **1:**125–134.

O'Rand, M. G., 1977a, Restriction of a sperm surface antigen's mobility during capacitation, *Dev. Biol.* **55:**260–270.

O'Rand, M. G., 1977b, The presence of sperm-specific surface isoantigens on the egg following fertilization, *J. Exp. Zool.* **212:**267–273.

O'Rand, M. G., 1979, Changes in sperm surface properties correlated with capacitation, in: *The Spermatozoa* (D. W. Faucett and J. M. Bedford, eds.), Urban & Schwarzenberg, Munich, pp. 195–204.

O'Rand, M. G., and Metz, C. B., 1976, Isolation of an "immobilizing antigen" from rabbit sperm membranes. *Biol. Reprod.* **14:**586–598.

O'Rand, M. G., and Porter, J. P., 1979, Isolation of a sperm membrane sialoglycoprotein autoantigen from rabbit testis, *J. Immunol.* **122:**1248–1254.

O'Rand, M. G., and Romrell, L. J., 1977, Appearance of cell surface auto- and isoantigens during spermatogenesis in the rabbit, *Dev. Biol.* **55**:347–358.

Orgebin-Crist, M. C., 1965, Passage of spermatozoa labelled with thymidine-^{3}H through the ducts of epididymis of the rabbit, *J. Reprod. Fertil.* **10**:241–251.

Orgebin-Crist, M. C., 1967, Maturation of spermatozoa in the rabbit epididymis: Fertilizing ability and embryonic mortality in does inseminated with epididymal spermatozoa, *Ann. Biol. Anim. Biochim. Biophys.* **7**:373–389.

Orgebin-Crist, M. C., 1969, Studies on the function of the epididymis, *Biol. Reprod. Suppl.* **1**:155–175.

Overstreet, J. W., and Bedford, J. M., 1974a, Transport, capacitation and fertilizing ability of epididymal spermatozoa, *J. Exp. Zool.* **189**:203–214.

Overstreet, J. W., and Bedford, J. M., 1974b, Importance of sperm capacitation for gamete contact in the rabbit, *J. Reprod. Fertil.* **39**:393–398.

Overstreet, J. W., and Bedford, J. M., 1974c, Comparison of the penetrability of the egg vestments in follicular oocytes, unfertilized and fertilized ova of the rabbit, *Dev. Biol.* **41**:185–192.

Overstreet, J. W., and Cooper, G. W., 1978, Sperm transport in the reproductive tract of the female rabbit. I. The rapid transit phase of transport, *Biol. Reprod.* **19**:101–114.

Overstreet, J. W., and Cooper, G. W., 1979a, The time and location of the acrosome reaction during sperm transport in the female rabbit, *J. Exp. Zool.* **209**:97–104.

Overstreet, J. W., and Cooper, G. W., 1979b, Effect of ovulation and sperm motility on the migration of rabbit spermatozoa to the site of fertilization, *J. Reprod. Fertil.* **55**:53–59.

Overstreet, J. W., and Hembree, W. C., 1976, Penetration of the zona pellucida of non-living human oocytes by human spermatozoa *in vitro*, *Fertil. Steril.* **27**:815–831.

Overstreet, J. W., and Katz, D. F., 1977, Sperm transport and selection in the female genital tract, in: *Development in Mammals*, Volume 2 (M. H. Johnson, ed.), North-Holland, Amsterdam, pp. 31–65.

Overstreet, J. W., Cooper, G. W. and Katz, D. F., 1978, Sperm transport in the reproductive tract of the female rabbit. II. The sustained phase of transport, *Biol. Reprod.* **19**:115–132.

Overstreet, J. W., Katz, D. F., and Johnson, L. L., 1980a, Motility of rabbit spermatozoa in the secretions of the oviduct, *Biol. Reprod.* **22**:1083–1088.

Overstreet, J. W., Yanagimachi, R., Katz, D. F., Hayashi, K., and Hanson, F. W., 1980b, Penetration of human spermatozoa into the human zona pellucida and the zona-free hamster egg: A study of fertile donors and infertile patients, *Fertil. Steril.* **33**:534–542.

Papahadjopoulos, D., 1978, Calcium-induced phase changes and fusion in natural and model membranes, in: *Cell Surface Reviews*, Volume 5 (G. Poste and G. L. Nicolson, eds.), Elsevier/North-Holland, Amsterdam, pp. 765–790.

Papahadjopoulos, D., Poste, G., and Vail, W. J., 1979, Studies on membrane fusion and model membranes, in: *Methods in Membrane Biology*, Volume 10 (E. D. Korn, ed.), Plenum Press, New York, pp. 1–121.

Pavlok, A., 1968, Fertilization of mouse ova *in vitro*. I. Effect of some factors on fertilization, *J. Reprod. Fertil.* **16**:401–408.

Pavlok, A., 1979, Interspecies interaction of zona-free ova with spermatozoa in mouse, rat and hamster, *Anim. Reprod. Sci.* **2**:395–402.

Pavlok, A., and McLaren, A., 1972, The role of cumulus cells and the zona pellucida in fertilization of mouse eggs *in vitro*, *J. Reprod. Fertil.* **29**:91–97.

Perreault, S., Zaneveld, L. J. D., and Rogers, B. J., 1980, Inhibition of fertilization in the hamster by sodium aurothiomalate, a hyaluronidase inhibitor, *J. Reprod. Fertil.* **60**:461–467.

Peterson, R. N., Bundman, D., and Freund, M., 1978a, Effect of ionophore induced calcium uptake and dibutyryl cyclic AMP on the acrosomal membrane of boar spermatozoa, *Fed. Proc.* **37**:380.

Peterson, R. N., Russell, L., Bundman, D., and Freund, M., 1978b, Presence of microfilaments and tubular structures in boar spermatozoa after chemically inducing the acrosome reaction, *Biol. Reprod.* **19:**459–466.

Peterson, R. N., Russell, L., Bundman, D., and Freund, M., 1979, Direct evidence for boar sperm plasma membrane receptors for the zona pellucida, *J. Cell Biol.* **83:**200a (FD 1006).

Phillips, D. M., 1972, Structure of the mammalian acrosome, *J. Ultrastruct. Res.* **38:**591–604.

Phillips, D. M., 1977, Surface of the equatorial segment of the mammalian acrosome, *Biol. Reprod.* **16:**128–137.

Phillips, D. M., and Shalgi, R. M., 1980a, Surface properties of the zona pellucida, *J. Exp. Zool.* **213:**1–8.

Phillips, D. M., and Shalgi, R., 1980b, Surface architecture of the mouse and hamster zona pellucida and oocyte, *J. Ultrastruct. Res.* **72:**1–12.

Pikó, L., 1967, Immunological phenomena in the reproductive process, *Int. J. Fertil.* **12:**377–383.

Pikó, L., 1969, Gamete structure and sperm entry in mammals, in: *Fertilization*, Volume 2 (C. B. Metz and A. Monroy, eds.), Academic Press, New York, pp. 325–403.

Pikó, L., and Tyler, A., 1964, Fine structural studies of sperm penetration in the rat, *Proc. Vth Int. Congr. Anim. Reprod. A. I. Trento* **2:**372–377.

Plachot, M., and Mandelbaum, J., 1978, Comparative study of extra- and intrafollicular hamster oocyte maturation, *Ann. Biol. Anim. Biochim. Biophys.* **18:**1237–1246.

Plattner, H., 1971, Bull spermatozoa: A re-investigation by freeze-etching using widely different cryofixation procedures, *J. Submicrosc. Cytol.* **3:**19–32.

Poole, A. R., Howell, J. I., and Lucy, J. A., 1970, Lysolecithin and cell fusion, *Nature (London)* **227:**810–814.

Poste, G., 1970, Virus-induced polykaryocytosis and the mechanism of cell fusion, *Adv. Virus Res.* **16:**303–356.

Poste, G., 1972, Mechanisms of virus-induced cell fusion, *Int. Rev. Cytol.* **33:**157–252.

Poulos, A., Voglmayr, J. K., and White, I. G., 1973, Phospholipid changes in spermatozoa during passage through the genital tract of the bull, *Biochim. Biophys. Acta* **306:**194–202.

Poulos, A., Brown-Woodman, P. D. C., White, I. G., and Cox R. I., 1975, Changes in phospholipids of ram spermatozoa during migration through the epididymis and possible origin of prostaglandin F_{2X} in testicular and epididymal fluid, *Biochim. Biophys. Acta* **388:**12–18.

Quinn, P. J., 1979, Failure of human spermatozoa to penetrate zona free mouse and rat ova *in vitro*, *J. Exp. Zool.* **210:**497–506.

Quinn, P. J., and White, I. G., 1967, The phospholipid and cholesterol content of epididymal and ejaculated ram spermatozoa and seminal plasma in relation to cold shock, *Aust. J. Biol. Sci.* **20:**1205–1215.

Rajalakshmi, H., and Prasad, M. R. N., 1969, Changes in sialic acid in the testis and epididymis of the rat during the onset of puberty, *J. Endocrinol.* **44:**379–385.

Reddy, J. M., Joyce, C., and Zaneveld, L. J. D., 1980, Role of hyaluronidase in fertilization: The antifertility activity of Myocrisin, a nontoxic hyaluronidase inhibitor, *J. Androl.* **1:**28–32.

Reyes, A., and Rosado, A., 1975, Interference with sperm binding to zona pellucida by blockage of –SH group, *Fertil. Steril.* **26:**201–202.

Reyes, A., Mercado, F., Goicoechea, B., and Rosado, A., 1976, Participation of membrane sulfhydryl groups in the epididymal maturation of human and rabbit spermatozoa, *Fertil. Steril.* **27:**1452–1458.

Rink, T. J., 1977, Membrane potential of guinea-pig spermatozoa, *J. Reprod. Fertil.* **51:**155–159.

Rodger, J. C., and Bedford, J. M., 1980, Gamete interaction in the marsupial: *Didelphis virginiana*, *J. Cell Biol.* **87:**137a.

Rogers, B. J., 1978, Mammalian sperm capacitation and fertilization *in vitro:* A critique of methodology, *Gamete Res.* **1:**165–223.

Rogers, B. J., and Garcia, L., 1979, Effect of cAMP on acrosome reaction and fertilization, *Biol. Reprod.* **21:**365–372.

Rogers, B. J., and Morton, B., 1973, ATP level in hamster spermatozoa during capacitation *in vitro*, Biol. Reprod. **9**:361–369.

Rogers, B. J., and Yanagimachi, R., 1975, Retardation of guinea pig sperm acrosome reaction by glucose: The possible importance of pyruvate and lactate metabolism in capacitation and the acrosome reaction, *Biol. Reprod.* **13**:568–575.

Rogers, B. J., and Yanagimachi, R., 1976, Competitive effect of magnesium on the calcium-dependent acrosome reaction in guinea pig spermatozoa, *Biol. Reprod.* **15**:614–619.

Rogers, B. J., Ueno, M., and Yanagimachi, R., 1977, Inhibition of hamster sperm acrosome reaction and fertilization by oligomycin, antimycin A and rotenone, *J. Exp. Zool.* **199**:129–136.

Rogers, B. J., Van Campen, H., Ueno, M., Lambert, H., Bronson, R., and Hale, R., 1979, Analysis of human spermatozoal fertilizing ability using zona-free ova, *Fertil. Steril.* **32**:664–670.

Romrell, L. J., and O'Rand, M. G., 1978, Capping and ultrastructural localization of sperm surface isoantigens during spermatogenesis, *Dev. Biol.* **63**:76–93.

Roomans, G. M., 1975, Calcium binding to the acrosomal membrane of human spermatozoa, *Exp. Cell Res.* **96**:23–30.

Rosado, A., Velázquez, A., and Lara-Ricalde, R., 1973, Cell polarography. II. Effect of neuraminidase and follicular fluid upon the surface characteristics of human spermatozoa, *Fertil. Steril.* **24**:349–354.

Rosado, A., Hicks, J. J., Reyes, A., and Blanco, I., 1974, Capacitation *in vitro* of rabbit spermatozoa with cyclic adenosine monophosphate and human follicular fluid, *Fertil. Steril.* **25**:821–824.

Rothschild, L., 1956, *Fertilization*, Methuen, London.

Russell, L., Peterson, R. N., and Freund, M., 1979a, Morphologic characteristics of the chemically induced acrosome reaction in human spermatozoa, *Fertil. Steril.* **32**:87–92.

Russell, L., Peterson, R. N., and Freund, M., 1979b, Direct evidence for formation of hybrid vesicles by fusion of plasma and outer acrosomal membranes during the acrosome reaction in boar spermatozoa, *J. Exp. Zool.* **208**:41–56.

Saling, P. M., and Storey, B. T., 1979, Mouse gamete interaction during fertilization *in vitro*, *J. Cell Biol.* **83**:544–555.

Saling, P. M., Storey, B. T., and Wolf, D. P., 1978, Calcium-dependent binding of mouse epididymal spermatozoa to the zona pellucida, *Dev. Biol.* **65**:515–525.

Saling, P. M., Sowinski, J., and Storey, B. T., 1979, An ultrastructural study of epididymal mouse spermatozoa binding to zonae pellucidae *in vitro:* Sequential relationship to the acrosome reaction, *J. Exp. Zool.* **209**:229–238.

Santos-Sacchi, J., and Gordon, M., 1980, Induction of the acrosome reaction in guinea pig spermatozoa by cGMP analogue, *J. Cell Biol.* **85**:798–803.

Santos-Sacchi, J., Gordon, M., and Williams, W. L., 1980, Potentiation of the cGMP induced guinea pig acrosome reaction by zinc, *J. Exp. Zool.* **213**:289–292.

Sato, K., 1979, Polyspermy-preventing mechanisms in mouse eggs fertilized *in vitro*, *J. Exp. Zool.* **210**:353–359.

Sato, K., and Blandau, R. J., 1979, Time and process of sperm penetration into cumulus-free mouse eggs fertilized *in vitro*, *Gamete Res.* **2**:295–304.

Scacciati, J. M., and Mancini, R. E., 1975, Soluble and insoluble antigens of human spermatozoa, *Fertil. Steril.* **26**:6–12.

Schatten, G., and Schatten, H., 1979, Pronuclear movements and fusion observed by video microscrope and isolation of the pronuclear apparatus, the structure responsible for the observed movements, *Biol. Reprod.* **20**(Suppl. 1):53a.

Schill, W. B., Heimburger, N., Schiessler, H., Stolla, R., and Fritz, 1975, Reversible attachment and localization of acid-stable seminal plasma acrosin-trypsin inhibitors on boar spermatozoa as revealed by the indirect immunofluorescent staining technique, *Hoppe-Seyler's Z. Physiol. Chem.* **356**:1473–1476.

Schwarz, M. A., and Koehler, J. K., 1979, Alterations in lectin binding to guinea pig spermatozoa accompanying *in vitro* capacitation and acrosome reaction, *Biol. Reprod.* **21**:1245–1309.

Scott, T. W., Voglmayr, J. K., and Setchell, B. P., 1967, Lipid composition and metabolism in testicular and ejaculated ram spermatozoa, *Biochem. J.* **102**:445–461.

SeGall, G. K., and Lennarz, W. L., 1979, Chemical characterization of the components of the jelly coat from sea urchin egg responsible for induction of the acrosome reaction *Dev. Biol.* **7**:33–48.

Shalgi, R., and Kraicer, P. F., 1978, Timing of sperm transport, penetration and cleavage in the rat, *J. Exp. Zool.* **204**:353–360.

Shalgi, R., and Phillips, D. M., 1980a, Mechanics of sperm entry in cyclic hamster, *J. Ultrastruct. Res.* **71**:154–161.

Shalgi, R., and Phillips, D. M., 1980b, Mechanics of *in vitro* fertilization in the hamster, *Biol. Reprod.* **23**:433–444.

Shams-Borhan, G., Huneau, D., and Fléchon, J. E., 1979, Acrosin does not appear to be bound to the inner acrosomal membrane of bull spermatozoa, *J. Exp. Zool.* **209**:143–150.

Shivers, C. A., 1979, Studies on the antigenicity of the zona pellucida, in: *Animal Models for Research on Contraception and Fertility* (N. Alexander, ed.), Harper & Row, New York, pp. 314–325.

Shivers, C. A., and Dudkiewicz, A. B., 1974, Inhibition of fertilization with specific antibodies, in: *Physiology and Genetics of Reproduction*, Part B (E. M. Coutinho and F. Fuchs, eds.), Plenum Press, New York, pp. 81–96.

Singh, J. P., Babcock, D. F., and Lardy, H. A., 1978, Increased Ca^{2+} influx is a component of sperm capacitation, *Biochem. J.* **172**:549–556.

Singh, J. P., Babcock, D. F., and Lardy, H. A., 1980, Induction of accelerated acrosome reaction in guinea pig sperm, *Biol. Reprod.* **22**:566–570.

Snider, D. R., and Clegg, E. D., 1975, Alteration of phospholipids in porcine spermatozoa during *in vivo* uterus and oviduct incubation, *J. Anim. Sci.* **40**:269–274.

Soupart, P., 1967, Studies on the hormonal control of rabbit sperm capacitation, *J. Reprod. Fertil. Suppl.* **2**:49–63.

Soupart, P., 1970, Leucocyte and sperm capacitation in the rabbit uterus, *Fertil. Steril.* **21**:724–756.

Soupart, P., 1972, Sperm capacitation: Methodology, hormonal control and search for a mechanism, in: *Biology of Mammalian Fertilization and Implantation* (K. S. Moghissi and E. S. E. Hafez, eds.), Thomas, Springfield, Ill., pp. 54–125.

Soupart, P., and Morgenstern, L. L., 1973, Human sperm capacitation and *in vitro* fertilization, *Fertil. Steril.* **24**:462–478.

Soupart, P., and Orgebin-Crist, M. C., 1966, Capacitation of rabbit spermatozoa delayed *in vivo* by double ligation of uterine horne, *J. Exp. zool.* **163**:311–318.

Soupart, P., and Strong, P. A., 1974, Ultrastructural observation on human oocytes fertilized *in vitro*, *Fertil. Steril.* **25**:11–44.

Soupart, P., and Strong, P. A., 1975, Ultrastructural observations on polyspermic penetration of zona pellucida-free human oocytes inseminated *in vitro*, *Fertil. Steril.* **36**:523–537.

Soupart, P., Anderson, M. L., Albert, D. H., Coniglio, J. G., and Repp, J. S., 1979, Accumulation, nature, and possible functions of the malachite green affinity material in ejaculated human spermatozoa, *Fertil. Steril.* **32**:450–454.

Srivastava, P. N., Akruk, S. R., and Williams, W. L., 1979, Dissolution of rabbit zona by sperm acrosomal extract: Effect of calcium, *J. Exp. Zool.* **207**:521–529.

Stackpole, C. W., and Devorkin, D., 1974, Membrane organization in mouse spermatozoa revealed by freeze-etching, *J. Ultrastruct. Res.* **49**:167–187.

Stambaugh, R., 1978, Enzymatic and morphological events in mammalian fertilization, *Gamete Res.* **1**:65–85.

Stambaugh, R., and Buckley, J., 1968, Zona pellucida dissolution enzymes of the rabbit sperm head, *Science* **161**:585–586.

Stambaugh, R., and Buckley, J., 1969, Identification and subcellular localization of the enzymes effecting penetration of the zona pellucida by rabbit spermatozoa, *J. Reprod. Fertil.* **19**:423–432.

Stambaugh, R., and Smith, M., 1978, Tubulin and microtubule-like structures in mammalian acrosome, *J. Exp. Zool.* **203**:135–141.

Stambaugh, R., Brackett, B. G., and Mastroianni, L., 1969, Inhibition of *in vitro* fertilization of rabbit ova by trypsin inhibitors, *Biol. Reprod.* **1**:223–227.

Stefanini, M., Oura, C., and Zamboni, L., 1969, Ultrastructure of fertilization in the mouse. II. Penetration of sperm into the ovum, *J. Submicrosc. Cytol.* **1**:1–23.

Stone, R. T., Foley, C. W., Thorne, J. G., and Huber, T. L., 1973, Effect of oviductal fluids on oxidative phosphorylation in spermatozoa, *Proc. Soc. Exp. Biol. Med.* **142**:64–67.

Summers, R. G., Talbot, P., Keough, E. M., Hylander, B. L., and Franklin, L. E., 1976, Ionophore A23187 induces acrosome reactions in sea urchin and guinea pig spermatozoa, *J. Exp. Zool.* **196**:381–385.

Suzuki, F., and Nagano, T, 1980, Epididymal maturation of rat spermatozoa studied by thin sectioning and freeze-fracture, *Biol. Reprod.* **22**:1219–1231.

Szollosi, D., 1965, The fate of sperm middle-piece mitochondria in the rat egg, *J. Exp. Zool.* **159**:367–378.

Szollosi, D., 1966, Time and duration of DNA synthesis in rabbit eggs after sperm penetration, *Anat. Rec.* **154**:209–212.

Szollosi, D., 1976, Oocyte maturation and paternal contribtuion to the embryos in mammals, in: *Current Topics in Pathology*, Volume 62 (E. Grundmann and W. H. Kirsten, eds.), Springer-Verlag, Berlin, pp. 9–27.

Szollosi, D., and Hunter, R. H. F., 1973, Ultrastructural aspects of fertilization in the domestic pig: Sperm penetration and pronucleus development, *J. Anat.* **116**:181–206.

Szollosi, D., and Hunter, R. H. F., 1978, The nature and occurrence of the acrosome reaction in spermatozoa of the domestic pig, *Sus scrota*, *J. Anat.* **127**:33–41.

Takahashi, Y. M., and Sugiyama, M., 1973, Relation between the acrosome reaction and fertilization in the sea urchin. I. Fertilization in Ca-free sea water with egg-water-treated spermatozoa, *Dev. Growth Differ.* **15**:261–267.

Talbot, P., and Franklin, L. E., 1974, Hamster sperm hyaluronidase. II. Its release from sperm *in vitro* in relation to the degenerative and normal acrosome reaction, *J. Exp. Zool.* **189**:321–332.

Talbot, P., and Franklin, L. E., 1976, Morphology and kinetics of the hamster sperm acrosome reaction, *J. Exp. Zool.* **198**:163–176.

Talbot, P., and Franklin, L. E., 1978a, Trypsinization increases lectin-induced agglutinability of uncapacitated guinea pig sperm, *J. Exp. Zool.* **204**:291–298.

Talbot, P., and Franklin, L. E., 1978b, Surface modification of guinea pig sperm during *in vitro* capacitation: An assessment using lectin-induced agglutination of living sperm, *J. Exp. Zool.* **203**:1–14.

Talbot, P., and Kleve, M. G., 1978, Hamster sperm cross react with antiactin, *J. Exp. Zool.* **204**:131–136.

Talbot, P., Summers, R. G., Hylander, B. L., Keough, E. M., and Franklin, L. E., 1976, The role of calcium in the acrosome reaction: An analysis using ionophore A23187, *J. Exp. Zool.* **198**:383–392.

Tamblyn, T. M., 1980, Identification of actin in boar epididymal spermatozoa, *Biol. Reprod.* **22**:727–734.

Tash, J. S., and Mann, T., 1973, Adenosine 3′:5′-cyclic monophosphate in relation to motility and senescence of spermatozoa, *Proc. R. Soc. London Ser. B* **184**:109–114.

Teichman, R. J., Cummins, J. M., and Takei, G. H., 1974, The *in vitro* incorporation of ^{14}C and ^3H choline into phospholipids of maturing rabbit spermatozoa and reproductive tract tissue, *Biol. Reprod.* **11:**644–653.

Temple-Smith, P. D., and Bedford, J. M., 1976, The features of sperm maturation in the epididymis of a marsupial, the brushtailed possum *Trichosurus vulpecula*, *Am. J. Anat.* **147:**471–500.

Terner, C., MacLaughlin, J., and Smith, B. R., 1975, Changes in lipase and phospholipase activities of rat spermatozoa in transit from the caput to the cauda epididymis, *J. Reprod. Fertil.* **45:**1–8.

Thadani, V. M., 1979, Injection of sperm heads into immature rat oocyte, *J. Exp. Zool.* **210:**161–168.

Thadani, V. M., 1980, A study of hetero-species sperm–egg interactions in the rat, mouse and deer mouse using *in vitro* fertilization and sperm injection, *J. Exp. Zool.* **212:**435–453.

Thibault, C., 1969, La fécondation chez les mammiferes, in: *Traité de Zoologie*, Volume 16 (P. Grasse, ed.), Masson, Paris, pp. 911–963.

Thibault, C., 1972, Physiology and physiopathology of the fallopian tube, *Int. J. Fertil.* **17:**1–13.

Thibault, C., 1973a, Sperm transport and storage in vertebrates, *J. Reprod. Fertil. Suppl.* **18:**39–53.

Thibault, C., 1973b, *In vitro* maturation and fertilization of rabbit and cattle oocytes, in: *The Regulation of Mammalian Reproduction* (S. J. Segal, R. Crozier, P. A. Corfman, and P. Condliff, eds.), Thomas, Springfield, Ill., pp. 231–240.

Thibault, C., and Gerard, M., 1970, Factear cytoplasmique nécessaire â la formation du pronucleus mâle dans l'ovocyte de lapine, *C. R. Acad. Sci.* **270:**2025–2026.

Thibault, C., Gerard, M., and Menezo, Y., 1975, Acquisition par l'ovocyte de lapine et de veau du facteur de décondensation du noyau du spérmatozoide fécondant (MPGF), *Ann. Biol. Anim. Biochim. Biophys.* **15:**705–714.

Thompson, R. S., Smith, D. M., and Zamboni, L., 1974, Fertilization of mouse ova *in vitro*: An electron microscopic study, *Fetil. Steril.* **25:**222–249.

Toyoda, Y., and Chang, M. C., 1968, Sperm penetration of rat eggs *in vitro* after dissolution of zona pellucida by chymotrypsin, *Nature (London)*, **220:**589–591.

Toyoda, Y., and Chang, M. C., 1974, Capacitation of epididymal spermatozoa in a medium with high K/Na ratio and cyclic AMP for the fertilization of rat eggs *in vitro*, *J. Reprod. Fertil.* **36:**125–134.

Tsunoda, Y., and Chang, M. C., 1976, Reproduction in rat and mice isoimmunized with homogenates of ovary or testis with epididymis, or sperm suspension, *J. Reprod. Fertil.* **46:**379–382.

Tsunoda, Y., and Sugie, T., 1979, Effect of antivitellus serum on fertilization in the mouse, *Biol. Reprod.* **21:**749–753.

Tung, K. S. K., Okada, A., and Yanagimachi, R., 1980, Sperm autoantibodies and fertilization. I. Effects of antisperm autoantibodies on rouleaux formation, viability, and acrosome reaction of guinea pig spermatozoa, *Biol. Reprod.* **23:**877–886.

Tzartos, S. J., 1979, Inhibition of *in vitro* fertilization of intact and denuded hamster eggs by univalent anti-sperm antibodies, *J. Reprod. Fertil.* **55:**447–455.

Uehara, T., and Yanagimachi, R., 1976, Microsurgical injection of spermatozoa into hamster eggs with subsequent transformation of sperm nuclei into male pronuclei, *Biol. Reprod.* **15:**467–470.

Uehara, T., and Yanagimachi, R., 1977, Behavior of nuclei of testicular, caput and cauda epididymal spermatozoa injected into hamster eggs, *Biol. Reprod.* **16:**315–321.

Usui, N., and Yanagimachi, R., 1976, Behavior of hamster sperm nuclei incorporated into eggs at various stages of maturation, fertilization and early development: The appearance and disappearance of factors involved in sperm chromatin decondensation in egg cytoplasm, *J. Ultrastruct. Res.* **57:**276–288.

Vacquier, V. D., 1979, The fertilizing capacity of sea urchin sperm rapidly decreases after induction of the acrosome reaction, *Dev. Growth Differ.* **21**:61–69.

Vacquier, V. D., and Moy, G. W., 1977, Isolation of bindin: The protein responsible for adhesion of sperm to sea urchin eggs, *Proc. Natl. Acad. Sci. USA* **74**:2456–2460.

Vacquier, V. D., Epel, D., and Douglas, L., 1972, Sea urchin eggs release protease activity at fertilization, *Nature (London)* **237**:34–36.

Vaidya, R. A., Bedford, J. M., Glass, R. H., and Morris, J. M., 1969, Evaluation of the removal of tetracycline fluorescence from spermatozoa as a test for capacitation in the rabbit, *J. Reprod. Fertil.* **19**:483–489.

Vaidya, R. A., Glass, R. W., Dandekar, P., and Johnson, K., 1971, Decrease in electrophoretic mobility of rabbit spermatozoa following intra-uterine incubation, *J. Reprod. Fertil.* **24**:299–301.

Vasseur, E., 1949, Chemical studies on the jelly coat of the sea urchin eggs, *Acta. Chem. Scand.* **2**:900–913.

Vierula, M., and Rajaniemi, H., 1980, Radioiodination of surface proteins of bull spermatozoa and their characterization by sodium dodecyl sulphate polyacrylamide gel eletrophoresis, *J. Reprod. Fertil.* **58**:483–489.

Vijayasarathy, S., Shivaji, S., Iqbai, M., and Balaram, P., 1980, Formyl-Met-Leu-Phe induces chemotaxis and acrosomal enzyme release in bull sperm, *FEBS Lett.* **115**:178–180.

Voglmayr, J. K., 1975, Metabolic changes in spermatozoa during epididymal transit, in: *Handbook of Physiology*, Section 7, Volume 5 (D. W. Hamilton and R. O. Greep, eds.), American Physiological Society, Washington, D.C., pp. 437–451.

Weil, A. J., 1965, The spermatozoa-coating antigen (SCA) of the seminal vesicle, *Ann. N. Y. Acad. Sci.* **124**:267–269.

Weil, A. J., and Rodenburg, J. M., 1962, The seminal vesicle as the source of the spermatozoa-coating antigen of seminal plasma, *Proc. Soc. Exp. Biol. Med.* **109**:567–570.

Weinman, D. E., and Williams, W. L., 1964, Mechanism of capacitation of rabbit spermatozoa, *Nature (London)* **203**:423–424.

Wenstrom, J. C., and Hamilton, D. W., 1980, Dolichol concentration and biosynthesis in rat testis and epididymis, *Biol. Reprod.* **23**:1054–1059.

White, I. G., 1973, Metabolism of spermatozoa with particular relation to the epididymis, in: *Advances in Biosciences*, Volume 10 (G. Raspe, ed.), Pergamon Press, New York, pp. 157–168.

Wislocki, G. B., 1949, Seasonal changes in the testes, epididymides and seminal vesicles of deer investigated by histochemical methods, *Endocrinology* **44**:167–189.

Wolf, D. P., 1977, Involvement of a trypsin-like activity in sperm penetration of zona-free mouse ova, *J. Exp. Zool.* **199**:149–156.

Wolf, D. P., 1978, The block to sperm penetration in zona-free mouse eggs, *Dev. Biol.* **64**:1–10.

Wolf, D. P., and Armstrong, P. B., 1978, Penetration of the zona-free mouse egg by capacitated epididymal sperm: Cinematographic observations, *Gamete Res.* **1**:39–46.

Wolf, D. P., and Hamada, M., 1977, Induction of zonal and egg plasma membrane blocks to sperm penetration in mouse eggs with cortical granule exudate, *Biol. Reprod.* **17**:350–354.

Wolf, D. P., Inoue, M., and Stark, R. A., 1976, Penetration of zona-free mouse ova, *Biol. Reprod.* **15**:213–221.

Wooding, F. B. P., and O'Donnell, J. M., 1971, A detailed ultrastructural study of the head membranes of ejaculated bovine sperm, *J. Ultrastruct. Res.* **35**:71–85.

Yanagimachi, R., 1966, Time and process of sperm penetration into hamster ova *in vivo* and *in vitro*, *J. Reprod. Fertil.* **11**:359–370.

Yanagimachi, R., 1969a, *In vitro* acrosome reaction and capacitation of golden hamster spermatozoa by bovine follicular fluid and its fractions, *J. Exp. Zool.* **170**:269–280.

Yanagimachi, R., 1969b, *In vitro* capacitation of hamster spermatozoa by follicular fluid, *J. Reprod. Fertil.* **18**:275–286.

Yanagimachi, R., 1970a, *In vitro* capacitation of golden hamster spermatozoa by homologous and heterologous blood sera, *Biol. Reprod.* **3**:147–153.

Yanagimachi, R., 1970b, The movement of golden hamster spermatozoa before and after capacitation, *J. Reprod. Fertil.* **23**:193–196.

Yanagimachi, R., 1972a, *In vitro* fertilization of guinea pig ova, *Anat. Rec.* **172**:430a.

Yanagimachi, R., 1972b, Fertilization of guinea pig eggs *in vitro*, *Anat. Rec.* **174**:9–20.

Yanagimachi, R., 1972c, Penetration of guinea-pig spermatozoa into hamster eggs *in vitro*, *J. Reprod. Fertil.* **28**:477–480.

Yanagimachi, R., 1975, Acceleration of the acrosome reaction and activation of guinea pig spermatozoa by detergents and other reagents, *Biol. Reprod.* **13**:519–526.

Yanagimachi, R., 1977, Specificity of sperm–egg interaction, in: *Immunobiology of Gametes* (M. Edidin and M. H. Johnson, eds.), Cambridge University Press, London, pp. 255–295.

Yanagimachi, R., 1978a, Sperm–egg association in mammals, in: *Current Topics in Developmental Biology*, Volume 12 (A. A. Moscona and A. Monroy, eds.), Academic Press, New York, pp. 83–105.

Yanagimachi, R., 1978b, Calcium requirement for sperm–egg fusion in mammals, *Biol. Reprod.* **19**:949–958.

Yanagimachi, R., and Mahi, C. A., 1976, The sperm acrosome reaction and fertilization in the guinea pig: A study *in vivo*, *J. Reprod. Fertil.* **46**:49–54.

Yanagimachi, R., and Noda, Y. D., 1970a, Ultrastructural changes in the hamster sperm head during fertilization, *J. Ultrastruct. Res.* **31**:465–485.

Yanagimachi, R., and Noda, Y. D., 1970b, Physiological changes in the post-nuclear cap region of mammalian spermatozoa: A necessary preliminary to the membrane fusion between sperm and egg cells, *J. Ultrastruct. Res.* **31**:486–493.

Yanagimachi, R., and Noda, Y. D., 1970c, Fine structure of the hamster sperm head, *Am. J. Anat.* **128**:367–388.

Yanagimachi, R., and Noda, Y. D., 1970d, Electron microscopic studies of sperm incorporation into golden hamster egg, *Am. J. Anat.* **128**:429–462.

Yanagimachi, R., and Teichman, R. J., 1972, Cytochemical demonstration of acrosomal proteinase in mammalian and avian spermatozoa by a silver proteinate method, *Biol. Reprod.* **6**:87–97.

Yanagimachi, R., and Usui, N., 1972, The appearance and disappearance of factors involved in sperm chromatin decondensation in the hamster egg, *J. Cell Biol.* **55**:293a.

Yanagimachi, R., and Usui, N., 1974, Calcium dependence of the acrosome reaction and activation of guinea pig spermatozoa *Exp. Cell Res.* **89**:161–174.

Yanagimachi, R., Noda, Y. D., Fujimoto, M., and Nicolson, G. L., 1972, The distribution of negative surface charges on mammalian spermatozoa, *Am. J. Anat.* **135**:497–520.

Yanagimachi, R., Nicolson, G. L., Noda, Y. D., and Fujimoto, M., 1973, Electron microscopic observations of the distribution of acidic anionic residues on hamster spermatozoa and eggs before and during fertilization, *J. Ultrastruct. Res.* **43**:344–353.

Yanagimachi, R., Yanagimachi, H., and Rogers, B. J., 1976, The use of zona-free animal ova as a test system for the assessment of the fertilizing capacity of human spermatozoa, *Biol. Reprod.* **15**:471–476.

Yanagimachi, R., Lopata, A., Odom, C. B., Bronson, R. A., Mahi, C. A., and Nicolson, G. L., 1979, Retention of biologic characteristics of zona pellucida in highly concentrated salt solution: The use of salt-stored eggs for assessing the fertilizing capacity of spermatozoa, *Fertil. Steril.* **31**:562–574.

Yanagimachi, R., Miyashiro, L. H., and Yanagimachi, H., 1980, Reversible inhibition of sperm–egg fusion in the hamster by low pH, *Dev. Growth Differ.* **22**:281–288.

Yanagimachi, R., Okada, A., and Tung, K. S. K., 1981, Sperm autoantigens and fertilization. II. Effects of anti-guinea pig autoantibodies on sperm-ovum interactions, *Biol. Reprod.* **24:**512-518.

Yang, C. H., and Srivastava, P. N., 1974, Purification and properties of aryl sulfatases from rabbit sperm acrosomes, *Proc. Soc. Exp. Biol. Med.* **145:**721-725.

Yang, W. H., Lin, L. L., Wang, J. R., and Chang, M. C., 1972, Sperm penetration through the zona pellucida and perivitelline space in the hamster, *J. Exp. Zool.* **179:**191-206.

Young, R. J., 1979, Rabbit sperm chromatin is decondensed by a thiol-induced proteolytic activity not endogenous to its nucleus, *Biol. Reprod.* **20:**1001-1004.

Young, W. C., 1931, A study of the function of the epididymis. III. Functional changes undergone by spermatozoa during their passage through the epididymis and vas deferens in the guinea pig, *J. Exp. Biol.* **8:**151-162.

Zamboni, L., 1971, *Fine Morphology of Mammalian Fertilization*, Harper & Row, New York.

Zamboni, L., 1972, Fertilization in the mouse, in: *Biology of Mammalian Fertilization and Implantation* (K. S. Moghissi and E. S. E. Hafez, eds.), Thomas, Springfield, Ill., pp. 213-262.

Zamboni, L., and Mastroianni, L., 1966, Electron microscopic studies on rabbit ova. I. The follicular oocytes, *J. Ultrastruct. Res.* **14:**95-117.

Zaneveld, L. J. D., 1976, Sperm enzyme inhibitors as antifertility agents, in: *Human Semen and Fertility Regulation in Men* (E. S. E. Hafez, ed.), Mosby, St. Louis, pp. 570-582.

Zaneveld, L. J. D., and Williams, W. I., 1970, A sperm enzyme that disperses the corona radiata and its inhibition by decapacitation factor, *Biol. Reprod.* **2:**363-368.

Zaneveld, L. J. D., Srivastava, P. N., and Williams, W. L., 1969, Relationship of a trypsin-like enzyme in rabbit spermatozoa to capacitation, *J. Reprod. Fertil.* **20:**337-339.

Zaneveld, L. J. D., Robertson, R. T., Kessler, M., and Williams, W. L., 1971, Inhibition of fertilization *in vivo* by pancreatic and seminal plasma trypsin inhibitors, *J. Reprod. Fertil.* **25:**387-392.

Zaneveld, L. J. D., Polakoski, K. L., Robertson, R. T., and Williams, W. L., 1975, Trypsin inhibitors and fertilization, in: *Proteinase and Biological Control* (H. Fritz and H. Tschesche, eds.), de Gruyter, New York, pp. 236-243.

Zirkin, B. R., and Chang, T. S. K., 1977, Involvement of endogenous proteolytic activity in thiol-induced release of DNA template restrictions in rabbit sperm nuclei, *Biol. Reprod.* **17:**131-137.

Zirkin, B. R., Chang, T. S. K., and Heaps, J., 1980, Involvement of an acrosin-like proteinase in the sulfhydryl-induced degradation of rabbit sperm nuclear protamine, *J. Cell Biol.* **85:**116-121.

6

THE MAMMALIAN EGG'S BLOCK
TO POLYSPERMY

DON P. WOLF

The eggs of most mammals at ovulation are metabolically relatively inert cells arrested in metaphase II of meiosis. In response to an activation stimulus normally provided by the fertilizing sperm but induced artificially by a number of parthenogenetic agents, the egg resumes meiosis, undergoes a cortical reaction, and becomes metabolically more active. Visible evidence for the resumption of meiosis involves the abstriction of a second polar body at approximately 30 min postactivation. In the cortical reaction, the egg undergoes the exocytotic release of its cortical granules, a process that results in formation of a new mosaic plasma membrane from the fusion of limiting cortical granule membranes with the egg plasma membrane. At the same time, cortical granule contents released into the perivitelline space come in contact with the egg plasma membrane and the zona pellucida. The cortical reaction and granule exocytosis are of primary interest to any discussion of polyspermy for cortical granule contents have been associated with polyspermy-preventing mechanisms in the eggs of animals of diverse species (for review, see Schuel, 1978, or Gulyas, 1980).

The operation of an effective block to multiple sperm penetration in mammals is critical to mammalian development, for the entry of more than one sperm leads to abnormal embryogenesis and early death. The cumulative effect of several factors, however, serves to limit this outcome in mammals: (1) the restricted number of sperm reaching the site of fertilization; (2) the

DON P. WOLF • Division of Reproductive Biology, Departments of Obstetrics and Gynecology, and Biochemistry and Biophysics, University of Pennsylvania School of Medicine, Philadelphia, Pennsylvania 19104.

protective effect of the egg's associated cumulus and corona cells; and (3) the egg's block to polyspermy responses per se—the zona reaction and the egg plasma membrane block to polyspermy. It is these latter two events that will command the attention of this review.

Our current concepts of the mammalian egg's block responses are derived largely from the pioneering studies of Austin and co-workers in the early 1950s (for review, see Austin and Bishop, 1957). These investigators recovered eggs from naturally mated animals and quantitated the incidence of multiple sperm penetration of the vitellus and of the zona pellucida. Upon examination of eggs from several species, it was concluded that blocks to polyspermy occur to varying degrees at two levels: the zona pellucida and the egg plasma membrane. Thus in one group of animals (hamster, dog, sheep), sperm were

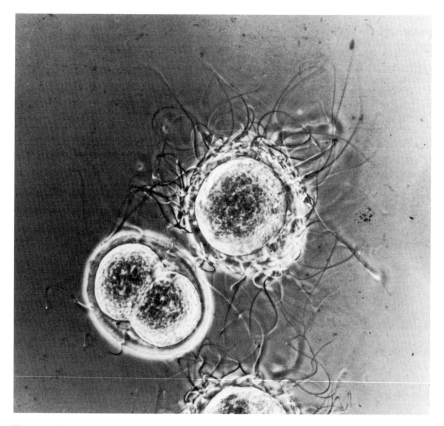

Figure 1. Capacitated sperm binding to zonae of unfertilized eggs and *in vivo*-produced two-cell embryos. The inability of sperm to bind to zonae surrounding fertilized eggs reflects the occurrence of a zona reaction.

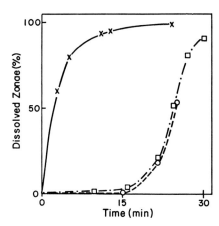

Figure 2. Solubility in mercaptoethanol of zonae surrounding unfertilized (X) and *in vitro* (○) or *in vivo* (□) produced two-cell embryos. The change in zona solubility at fertilization is referred to as zona hardening. (Taken from Inoue and Wolf, 1974. Published with permission.)

never seen in the perivitelline space, supporting the existence of a primary block at the zona level. In a second group (rabbit, pocket gopher, and probably mole), multiple sperm were recovered in the perivitelline space of monospermic embryos, necessitating the presence of a primary block at the level of the egg plasma membrane. In addition, a third group was defined as intermediate between the two extremes with occasional perivitelline space sperm (mouse, rat, guinea pig, ferret, cat).

Zona Reaction

The zona reaction, for discussion purposes, can be separated conveniently into two components: (1) a change that dramatically reduces sperm binding to and penetration of this structure effected through alterations in zonae sperm receptors (Figure 1); and (2) a change in physicochemical properties that results in increased zonae resistance to dissolution, i.e., zona hardening (Figure 2). Over the years, considerable attention has been devoted to zona hardening, as it is easy to monitor *in vitro* with a dissecting microscope, and the effects of various chemical (e.g., disulfide bond-reducing agents, low pH), enzymatic (proteases), and physical (heat) agents have been described (for summary, see Inoue and Wolf, 1975a; or Gwatkin, 1977). It should be stressed that these two components of the zona reaction are not necessarily indicative of the same event, for they can be separated from each other in at least three cases; a molecular basis for the separation is discussed below. For the rabbit, zona hardening has been reported to occur (Gould *et al.*, 1971) in a species that does not show a zona block, i.e., in the absence of changes in zona penetrability (Bedford and Cross, 1978). Conversely, in the hamster, dramatic changes in zona penetrability occur, at least in eggs recovered from natural matings, in the absence of demonstrable zona hardening (Chang and Hunt, 1956; Inoue and Wolf, 1975b; Gwatkin, 1977); and in the mouse, where both responses have been observed, a separation can be made based on temporal considerations. As indicated in Figure 3, in data derived from Inoue and Wolf (1975b) and Nicosia *et al.* (1977), zona hardening is observed in the mouse within 1–2 hr of penetration, while changes in sperm binding to the zonae are not seen until 6–10 hr after fertilization *in vivo*.

In considering molecular events involved in the zona reaction, a brief discussion of the nature of this acellular structure is appropriate (Figure 4). Histochemical studies that earlier indicated that zonae contained carbohydrate and protein have been corroborated and extended recently by direct chemical analysis, and we now know that zonae are comprised of 70–80% protein and 20% carbohydrate (Dunbar *et al.*, 1980). Zona glycoproteins are probably asymmetrically distributed, as evidenced by differential lectin reactivity (Nicolson *et al.*, 1975; Dunbar *et al.*, 1980) and in some species by the presence of histochemically distinct layers within the zona (Wartenberg and Stegner, 1960). Marked changes in zona morphology following fertilization comparable to fertilization envelope formation in lower animals (Grey *et al.*, 1974) have not been reported, although Baranska *et al.* (1975) did describe changes in ruthenium red staining in the mouse when zonae of unfertilized and fertilized eggs were compared. The characterization of isolated zonae has been hindered by the limited availability of starting material; however, two approaches are presently being used to overcome this problem: isolation of large numbers of ovarian oocytes by sieving techniques in the pig (Dunbar *et al.*, 1980) and cow (Gwatkin *et al.*, 1979) and in the mouse isolation of a few zonae by manual methods followed by the attachment of a radioactive tag

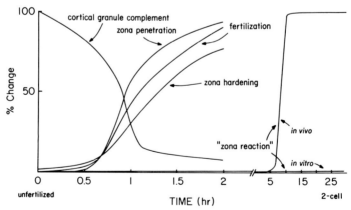

Figure 3. Kinetics of cortical granule loss, zona hardening, and zona sperm binding changes in the mouse. (Data derived from Inoue and Wolfe, 1975, and Nicosia *et al.*, 1977. Published with permission.)

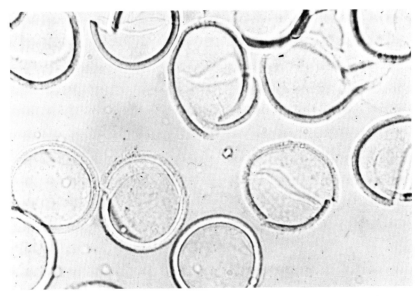

Figure 4. Zonae pellucidae isolated from cumulus-dispersed mouse eggs by mouth-operated micropipets.

([^{125}I]iodo sulfanilic acid) (Bleil and Wasserman, 1980a,b). The electrophoretic characterization of dissociated zonae components was initiated several years ago, and in one case (Repin and Akimova, 1976), differences in polypeptide patterns for zonae of unfertilized and fertilized mouse eggs were reported; however, this finding has not been corroborated by recent studies (Bleil and Wassarman, 1980b). In general, by polyacrylamide gel electrophoresis in dissociating solvents, zonae can be resolved into several major polypeptide bands whose mobility does not change at fertilization. Apparent molecular weights of 200,000, 120,000, and 83,000 were reported by Bleil and Wassarman (1980a,b) for zona pellucida proteins 1, 2, and 3, respectively in the mouse. Based on the behavior of similar glycoproteins, it would appear likely that each of these bands contains a family of glycoproteins homogeneous in polypeptide backbone but heterogeneous in oligosaccharide side chains.

Much of the species specificity controlling sperm–egg interaction in mammals resides with the zona pellucida, probably effected through species-specific sperm receptors. Sperm binding to the zona requires calcium (Saling *et al.*, 1978) and is sensitive to proteolysis (Hartmann and Gwatkin, 1971), to various plant lectins, and to antibodies directed against zonae (Dunbar and Raynor, 1980), consistent with the presence of a receptor that is glycoprotein in nature. Sperm receptor activity has been demonstrated in solubilized preparations of hamster (Gwatkin *et al.*, 1976) and mouse zonae (Bleil and

Wassarman, 1980a), by competition assays where fertilization or sperm binding to the zona is inhibited by solubilized receptor. Bleil and Wassarman (1980b) more recently showed that zonae from two-cell embryos no longer contained receptor activity, consistent with the occurrence of a zona reaction at fertilization. They associated this activity with an 83,000-dalton zona component (ZP 3) isolated from solubilized zonae of unfertilized eggs.

Zona Reaction Mechanisms

As alluded to earlier, cortical granules were implicated in the mammalian egg's block responses at the time of their original description in hamster eggs (Austin, 1956). Their formation, distribution, and chemical composition in mammals have been reviewed recently by Gulyas (1980). Parenthetically, the hamster provided a fortuitous choice in these early studies as the granules in this species are rather large and can be seen with a phase microscope; attempts to visualize granules at the light microscopic level in other laboratory animals have met with only limited success (Nitsch et al., 1977). Cortical granules disappear at fertilization in all mammalian species studied to date, although the reaction is probably slow compared with marine invertebrate eggs. A temporal correlation is apparent between cortical granule loss and establishment of a zona block to penetration (Szollosi, 1967), at least in the hamster. Barros and Yanagimachi in 1972 estimated that a zona block occurred within 15 min of sperm attachment to the vitellus or within 10–20 min of cortical granule release. In the electrically activated hamster egg (Gwatkin et al., 1973), granule loss and the loss of fertilizability occurred in 50% of the eggs within 8 and 16 min of stimulation, respectively, leading to a block time estimate of 8 min. The kinetics of cortical granule release are similar, albeit somewhat slower in mouse (Wolf et al., 1976; Nicosia et al., 1977; Fukuda and Chang, 1978) and rabbit eggs (Fraser et al., 1972). However, in these species, a tight correlation between granule release and zona reaction is either not anticipated (rabbit) or not observed (mouse) (see Figure 3). Based on continuous observations of mouse eggs, Sato (1979) noted a decline in the frequency of sperm passage through the zona within 1 min of initial sperm–egg fusion. Sato suggested that the zona reaction in the mouse is completed within 5 min; however, he did not specify the visible indicators that were used as evidence of "initial sperm–egg fusion," the beginning point in his time measurements, and he did not report sperm–egg interactions under comparable conditions with control, unfertilized eggs.

Direct evidence for cortical granule involvement in the zona reaction was presented in a landmark paper by Barros and Yanagimachi in 1971 when egg activation products were recovered from zona-free hamster eggs. These supernatant fractions, presumed to contain the extruded contents of the egg's cortical granules, were capable of rendering zonae of test eggs resistant to penetration, a response functionally similar to the zona reaction. As activation products were recovered from inseminated eggs, the authors demonstrated that supernatant solutions from sperm controls were inactive. Unequivocal association of this activity with the egg was provided by the studies of Gwatkin *et al.* (1973), where egg activation products were isolated from both fertilized and electrically activated eggs, the latter, of course, not requiring sperm. As characterized by Gwatkin *et al.* (1973), egg activation products were (1) active on both hamster and mouse eggs, (2) heat labile, and (3) neutralized by trypsin inhibitors, leading to a tentative identification of the active component as a trypsinlike protease. Egg activation products have also been isolated from inseminated zona-free mouse eggs and shown to be active in reducing the penetration of intact eggs (Wolf and Hamada, 1977). This activity, also neutralized by trypsin inhibitors, was so labile at 4° C as to preclude biochemical characterization. In summary, evidence currently supports the existence of a cortical granule trypsinlike protease that effects a change in the sperm binding properties of zonae through the alteration of a specific sperm receptor. It is appropriate to note, however, that unlike the marine invertebrate system, trypsinlike enzymes have not yet been isolated or characterized from mammalian cortical granules.

A second cortical granule activity has been implicated in the zona hardening reaction, namely, an ovoperoxidase (Gulyas and Schmell, 1980; Schmell and Gulyas, 1980). By TEM histochemical techniques, peroxidase activity was associated with intact cortical granules in unfertilized mouse eggs and with the egg surface, zona pellucida, and particulate material in the perivitelline space in artificially activated eggs. Furthermore, the peroxidase inhibitors, phenylhydrazin and sodium sulfite as well as some tyrosine analogues, were capable of inhibiting zona hardening. The authors concluded that the hardening reaction involves ovoperoxidase-catalyzed formation of dityrosine residues in analogy to the hardening reaction mechanism described in sea urchin eggs (Foerder and Shapiro, 1977; Hall, 1978).

Egg Plasma Membrane Block

Monospermic embryos recovered from natural matings in a few species and from *in vitro* inseminations in many species usually contain sperm in the perivitelline space, necessitating a block to polyspermy at the egg plasma membrane. In the rabbit, which falls into this category, the absence of a zona reaction has been documented experimentally: populations of fertilized and unfertilized eggs instilled into the oviducts of inseminated animals showed comparable frequencies of zona penetration (Overstreet and Bedford, 1974). *In vitro* studies on the block to polyspermy have involved almost exclusively

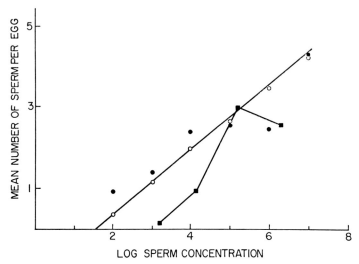

Figure 5. Relationship between sperm concentration and polyspermy. The mean number of sperm recovered at each inseminating concentration was calculated for zona-free eggs (●) and corrected for differences in sperm preparations by an analysis of covariance (○). Comparable uncorrected values are included for zona-intact eggs (■). (Taken from Wolf, 1978.)

the use of zona-free eggs of mice, and it is significant to note that insemination of such eggs with "normal" concentrations (10^5 cells/ml) of epididymal sperm results in very high levels of polyspermy, the degree of polyspermy being directly related to sperm concentration (Figure 5). As a consequence, the response under study is more appropriately termed a bock to multiple or unlimited sperm penetration. In early studies in the mouse (Pavlok and McLaren, 1972) and rat (Toyoda and Chang, 1968; Niwa and Chang, 1975), evidence for a block came from the observation that the penetration of zona-free eggs was limited and that polyspermy levels were often comparable to those of zona-intact controls. Limitations in sperm quality or number were largely ignored in these studies, and proteases were used in zona removal, a procedure that is not without consequences, at least in the mouse (Wolf *et al.*, 1976). The block response has more recently been studied in mechanically denuded zona-free eggs of the mouse, where reinsemination experiments have estimated that a block time occurs 40 min after initial sperm penetration (Wolf, 1978). As in the case of the zona reaction, species specificity is apparent in the block response of the egg plasma membrane. The hamster does not show a block at this level, as evidenced by the observation that capacitated sperm in this species are capable of penetrating zona-free eggs at both pronuclear and early cleavage stages (Usui and Yanagimachi, 1976).

As a correlate of the egg plasma membrane block, changes in capacitated sperm binding to the egg at fertilization have been studied in the mouse (Wolf and Hamada, 1979). Although a sperm receptor as such has not been characterized in the egg plasma membrane, species specificity is expressed in sperm–zona–free egg interactions in most mammals; one notable exception to this rule is the hamster (Hanada and Chang, 1972, 1976), where the zona-free egg has gained widespread popularity as a surrogate in the testing of sperm fertilizing capacity (Yanagimachi *et al.*, 1976). In the capacitated sperm binding studies with mouse eggs mentioned above, not only were differences apparent in the number of sperm bound to unfertilized and to fertilized eggs but also in their respective ability to respond to a challenge exposure to sperm. The kinetics of sperm penetration of and sperm detachment from the vitellus are depicted in Figure 6 where a cause-and-effect relationship between these events is suggested.

Documented changes in the functional properties of the egg membrane at fertilization include alterations in membrane permeability to sodium and potassium (Powers and Tupper, 1977), to glycerol (Jackowski *et al.*, 1980), and in electrical potential (Powers and Tupper, 1974). Physical correlates to such changes may well involve alterations in membrane fluidity and the lateral diffusion of membrane constituents. Adding to the already complex situation, the unfertilized-to-fertilized transformation probably involves not only changes in preexisting membranes but also the formation of new membranes through addition of sperm membrane (Gabel *et al.*, 1979), cortical granule membrane, and the loss of membrane in the second polar body. Additionally, asymmetry in the unfertilized mouse egg surface has been documented by fluorescent Con A binding (Eager *et al.*, 1976) as well as by TEM (Nicosia *et*

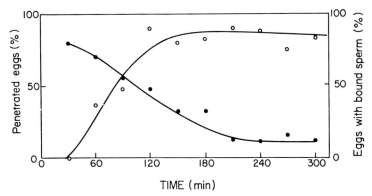

Figure 6. Kinetics of capacitated sperm penetration of and binding to unfertilized zona-free mouse eggs. Penetration (○); binding (●). Eggs were inseminated with approximately 10^4 sperm/ml. (Taken from Wolf and Hamada, 1979.)

al., 1977) and SEM (Nicosia *et al.*, 1978; Jackowski and Dumont, 1979) analysis. Lectin binding, its concentration and distribution, has been employed in efforts to monitor the distribution of macromolecular components in membranes, and fertilization-dependent changes in Con A binding have been reported in the rabbit (Gordon *et al.*, 1975). Comparable responses in lectin binding have not been observed in the mouse (Pienkowski, 1974) or hamster egg (Yanagimachi, 1977). Moreover, unfertilized mouse eggs, which cannot be agglutinated by Con A, are agglutinated by Con A after fertilization, parthenogenetic activation, or exposure to Pronase (Pienkowski, 1974), and it has been speculated that this greater agglutinability reflects increased mobility of surface components (Solter, 1977). In contrast, using single-cell photobleaching techniques, Johnson and Edidin (1978) concluded that the apparent lateral diffusion rate of surface membrane lipids and proteins decreased dramatically after fertilization in the mouse. The species specificity apparent in these studies and the fragmentary nature of the results obviously do not yet allow the establishment of cause-and-effect relationships or an association of membrane function with changes in membrane physical properties. Most of the work described here involved the use of zona-free mouse eggs, a species in which the egg plasma membrane block may be secondary to a zona reaction; consequently, the establishment of a more appropriate model such as the rabbit seems warranted.

Block to Polyspermy Mechanisms

A role for cortical granules in the egg plasma membrane block to polyspermy has been postulated by several authors. The evidence basically is that the frequency of polyspermic fertilization can be increased experimentally by manipulations that either partially or completely inhibit the cortical reaction (for references, see Gulyas, 1980). In the rabbit, for instance, artificially activated eggs that retain granules remain fertile and are monospermic, while aged eggs that lose granules become polyspermic (Fléchon *et al.*, 1975). [Unfortunately, not all authors agree that aged rabbit eggs lose granules (Longo, 1974; Oh and Bracket, 1975).] On the other hand, in inbred strains of mice with differing fertilities, low cortical granule complements have been associated with low fertility; the rationale in this case is that the reduced number of granules is indicative of premature granule release (for which there is independent evidence; Wabik-Sliz, 1979) and subsequent fertility impairment (Kaleta, 1979). Wolf and Hamada (1977) reported that preexposure of zona-free mouse eggs to a crude preparation of cortical granule exudate decreased the mean number of sperm penetrating these eggs, consistent with a cortical granule involvement in the plasma membrane block; however, the decrease, although statistically significant, was limited and the granule preparation was impure, a fact that may be especially significant in view of the sensitivity of the plasma membrane in this species to protease alteration (Wolf et al., 1976). The role of cortical granules in the plasma membrane block in other mammals is unclear. Results concerning the fertility of zona-free hamster eggs, while variable (Gwatkin et al., 1976; Hirao and Yanagimachi, 1978), are not relevant, as a plasma membrane block is not expressed in this species. In the rabbit, an increased concentration of negatively charged groups was detected on the surface of the fertilized egg, and the authors suggested cortical granule involvement (Cooper and Bedford, 1971).

Evidence against a cortical granule role in the plasma membrane block comes from a study with zona-free mouse eggs in which premature loss of cortical granules was triggered by ionophore exposure or by mechanical stimulation (Wolf et al., 1979). Egg exposure to ionophore resulted in a 50% loss of granules, as quantitated by TEM examination of thin sections, while complete granule loss accompanied mechanically induced egg activation. The fertility of these activated eggs was identical to that of controls as measured by the percentage of eggs penetrated and by the mean number of sperm per egg (Table I); moreover, ionophore-treated eggs subsequently underwent a normal sperm-induced block response, leading the authors to conclude that cortical granules are not involved in the plasma membrane block in the mouse.

In the absence of cortical granule involvement, a plasma membrane block may be electrically mediated. Rapid sperm-triggered depolarization of the plasma membrane is a common response of eggs of many lower vertebrates and invertebrates, and voltage clamp experiments have demon-

Table I
Penetration Characteristics of Activated Zona-Free Mouse Eggs[a]

Activation stimulus		Penetrated (%)	Polyspermic (%)	Mean number sperm/ egg
Mechanical removal of zonae	Control eggs[b]	81 (73/90)[c]	38 (28/73)	1.38
	Experimental[d]	87 (34/39)	47 (16/34)	1.74
Pretreatment with ionophore	Control eggs[b]	100 (64/64)	88 (56/64)	3.41
	Experimental[e]	100 (116/116)	91 (106/116)	3.37

[a]Taken from Wolf et al. (1979).
[b]Unactivated zona-free eggs inseminated in culture medium.
[c]The number of eggs is shown in parentheses.
[d]Eggs extruding second polar bodies within 30 min of zona removal and therefore classified as activated.
[e] Eggs exposed to $\geqslant 1.8\mu$M A23187 for at least 10 min at 37° C and then inseminated with 10^5 sperm/ml within 50 min.

strated that a block to sperm penetration may be associated with this event (Hagiwara and Jaffe, 1979). The electrophysiological properties of mammalian eggs have been characterized (Okamoto *et al.*, 1977); however, we do not yet know if an electrically mediated block exists in mammals. A clarification is expected soon, however, as the role of plasma membrane electrical properties in the fertilizability of rabbit eggs is under active investigation (McCulloh and Levitan, personal communication). Another non-cortical-granule-mediated mechanism has recently been described in mammals whereby zona-free mouse eggs cope with the polyspermic condition by abstricting supernumerary sperm in cytoplasmic blobs (Yu and Wolf, 1981). Little is currently known about the physiological significance or the generality of this process, but this observation does serve to enhance our awareness of other as yet undefined mechanisms by which the mammalian egg controls its own penetration.

Conclusions

The mammalian egg controls its own penetration by sperm at two levels: the zona pellucida and the egg plasma membrane. Changes in the zona pellucida that comprise a zona reaction are probably cortical granule mediated, involving alterations in the sperm binding capacity and/or in the solubility of this acellular structure. The former response involves a trypsin like protease (released upon cortical granule exocytosis) that alters sperm receptors in the zona pellucida; the latter response, zona hardening, may involve an ovoperoxidase-catalyzed formation of dityrosine residues.

Cortical granule involvement in the egg plasma membrane block appears unlikely and while a number of correlates to the block have been described, we are left without a sound explanation for this egg response. One possibility under active exploration is an electrically mediated block.

One of the major concerns in formulating unifying hypotheses for the mammalian eggs block to polyspermy responses remains the high degree of species specificity observed in the common laboratory animals that have been characterized to date. Thus, while we are beginning to understand responses of the mouse, rabbit, and hamster egg, a large totally unexplored area awaits attention.

ACKNOWLEDGMENT

This work was supported by NIH Grant HD-06274.

References

Austin, C. R., 1956, Cortical granules in hamster eggs, *Exp. Cell Res.* **10**:533–540.
Austin, C. R., and Bishop, M. W. H., 1957, Fertilization in mammals, *Biol. Rev.* **32**:296–349.

Baranska, W., Konwinski. M., and Kujawa, M., 1975, Fine structure of the zona pellucida of unfertilized egg cells and embryos, *J. Exp. Zool.* **192**:193–202.

Barros, C., and Yanagimachi, R., 1971, Induction of the zona reaction in golden hamster eggs by cortical granule material, *Nature (London)* **233**:268–269.

Barros, C., and Yanagimachi, R., 1972, Polyspermy-preventing mechanisms in the golden hamster egg, *J. Exp. Zool.* **180**:251–266.

Bedford, J. M., and Cross, N. L., 1978, Normal penetration of rabbit spermatozoa through a trypsin- and acrosin-resistant zona pellucida, *J. Reprod. Fertil.* **54**:385–392.

Bleil, J. D., and Wassarman, P. M., 1980a, Structure and function of the zona pellucida: Identification and characterization of the proteins of the mouse oocyte's zona pellucida, *Dev. Biol.* **76**:185–202.

Bleil, J. D., and Wassarman, P. M., 1980b, Mammalian sperm–egg interaction: Identification of a glycoprotein in mouse egg zonae pellucidae possessing receptor activity for sperm, *Cell* **20**:873–882.

Chang, M. C., and Hunt, D. M., 1956, Effects of proteolytic enzymes on the zona pellucida of fertilized and unfertilized mammalian eggs, *Exp. Cell Res.* **11**:497–499.

Cooper, G. W., and Bedford, J. M., 1971, Charge density change in the vitelline surface following fertilization of the rabbit egg, *J. Reprod. Fertil.* **25**:431–436.

Dunbar, B. S., and Raynor, B. D., 1980, Characterization of porcine zona pellucida antigens, *Biol. Reprod.* **22**:941–954.

Dunbar, B. S., Wardrip, N. J., and Hedrick, J. L., 1980, Isolation, physicochemical properties, and macromolecular composition of zona pellucida from porcine oocytes, *Biochemistry* **19**:356–365.

Eager, D. D., Johnson, M. H., and Thurley, K. W., 1976, Ultrastructural studies on the surface membrane of the mouse egg, *J. Cell Sci.* **22**:345–353.

Fléchon, J.-E., Huneau, D., Solari, A., and Thibault, C., 1975, Réaction corticale et blocage de la polyspermie dans l'oeuf de lapine, *Ann. Biol. Anim. Biochim. Biophys.* **15**:9–18.

Foerder, C. A., and Shapiro, B. M., 1977, Release of ovoperoxidase from sea urchin eggs hardens the fertilization membrane with tyrosine crosslinks, *Proc. Natl. Acad. Sci. USA* **79**: 4214–4218.

Fraser, L. R., Dandekar, P. V., and Gordon, M. R. 1972, Loss of cortical granules in rabbit eggs exposed to spermatozoa *in vitro*, *J. Reprod. Fertil.* **29**:295–297.

Fukuda, Y., and Chang, M. C., 1978, The time of cortical granule breakdown and sperm penetration in mouse and hamster eggs inseminated *in vitro*, *Biol. Reprod.* **19**:261–266.

Gabel, C. A., Eddy, E. M., and Shapiro, B. M., 1979, After fertilization, sperm surface components remain as a patch in sea urchin and mouse embryos, *Cell* **18**:207–215.

Gordon, M., Fraser, L. R., and Dandekar, P. V., 1975, The effect of ruthenium red and concanavalin A on the vitelline surface of fertilized and unfertilized rabbit ova, *Anat. Rec.* **181**:95–112.

Gould, K., Zaneveld, L. J. D., Srivastava, P. N., and Williams, W. L., 1971, Biochemical changes in the zona pellucida of rabbit ova induced by fertilization and sperm enzymes, *Proc. Soc. Exp. Biol. Med* **136**:6–10.

Grey, R. D., Wolf, D. P., and Hedrick, J. L., 1974, Formation and structure of the fertilization envelope in *Xenopus laevis*, *Dev. Biol.* **36**:44–61.

Gulyas, B. J., 1980, Cortical granules of mammalian eggs, *Int. Rev. Cytol.* **63**:357–392.

Gulyas, B. J., and Schmell, E. D., 1980, Ovoperoxidase activity in ionophore treated mouse eggs. I. Electron microscopic localization, *Gamete Res.* **3**:267.

Gwatkin, R. B. L., *Fertilization Mechanisms in Man and Mammals*, Plenum Press, New York.

Gwatkin, R. B. L., Williams, D. T., Hartmann, J. F., and Kniazuk, M., 1973, The zona reaction of hamster and mouse eggs: Production *in vitro* by a trypsin-like protease from cortical granules, *J. Reprod. Fertil.* **32**:259–265.

Gwatkin, R. B. L., Rasmusson, G. H., and Williams, D. T., 1976, Induction of the cortical reaction in hamster eggs by membrane-active agents, *J. Reprod. Fertil.* 47:299–303.

Gwatkin, R. B. L., Williams, D. T., and Meyenhofer, M., 1979, Isolation of bovine zonae pellucidae from ovaries with collagenase: Antigenic and sperm receptor properties, *Gamete Res.* 2:187–192.

Hagiwara, S., and Jaffe, L. A., 1979, Electrical properties of egg cell membranes, *Annu. Rev. Biophys. Bioeng.* 8:385–416.

Hall, H. G., 1978, Hardening of the sea urchin fertilization envelope by peroxidase-catalyzed phenolic coupling of tyrosines, *Cell* 15:343–355.

Hanada, A., and Chang, M. C., 1972. Penetration of zona-free rat eggs by spermatozoa of different species, *Biol. Reprod.* 6:300–309.

Hanada, A., and Chang, M. C., 1976, Penetration of hamster and rabbit zona-free eggs by rat and mouse spermatozoa with special reference to sperm capacitation, *J. Reprod. Fertil.* 46:239–241.

Hartmann, J. F., and Gwatkin, R. B. L., 1971, Alteration of sites on the mammalian sperm surface following capacitation, *Nature (London)* 234:479–481.

Hirao, Y., and Yanagimachi, R., 1978, Effects of various enzymes on the ability of hamster egg plasma membranes to fuse with spermatozoa, *Gamete Res.* 1:3–12.

Inoue, M., and Wolf, D. P., 1974, Comparative solubility properties of the zonae pellucidae of unfertilized and fertilized mouse ova, *Biol. Reprod.* 11:558–565.

Inoue, M., and Wolf, D. P., 1975a, Fertilization-associated changes in the murine zona pellucida: A time sequence study, *Biol. Reprod.* 13:546–551.

Inoue, M., and Wolf, D. P., 1975b, Comparative solubility properties of rat and hamster zonae pellucidae, *Biol. Reprod.* 12:535–540.

Jackowski, S., and Dumont, J. N., 1979, Surface alterations of the mouse zona pellucida and ovum following *in vivo* fertilization: Correlation with the cell cycle, *Biol. Reprod.* 20:150–161.

Jackowski, S., Leibo, S. P., and Mazur, P., 1980, Glycerol permeabilities of fertilized and unfertilized mouse ova, *J. Exp. Zool.* 212:329–341.

Johnson, M., and Edidin, M., 1978, Lateral diffusion in plasma membrane of mouse egg is restricted after fertilization, *Nature (London)* 272:448–450.

Kaleta, E., 1979, Sperm penetration *in vitro* into ovarian and tubal oocytes from mice of the inbred KE and C57 strains, *Gamete Res.* 2:99–104.

Longo, F. J., 1974, Ultrastructural changes in rabbit eggs aged *in vivo*, *Biol. Reprod.* 11:22–39.

Nicolson, G. L., Yanagimachi, R., and Yanagimachi, R., 1975, Ultrastructural localization of lectin-binding sites on the zonae pellucidae and plasma membranes of mammalian eggs, *J. Cell Biol.* 66:263–274.

Nicosia, S. V., Wolf, D. P., and Inoue, M., 1977, Cortical granule distribution and cell surface characteristics in mouse ova, *Dev. Biol.* 57:56–74.

Nicosia, S. V., Wolf, D. P., and Mastroianni, L., Jr. 1978, Surface topography of mouse eggs before and after insemination, *Gamete Res.* 1:145–155.

Nitsch, B., Brück, H.-J., and Palm, S., 1977, Simple methods for observing cortical granules in living mammalian eggs, *Experientia* 33:1252–1253.

Kiwa, K., and Chang, M. C., 1975, Requirement of capacitation for sperm penetration of zona-free rat eggs, *J. Reprod. Fertil.* 44:305–308.

Oh, Y. K., and Brackett, B. G., 1975, Ultrastructure of rabbit ova recovered from ovarian follicles and inseminated *in vitro*, *Fertil. Steril.* 26:665–685.

Okamoto, H., Takahashi, K., and Yamashita, N., 1977, Ionic currents through the membrane of the mammalian oocyte and their comparison with those in the tunicate and sea urchin, *J. Physiol.* 267:465–495.

Overstreet, J. W., and Bedford, J. M., 1974, Comparison of the penetrability of the egg vestments in follicular oocytes, unfertilized and fertilized ova of the rabbit, *Dev. Biol.* 41:185–192.

Pavlok. A., and McLaren, A., 1972, The role of cumulus cells and the zona pellucida in fertilization of mouse eggs *in vitro*, *J. Reprod. Fertil.* **29**:91-97.

Pienkowski, M., 1974, Study of the growth regulation of preimplantation mouse embryos using concanavalin A, *Proc. Soc. Exp. Biol. Med.* **145**:464-469.

Powers, R. D., and Tupper, J. T., 1974, Some electrophysiological and permeability properties of the mouse egg, *Dev. Biol.* **38**:320-331.

Powers, R. D., and Tupper, J. T., 1977, Developmental changes in membrane transport and permeability in the early mouse embryo, *Dev. Biol.* **56**:305-315.

Repin, V. S., and Akimova, I. M., 1976, Microelectrophoretic analysis of protein composition of zonae pellucidae of mammalian oocytes and zygotes, *Biochemistry (USSR)* **41**:39-45.

Saling, P. M., Storey, B. T., and Wolf, D. P., 1978, Calcium-dependent binding of mouse epididymal spermatozoa to the zona pellucida, *Dev. Biol.* **65**:515-525.

Sato, K., 1979, Polyspermy-preventing mechanisms in mouse eggs fertilized *in vitro*, *J. Exp. Zool.* **210**:353-359.

Schmell, E. D., and Gulyas, B. J., Ovoperoxidase activity in ionophore treated mouse eggs. II. Evidence for the enzyme's role in hardening the zona pellucida, *Gamete Res.* **3**:279.

Schuel, H., 1978, The role of cortical granules in fertilization, *Gamete Res.* **1**:299-382.

Solter, D., 1977, Organization and the antigenic properties of the egg membrane, in: *Immunobiology of Gametes* (M. Edidin and M. H. Johnson, eds.), Cambridge University Press, London, pp. 207-234.

Szollosi, D., 1967, Development of cortical granules and the cortical reaction in rat and hamster eggs, *Anat. Rec.* **159**:431-446.

Toyoda, Y., and Chang, M. C., 1968, Sperm penetration of rat eggs *in vitro* after dissolution of zona pellucida by chymotrypsin, *Nature (London)* **220**:589-591.

Usui, N., and Yanagimachi, R., 1976, Behavior of hamster sperm nuclei incorporated into eggs at various stages of maturation, fertilization and early development, *J. Ultrastruct. Res.* **57**:276-288.

Wabik-Sliz, B., 1979, Number of cortical granules in mouse oocytes from inbred strains differing in efficiency of fertilization, *Biol. Reprod.* **21**:89-97.

Wartenberg, H., and Stegner, H. E., 1960, Über die elektronenmikroskopische Feinstruktur des Menschlichen Ovarialeis, *Z. Zellforsch. Mikrosk. Anat.* **52**:450-474.

Wolf, D. P., 1978, The block to sperm penetration in zona-free mouse eggs, *Dev. Biol.* **64**:1-10.

Wolf, D. P., and Hamada, M., 1977, Induction of zonal and oolemmal blocks to sperm penetration in mouse eggs with cortical granule exudate, *Biol. Reprod.* **17**:350-354.

Wolf, D. P., and Hamada, M., 1979, Sperm binding to the mouse egg plasmalemma, *Biol. Reprod.* **21**:205-211.

Wolf, D. P., Inoue, M., and Stark, R. A., 1976, Penetration of zona-free mouse eggs, *Biol. Reprod.* **15**:213-221.

Wolf, D. P., Nicosia, S. V., and Hamada, M., 1979, Premature cortical granule loss does not prevent sperm penetration of mouse eggs, *Dev. Biol.* **71**:22-32.

Yanagimachi, R., 1977, Specificity of sperm–egg interactions, in: *Immunobiology of Gametes* (M. Edidin and M. H. Johnson, eds.), Cambridge University Press, London, pp. 255-295.

Yanagimachi, R., Yanagimachi, H., and Rogers, B. J., 1976, The use of zona-free animal ova as a test-system for the assessment of the fertilizing capacity of human spermatozoa, *Biol. Reprod.* **15**:471-476.

Yu. S.-F., Wolf, D. P., 1981, Polyspermic mouse eggs can dispose of supernumerary sperm, *Dev. Biol.* **82**:203-210.

7

GAMETE INTERACTION IN THE SEA URCHIN
A Model for Understanding the Molecular Details of Animal Fertilization

ALINA C. LOPO and VICTOR D. VACQUIER

Fertilization is the fusion of a sperm with an egg, resulting in the restoration of the diploid condition and the activation of the metabolically dormant egg, setting the zygote on the pathway to cleavage, organogenesis, and formation of an adult. Fertilization has been studied extensively for over 100 years because of curiosity about the mechanism that gives rise to a new generation. More recently, research on fertilization has become important because of the obvious applications to problems of fertility control. Fertilization also provides an excellent model system to study a variety of cellular phenomena. It is particularly useful as a model for studying cell adhesion and membrane fusion. Fertilization is a rare example of a natural fusion of the plasma membranes of two cells (reviewed in Epel and Vacquier 1978; others are myoblast fusion and fusion of placental trophoblast cells). In addition to the fusion of two plasma membranes, there are two exocytotic events associated with fertilization. One is the fusion of the sperm acrosome granule membrane with the overlying sperm plasma membrane; the second is the massive exocytosis of egg cortical granules seconds after sperm–egg fusion (Epel and Vacquier, 1978). Finally, fertilization is also an excellent model for the study of the biochemical activation of two cells. The sperm undergoes an activation in response to the external egg investments, involving ion fluxes, an increase in

ALINA C. LOPO • Department of Anatomy, University of California Medical Center, San Francisco, California 94143. **VICTOR D. VACQUIER** • Marine Biology Research Division, Scripps Institution of Oceanography, University of California, San Diego, La Jolla, California 92093.

respiration, and a change in cell shape involving the polymerization of actin (Tilney et al., 1973). The egg undergoes a dramatic metabolic activation, involving a variety of physiological changes such as ion fluxes, membrane fluidity changes, a membrane depolarization, increases in nucleoside and amino acid transport, and a marked increase in macromolecular synthesis (Epel, 1978).

The versatility of fertilization as a model to study a variety of cellular phenomena has led to an information explosion in the field during the last 10 years. Most of this research has used the gametes of invertebrates, most notably the sea urchin. There are many reasons for this popularity. Sea urchins are readily available in the intertidal and subtidal zones of all continents, and have minimal maintenance requirements. The sexes are separate, and fertilization is external; therefore the gametes can be easily

Table I
Biochemical Events Common to Sea Urchin and Mammalian Fertilization

1. The sperm membranes contain species-specific proteins involved in "recognition" of the egg surface prior to the acrosome reaction (Lopo and Vacquier, 1980b; Peterson et al., 1980).
2. Occurrence of an acrosome reaction (Dan, 1952; Austin, 1966).
3. Calcium is necessary for the induction of the acrosome reaction (Dan, 1954; Yanagimachi and Usui, 1974; Collins, 1976; Decker et al., 1976; Summers et al., 1976; Talbot et al., 1976).
4. Cyclic nucleotide metabolism is altered in sperm during the acrosome reaction (Garbers and Kopf, 1980).
5. A protease is exposed as a result of the acrosome reaction (Levine et al., 1978; Levine and Walsh, 1979, 1980; Meizel, 1972, 1978; Lui and Meizel, 1979).
6. Sperm binding is to receptors on the extracellular egg coat: the vitelline layer in sea urchins and the zona pellucida in mammal (Aketa, 1967; Tsuzuki and Aketa, 1969; Aketa et al., 1972; Tsuzuki et al., 1977; Epel and Vacquier, 1978; Glabe and Lennarz, 1979; Dunbar et al., 1980).
7. The attachment of sperm to eggs after the acrosome reaction exhibits species specificity (Hanada and Chang, 1972; Yanagimachi, 1972, 1977, 1978; Summers and Hylander, 1976; Kinsey et al., 1980).
8. "Sperm receptor" glycoproteins can be isolated from both the zona pellucida (Bleil and Wassarman, 1980a,b) and the vitelline layer (Schmell et al., 1977; Glabe and Vacquier, 1978; Dunbar et al., 1980).
9. A calcium transient in the egg triggers the cortical granule reaction after sperm–egg fusion has occurred (Gilkey et al., 1977; Fulton and Whittingham, 1978; Zucker et al., 1978).
10. A trypsinlike protease released from cortical granules destroys the sperm-binding capacity of the sea urchin vitelline layer (Vacquier et al., 1973; Carroll and Epel, 1975) and the mammalian zona pellucida (Barros and Yanagimachi, 1971; Gwatkin et al., 1973).
11. A peroxidase released from cortical granules hardens the vitelline layer (Foerder and Shapiro, 1977; Hall, 1978) and the zona pellucida (Schmell and Gulyas, 1980) by catalyzing the formation of di- and tri-tryosine cross-links between component proteins.
12. Fusion of sperm and egg results in activation of the new synthetic machinery of the egg and in cell division (Epel, 1978).
13. Sea urchin and mammalian sperm have cross-reacting surface antigens (Lopo and Vacquier, 1980c).

manipulated *in vitro*. Gamete interaction occurs synchronously in a time span of seconds. The large quantities of gametes, which are released in milliliter amounts, and the synchrony of development following fertilization have permitted biochemical analysis of the events of fertilization and early development (for reviews on sea urchin fertilization and early development, see Loeb, 1916; Lillie, 1919; Monroy, 1965; Metz and Monroy, 1967; Giudice, 1973; Czihak, 1975; Epel, 1978; Epel and Vacquier, 1978; Metz, 1978; Vacquier, 1979b, 1980). Finally, the many features that echinoderm and mammalian fertilization have in common (Table I) make the study of sea urchin fertilization relevant to the study of fertilization in higher organisms.

Fertilization in the Sea Urchin

The Sea Urchin Egg

The sea urchin egg differs from most animal eggs in that it completes meiosis before being released into the sea. It is therefore haploid, and its pronucleus is in interphase at the moment of fertilization. A plasma membrane bounds the perfectly spherical egg, and external and tightly apposed to it lies the vitelline layer, an extracellular glycoprotein coat 100–300 Å in diameter (Runnstrom, 1966; Glabe and Vacquier, 1977b; Kidd, 1978; Chandler and Heuser, 1980), bearing receptors for sperm on its external surface. Surrounding the entire egg is a second, almost transparent jelly coat, 30–50 μm in diameter. The jelly coat contains two major high-molecular-weight components, a fucose sulfate-rich polymer and a sialoprotein (SeGall and Lennarz, 1979).

The Sea Urchin Sperm

The sperm of the sea urchin is comprised of three parts: a head, midpiece, and tail, all limited by a plasma membrane. The nucleus, containing highly condensed chromatin, is the dominant structure in the head. Immediately anterior to it, at the apex of the sperm, lies the membrane-bound acrosome granule, subjacent to the plasma membrane. At the anterior end of the nucleus is a depression known as the nuclear fossa or subacrosomal space; research in other echinoderms indicates that this depression is filled with unpolymerized actin (Tilney *et al.*, 1973). The sperm is propelled through the sea by a typical eukaryotic flagellum that extends posteriorly from the nucleus. Energy for the movement is provided by a single large mitochondrial derivative that surrounds the base of the tail in the midpiece region of the sperm. When sperm are released from the male, they are in a highly concentrated, anoxic suspension and consequently are immotile. They begin swimming immediately upon dilution into normally oxygenated seawater.

When Sperm Meets Egg

In sea urchins, fertilization encompasses the period from the initial approach of the sperm toward the egg to the time of fusion of male and female pronuclei (30 min). This period may be divided into several steps, each a prerequisite to the next. First, the surface of the sperm plasma membrane contacts the extracellular jelly coat of the egg. In response to this interaction the sperm undergoes the acrosome reaction, a series of complex ionic events (Schackmann *et al.*, 1978; Schackmann and Shapiro, 1981) resulting in the extension of the acrosome process and exposure of a sperm-egg binding

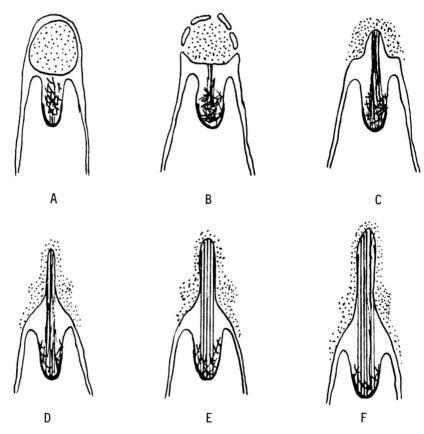

Figure 1. The acrosome reaction in sea urchin sperm. On contact with egg jelly, multiple fusion sites appear between the plasma membrane and the acrosome granule membrane, and g-actin in the nuclear fossa begins to polymerize (A,B). Fusion of the plasma and acrosome granule membranes exposes the acrosomal contents (C). The plasma membrane is now continuous with the inner acrosomal membrane (C). The actin continues to polymerize (C–F) into filaments that form a short acrosome process about 1μm in length. As the process becomes longer it pierces and becomes coated with the acrosome granule contents (F). (Adapted from Dan, 1967.)

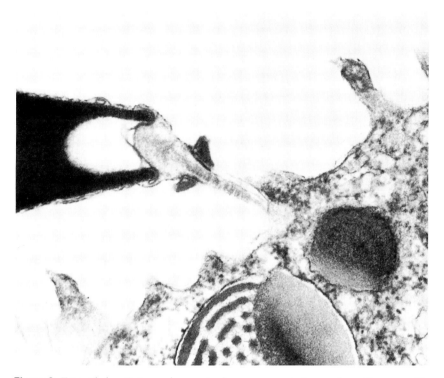

Figure 2. Transmission electron micrograph of acrosome-reacted sperm bound to an egg. The sperm is attached by the tip of the bindin-coated acrosome process, × 29,000. (Unpublished photograph courtesy of G. W. Moy and V. D. Vacquier.)

protein, bindin (Figure 1). The sperm attaches to the vitelline layer by the interaction of bindin, which covers the surface of the acrosome process, with the bindin receptor glycoprotein on the external surface of the egg vitelline layer (Figure 2). By an unknown process, the acrosome process penetrates the vitelline layer and the plasma membranes of the two cells fuse (reviewed in Epel and Vacquier, 1978). The egg then draws the motionless sperm into its cortical cytoplasm. Once in the egg cytoplasm the sperm nucleus undergoes several structural changes and migrates to the egg center (Schatten and Schatten, 1980), where it meets and fuses with the egg pronucleus (Longo and Kunkle, 1978; Mar, 1980).

The Plasma Membrane of Sea Urchin Sperm

Identification of Surface Proteins

The sperm is a highly specialized cell with only one function and its membrane must reflect this specialization. The sperm plasma membrane is a prime participant in the initiation of the fertilization process. A component of egg jelly interacts with the sperm membrane to induce the acrosome reaction, a necessary event for successful binding of sperm to the egg. Although in recent years considerable progress has been made in our understanding of the ultrastructure and mechanism of the acrosome reaction (Dan, 1956, 1967; Colwin and Colwin, 1967; Tilney *et al.*, 1973, 1978, 1979; Tilney, 1976a,b; Collins, 1976; Collins and Epel, 1977; Decker *et al.*, 1976; Schackmann *et al.*, 1978; Schackmann and Shapiro, 1981), there is no information on the initial molecular step triggering this dramatic response of the sperm. A receptor for egg jelly may exist on the plasma membrane of sea urchin sperm, because under natural conditions sperm do not undergo the acrosome reaction unless contact is made with the egg jelly. Although the chemical composition of jelly from different species is nearly identical, egg jelly can be highly species-specific with respect to induction of the acrosome reaction (Kinsey *et al.*, 1980).

Until recently, there has been little information on the composition of the plasma membrane of sea urchin sperm. Using fluorescently labeled lectins, Aketa (1975) showed that there is nonuniform binding of FITC–concanavalin A (Con A) to the surface of *Anthocidaris crassispina* sperm. FITC–Con A binds primarily to the anterior apex and midpiece of the sperm. In addition, univalent Con A blocks fertilization. This interaction appears to be species specific, because Con A neither binds to *Hemicentrotus pulcherrimus* sperm nor renders these sperm infertile. This suggests that species-specific carbohydrate sequences on the sperm membrane are responsible for some initial recognition step between sperm and egg.

Using a radioiodinated derivative of FITC, $[^{125}I]$diiodo-FITC, Gabel *et al.* (1979) labeled *Strongylocentrotus purpuratus* sperm. Sperm bound the fluorescent label nonuniformly, most of the fluorescence being associated with the midpiece (Gabel *et al.*, 1979). Because the label is also radioactive, the components associated with the fluorescence could be identified by gel electrophoresis. Autoradiograms of SDS gels of the labeled sperm showed that much of the label was associated with a polypeptide of molecular weight 35,000–37,000, and several low-molecular-weight peptides migrating just behind the dye front. The amount of label associated with the different peptides unfortunately was not quantitated. Differential extraction of the labeled sperm using 3.3% Triton X-100 indicated that several polypeptides of higher molecular weight were also labeled. The Triton-extractable material, representing the plasma membrane of the cell plus soluble protein, acrosome granule membrane, and mitochondrial contents, contained labeled bands migrating at molecular weights 55,0000, 47,000, 30,000 and 24,000 (Gabel *et al.*, 1979). When the Triton-insoluble material, including the nucleus, acrosome granule, and axoneme, was separated by gel electrophoresis, it contained the same labeled material that appeared when whole sperm were separated on a gel, suggesting there was internal labeling. It is likely that because of the high solubility of FITC in sea urchin sperm lipids (25% of the total label is in chloroform/methanol-soluble material), labeling of internal proteins occurred. Since anti-diiodo-FITC is available (Gabel *et al.*, 1979), this question may be easily answered by electron microscopic localization experiments with sea urchin sperm.

We have recently used a different approach to study the sea urchin sperm surface. Working by analogy from other membrane systems, we first identified proteins on the surface of *S. purpuratus* sperm and then produced rabbit antibodies against these components in an effort to assign a function in fertilization to them. Using radioiodination, several components from the

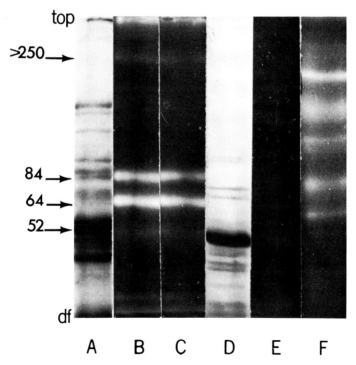

Figure 3. SDS–7.5% polyacrylamide gel electrophoresis of sperm proteins. (A) 1% Triton X-100 extract of *Strongylocentrotus purpuratus* sperm. The major labeled components are indicated by arrows and molecular weight ($\times 10^{-3}$). Coomassie blue stain. (B) Autoradiogram of Triton X-100 extract from sperm radioiodinated using the lactoperoxidase procedure. (C) Auto-radiogram of Triton X-100 extract from sperm labeled using Iodo-Gen. (D) Demembranated sperm flagella. Coomassie blue stain. (E) Autoradiogram of sperm trypsinized following radioiodination. (F) Autoradiogram of Triton X-100 extract from sperm labeled with 0.1% Triton X-100 included in the reaction medium. All channels are 5×10^5 cpm. (Reproduced with permission of Academic Press from Lopo and Vacquier, 1980a).

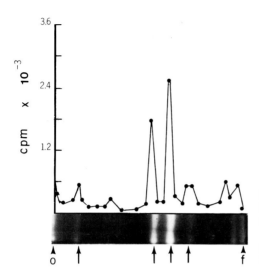

Figure 4. Distribution of radioactivity in ^{125}I-labeled sperm. Almost 75% of the radioactivity is in two peaks corresponding to 84K and 64K. (Reproduced with permission of Academic Press from Lopo and Vacquier, 1980a.)

sperm surface were identified (Figure 3; Lopo and Vacquier, 1980a). Analysis of the ^{125}I-labeled sperm using SDS–polyacrylamide gel electrophoresis showed that the ^{125}I was distributed primarily among four proteins of molecular weights 250,000, 84,000, 64,000 and 52,000. There was also a very small amount of label at molecular weight 130,000 and some low-molecular-weight material immediately behind the gel front. Most of the label incorporated into protein was associated with the 84K (28% of the label) and 64K (46% of the label) components (Figure 4). Interestingly, although both molecules contained much of the label, they were relatively minor components of the 1% Triton X-100 extract of whole sperm (Lopo and Vacquier, 1980a).

This very unusual iodination pattern led to a more extensive investigation of the 84K and 64K components. Antiserum against each of these glycoproteins was raised in rabbits by cutting out each band from a polyacrylamide gel, homogenizing the gel piece in saline, and injecting it into rabbits. The resulting antisera (anti-84K and anti-64K) agglutinated whole and living sperm (Figure 5). From electron microscope–immunoperoxidase localization, both antigens appeared to be distributed over the entire sperm surface (Figure 6). The critical question of whether 84K and 64K had a role in the induction of the acrosome reaction by egg jelly was tested by incubating Fab fragments from anti-84K or anti-64K with living sperm, adding egg jelly, and scoring acrosome-reacted sperm under phase contrast. The results (Figure 7) indicated that anti-84K Fab blocked the egg-jelly-induced acrosome reaction. The preimmune serum had no effect. To ascertain that the mechanism of the acrosome reaction was not disturbed by the antiserum

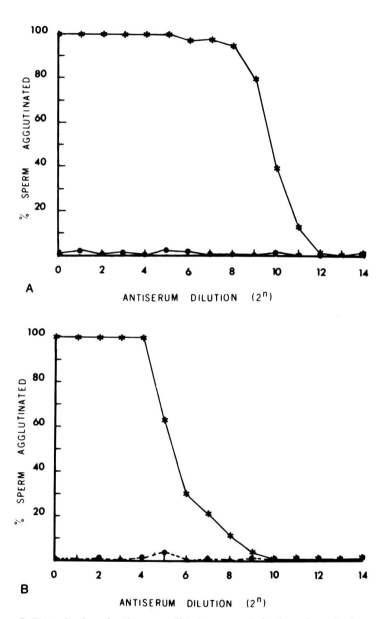

Figure 5. Determination of antiserum-mediated sperm agglutination using a Coulter counter assay. A 100-μl aliquot was counted and the number of unagglutinated sperm expressed as percentages. (A) Anti-64K; (B) anti-84K; (*) antiserum; (●) preimmune serum. (Reproduced with permission of Academic Press from Lopo and Vacquier, 1980b.)

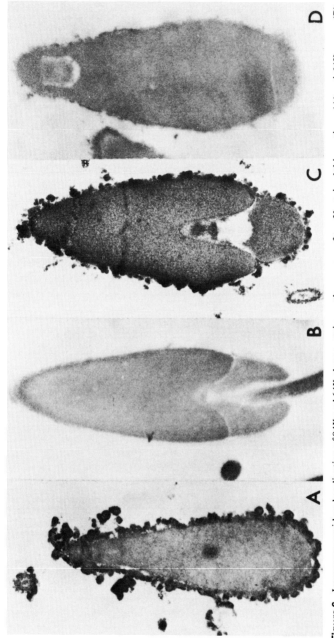

Figure 6. Immunoperoxidase localization of 84K and 64K glycoproteins on the sperm surface. Unstained thin sections. (A) anti-64K serum; (B) anti-64K preimmune serum; (C) anti-84K serum; (D) anti-84K preimmune serum. The globular electron–dense Hanker–Yates reaction product is evident in A and C and completely absent in B and D; × 25,000. (Reproduced with permission of Academic Press from Lopo and Vacquier, 1980b.)

binding, the acrosome reaction was artificially induced by additions of 1 M NH₄OH to elevate the pH to 9, or treatment with the calcium ionophore A23187. In both cases the sperm treated with anti-84K Fab reacted, suggesting that the egg-jelly-induced acrosome reaction had been blocked by a surface phenomenon. The anti-64K Fab fragments did not block the jelly-induced acrosome reaction or fertilization (Figures 7 and 8; Lopo and Vacquier, 1980b). This does not preclude a function in fertilization for 64K, as it could merely reflect the absence of antibody activity against critical determinants in the glycoprotein.

What role might the 84K sperm membrane glycoprotein play in the induction of the acrosome reaction? One possibility is that 84K is the molecule involved in the interaction of the sperm surface with the egg jelly fucose sulfate polymer to induce the acrosome reaction. This question could be tested by constructing an affinity surface using 84K and studying its interaction with the purified components of egg jelly. An alternative possibility is that 84K is a component involved in one of the ion movements leading to the extension of the acrosome filament (Tilney *et al.*, 1973, 1978; Schackmann *et al.*, 1978; Schackmann and Shapiro, 1981). We believe that the 84K glycoprotein is the first sperm surface component implicated in the induction of the acrosome reaction.

A slightly different approach has been taken by Cross (personal communication) to characterize the sea urchin sperm plasma membrane. Flagella from radioiodinated *S. purpuratus* sperm were used to obtain a subcellular fraction containing plasma membranes (Gray and Drummond, 1976). Gel electrophoresis revealed over 20 Coomassie blue-positive components. Five species of molecular weights 200,000, 149,000, 120,000 77,000, and 59,000 proved to be glycoproteins (by PAS staining) that were externally disposed (by lactoperoxidase-catalyzed radioiodination). The 200K, 77K, and 59K components isolated by the Cross technique apparently correspond to those identified in our study (Lopo and Vacquier, 1980a) as 250K, 84K, and 64K. The difference in molecular weight is likely due to the use of gradient gels by Cross and 7.5% gels by us. The technique used to isolate sperm plasma membranes in the Cross experiments is useful because it enriches the preparation with the molecular species of interest, facilitating their isolation.

Swarming Response of Sperm

When exposed to solubilized egg jelly the sperm of many sea urchin species undergo a behavioral response known as swarming, cluster formation (Loeb, 1916), or isoagglutination (Loeb, 1916; Lillie, 1919; Collins, 1976; Epel, 1978; Metz, 1978). This bizarre response of sperm to egg jelly has been known for many years (Loeb, 1916; Lillie, 1919) and formed the basis for the

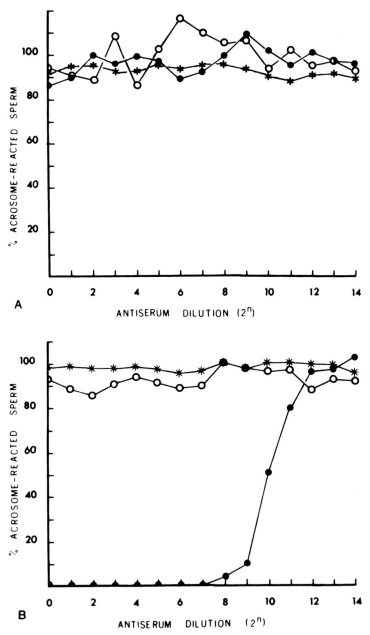

Figure 7. Effect of immune Fab fragments on the jelly-induced acrosome reaction. (A) Anti-64K Fab; (B) anti-84K Fab. (O) Preimmune Fab; (●) experimental Fab; (∗) pH-induced acrosome reaction. *S. purpuratus* sperm and antisera. These assays were done using limiting concentrations of sperm. The control data were normalized to 100%. (Reproduced with permission of Academic Press from Lopo and Vacquier, 1980b.)

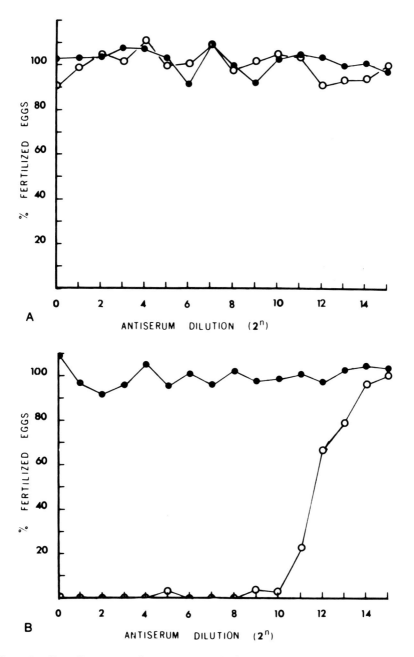

Figure 8. Effect of immune Fab fragments on fertilization. (A) Anti-64K Fab; (B) anti-84K Fab. (●) Preimmune Fab; (O) immune Fab. An egg was considered fertilized if the fertilization envelope was visible 10 min postinsemination. (Reproduced with permission of Academic Press from Lopo and Vacquier, 1980b.)

fertilizin–antifertilizin theory of Lillie (later modified by Tyler, 1949), who considered the phenomenon an isoagglutination (Lillie, 1915, 1919; Tyler, 1949; see also Vacquier, 1979a,b, and Vacquier *et al.*, 1979, for discussion of the Lillie–Loeb controversy). During swarming, actively swimming sperm aggregate into very dense spherical clumps that may be as large as 2–4 mm (Loeb, 1916; Lillie, 1919; Collins, 1976). After a period of time varying from 30 sec to 10 min, depending on the age of the sperm and the jelly concentration, the swarms spontaneously disperse. Sperm that have swarmed lose their fertilizing capacity and fail to swarm again when fresh jelly is added.

Collins (1976) investigated swarming and concluded that it is not a true agglutination (see also Loeb, 1916). The cells do not become physically linked because the clusters cannot be fixed (Loeb, 1916; Collins, 1976). Cluster formation is reversibly inhibited by inclusion of respiratory inhibitors in the medium (Lillie, 1919; Loeb, 1916; Collins, 1976), showing that the process depends on motility. Sperm mixed with jelly in calcium-free seawater (Dan, 1954; Collins, 1976) will swarm, although they will not undergo the acrosome reaction.

An involvement of chemotaxis in the swarming response of sea urchin sperm has been postulated but never demonstrated (Lillie, 1919; Collins, 1976). A role for chemoattractants in sperm–egg interaction has been described in coelenterates (Miller, 1966, 1979a,b; Miller and Tseng, 1974; Miller and Brokaw, 1970), tunicates (Miller, 1975), and brown algae (Müller *et al.*, 1979). Lopo *et al.*, (1977) demonstrated the possible existence of a secondary chemoattractant that may be responsible for the formation and maintenance of the swarms following the initial interaction between sperm and egg jelly. Their results suggest that at least in *Arbacia punctulata* the swarming sperm release a substance that acts as a secondary chemoattractant. The nature of the signal was investigated but not discovered. Lopo and Epel (unpublished results), using the same assay system, found that secondary chemotaxis was not demonstrable in *S. purpuratus* sperm by this procedure. One possible explanation for this discrepancy is that the chemotactic molecule in *S. purpuratus* might be too large to pass through the filters used in the assay.

Another poorly understood aspect of the swarming reaction of sea urchin sperm is its spontaneous reversibility. Tyler (1949) and Metz (1967) explained this reversibility as the result of the modification of the agglutinating substance of jelly (fertilizin) by sperm from a multivalent form to a univalent form. The multivalent form, in a manner analogous to agglutination by immunoglobulins, presumably links cells together into aggregates (Tyler, 1949). During swarming, the sperm somehow break up the multivalent fertilizin (egg jelly) into univalent form. The univalent form binds to the sperm surface, filling all available receptors, but is unable to agglutinate sperm. Hathaway and Metz (1962) presented evidence that ^{35}S-labeled jelly remains bound to sperm that have deagglutinated. However, the recent data of SeGall and Lennarz (1979) on isolation of the fucose sulfate-rich fraction from egg jelly show that this material induces the acrosome reaction but not agglutination in sperm. This finding suggests that the radioactivity is bound to receptors involved in the acrosome reaction but not in swarming. Although SeGall and Lennarz (1979) have not analyzed the biological activity of the sialoprotein component of egg jelly, there is a report (Isaka et al., 1970) that swarming is associated with the sialoprotein fraction from fractionated egg jelly in Japanese sea urchins. Further analysis of this phenomenon will require a more complete characterization of the swarm-inducing substance from egg jelly. The swarm-inducing substance from egg jelly of the starfish *Asterias amurensis* has been isolated and characterized (Uno and Hoshi, 1978). Chemical analysis indicates that it is a saponin. However, unlike sea urchin sperm, the swarming of starfish sperm is irreversible and the clusters can be preserved by fixatives, suggesting the nature of the response in asteroids is different from echinoids.

What role does sperm swarming have in fertilization? Lillie (1919) believed that the agglutinating substance, "fertilizin," was modified by the sperm to a form that could induce activation of the egg. However, sperm need not swarm in order to fertilize; sperm of at least one species, *Lytechinus pictus*, do not swarm at all. However, *S. purpuratus* sperm will swarm in *Lytechinus* egg jelly (Collins, 1976), suggesting again that the swarming factor may be released by sperm.

Sperm-Specific Surface Antigenicity Common to Seven Animal Phyla

During our studies on the sea urchin sperm membrane, we raised an antiserum that displayed unusual reactivity. This antiserum cross-reacted with the surface of sperm of 28 species from seven animal phyla. To this date we have not found a negative cross-reaction.

The antiserum was prepared by injecting whole glutaraldehyde-fixed *S. purpuratus* sperm into a virgin female rabbit. The whole serum of course had multiple specificities directed against sperm, but following absorption with sea urchin somatic cells and minced ovary there remained a specific reactivity for the sperm surface. This reactivity could be totally eliminated by absorption with fixed or living *S. purpuratus* sperm. We tested this sperm-specific antiserum (SSA) for reactivity with sperm of other species and found that it reacted to some degree with sperm of every species we tested (Table II). Activity was assayed by the immunoperoxidase reaction using Hanker–Yates reagent and by indirect immunofluorescence (Figure 9). Every nonsperm cell tested gave a negative reaction with SSA.

Because of the unusual reactivity of the serum, we carried out an

Table II

Reaction of SSA Prepared against *Strongylocentrotus purpuratus*
Sperm with Sperm of Other Species[a]

Phylum Coelenterata	Phylum Echinodermata
Class Anthozoa	Class Echinoidea
Metridium senile fibriatum	*S. purpuratus*
Phylum Annelida	*S. franciscanus*
Class Polychaeta	*S. pallidus*
Family Spionidae (1 species)	*S. droebachiensis*
Family Polynoidae (1 species)	*Lytechinus pictus*
Phylum Mollusca	*Arbacia punctulata*
Class Amphineura	*Tripneustes gratilla*
Cryptochiton stelleri	*Dendraster excentricus*
Class Gastropoda	Class Ophiuroidea
Acmaea sp.	*Ophioplocus esmarkii*
Class Pelecypoda	Class Asteroidea
Macoma nasuta	*Patiria miniata*
Phylum Echiuroidea	Phylum Chordata
Urechis caupo	Class Urochordata
Phylum Arthropoda	*Styela clava*
Class Crustacea	*S. plicata*
Cancer antennarius	*Ciona intestinalis*
Pinnixa tubicola	Class Osteichthyes
Class Merostomata	*Salmo* sp.
Limulus polyphemus	Class Amphibia
	Rana pipiens
	Class Aves
	Meleagris gallopavo
	Class Mammalia
	Mesocricetus auratus
	Rattus norvegicus

[a] Reactivity of the SSA was assayed by indirect immunofluorescence or by the immunofluorescence or by the immunoperoxidase procedure. The sperm were fixed in either 3%
glutaraldehyde or formaldehyde. Preimmune serum did not react (Lopo and Vacquier,
1980c).

extensive series of controls to establish that the observed activity was not an
artifact. A glutaraldehyde-hapten effect was ruled out because (1) the SSA
also reacted with living and formaldehyde-fixed sperm; (2) two other sera
were raised, one using whole, unfixed sea urchin sperm and one against a 1%
Triton X-100 extract of living sea urchin sperm, and both had identical
reactivity to the initial SSA; and (3) the SSA activity could be absorbed out by
living or formaldehyde-fixed sperm. The latter point also showed that the
activity was associated with the surface (Lopo and Vacquier, 1980c). Other
controls to establish that the SSA activity was not an artifact included
determining that the activity was not due to Freund's adjuvant (Russo *et al.*,
1975), or to nonspecific binding of the Fc region of antibodies (Allen and

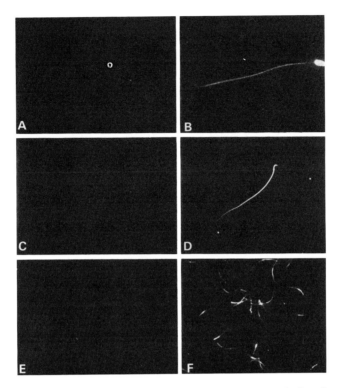

Figure 9. Reactivity of SSA with sperm of three species visualized by indirect immunofluorescence. (A,B) Sea urchin, (C,D) rat; (E,F) turkey. (A,C,E) Preimmune serum; (B,D,F) immune serum (SSA). The fluorescence appears over the entire sperm surface. (Reproduced with permission of Macmillan Journals from Lopo and Vacquier, 1980c.)

Bourne, 1978). Recognition of an accessory male gland secretion by SSA was also ruled out. The activity we observed was not due to cross-reacting antigens of mammalian sperm, preimplantation embryos, or the central nervous system (Schachner *et al.*, 1975; Solter and Schachner, 1976; Chaffee and Schachner, 1978), because rat brain did not cross-react and did not absorb the activity.

We excluded the possibility that the SSA was H-Y antigen (Wachtel, 1977a,b; Silvers and Wachtel, 1977) in three ways. First, absorbing the serum with sea urchin male somatic cells did not decrease or eliminate the activity. Second, extensive absorption of the serum with male rat spleen cells (Goldberg *et al.*, 1971) did not remove the activity. Finally, and most convincingly, turkey sperm gave a positive response. In birds the female is the heterogametic sex, and therefore the bearer of H-Y antigen (Ohno, 1979).

We do not know what function this cross-reactive determinant(s)

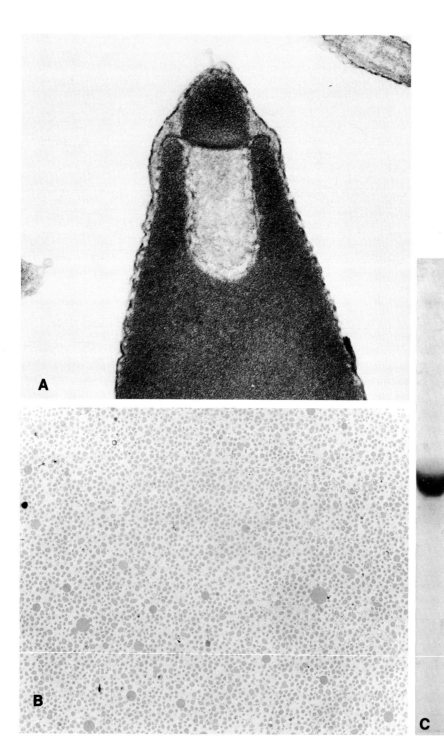

common to the surface of animal sperm may have. It (they) could be a differentiation antigen that appears during spermatogenesis. These results are intriguing because a common sperm-surface antigenicity has broad implications for the development of immunocontraceptive methods. We are presently performing immunoprecipitation studies to determine the number of specificities recognized by the SSA.

Isolation of Acrosome Granules and Identification of Bindin as the Major Component Involved in Sperm Adhesion

Isolation of Bindin from Sea Urchin Sperm

When echinoderm sperm are exposed to egg jelly they undergo the acrosome reaction (Figure 1). This event was first described by Popa (1927), but the significance of his observations was not understood until reinterpreted by Jean Clark Dan (1952, 1954) some years later.

The first visible change in sperm undergoing the acrosome reaction is the formation of several fusion sites between the acrosome granule and the overlying plasma membrane (Summers *et al.*, 1975) that expose the contents of the granule. As this fusion progresses, material presumed to be unpolymerized g-actin, or profilactin (Tilney *et al.*, 1973) stored in the subacrosomal space, polymerizes into filamentous f-actin and forms a bundle of microfilaments anchored to a specialized region of the outer surface of the nuclear envelope (Tilney, 1976a,b, 1978; Tilney and Mooseker, 1976). As the microfilament bundle extends, it pierces the now-exposed acrosome granule and becomes coated with the granule contents. The resulting acrosome-reacted sperm bears a process approximately 1 μm long, covered in its entirety by the contents of the acrosome granule (Moy and Vacquier, 1979).

Popa (1927) correctly assumed that adhesion of sperm to other objects was mediated by the contents of the granule. This assumption was later supported by work on the fine structure of sperm–egg adhesion, showing that the granule material coating the acrosome process is localized at the point of attachment of sperm to egg (reviewed in Summers *et al.*, 1975). Vacquier and Moy (1977) isolated the acrosome granules of *S. purpuratus* sperm and demonstrated that the major component is a single protein of molecular weight 30,500 ("bindin") (Figure 10C). The isolated acrosome granules

---

Figure 10. (A) Transmission electron micrograph of *S. purpuratus* sperm. Note acrosome granule at tip of sperm. × 44,000. (Unpublished photograph courtesy of V. D. Vacquier and G. W. Moy.) (B) Transmission electron micrograph of acrosome granules isolated from *S. purpuratus* sperm. × 2220. (Unpublished photograph courtesy of V. D. Vacquier and G. W. Moy.) (C) SDS electrophoresis in 12.5% polyacrylamide gel of isolated acrosome granule material reveals a single component of molecular weight 30,500. (From Vacquier and Moy, 1977.)

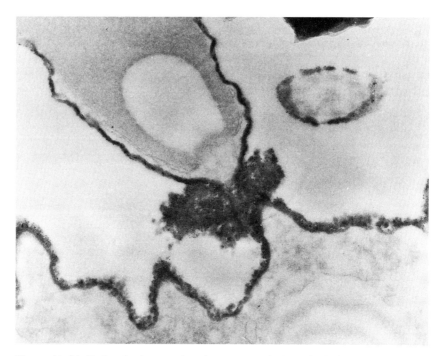

Figure 11. Bindin localized at the site of sperm–egg binding. Bindin is seen on the sperm membrane and on the egg surface adjacent to the site of sperm attachment; × 79,000. (Unpublished photograph courtesy of G. W. Moy and V. D. Vacquier.)

closely resemble those in intact sperm in size and morphology (Figure 10A and B). Antibody raised against electrophoretically purified bindin was used to show that the material localized in the acrosome process and at the site of sperm–egg attachment (Figure 11). The antibody also showed that bindin is not exposed at the sperm surface until after the acrosome reaction, furnishing additional evidence that the acrosome reaction is required for successful fertilization (Moy and Vacquier, 1979). In addition, Glabe and Vacquier (1977a) and Glabe and Lennarz (1979) showed that bindin is a species-specific agglutinin of unfertilized sea urchin eggs (Figure 12). Based on this evidence bindin has been proposed to be the mediator of species-specific sperm–egg adhesion.

A partial characterization of bindin from *S. purpuratus* and *S. franciscanus* indicates that the two molecules have very similar amino acid compositions. The only species difference is in the number of aspartic acid and proline residues (Bellet *et al.*, 1977). There is also a large number of coincident spots in the peptide maps of the two species (Bellet *et al.*, 1977), and a high degree of homology in the known amino acid sequence (first 45 residues;

Vacquier and Moy, 1978). Antibody to *S. purpuratus* bindin cross-reacts with the acrosome granule of all species of the class Echinoidea but not with members of other echinoderm classes (Moy and Vacquier, 1979).

Levine *et al.* (1978; Levine and Walsh, 1979, 1980) recently demonstrated the presence of an acrosinlike protease exposed after the induction of the acrosome reaction of sea urchin sperm. Eighty percent of the protease activity associated with *S. purpuratus* sperm is exposed following treatment with egg jelly. The enzyme is bound to the cell and is not released to the medium. Levine *et al.* (1978; Levine and Walsh, 1979, 1980) proposed that the enzyme is the sea urchin counterpart to mammalian acrosin. Using immunoelectron microscopy, Green and Summers (1980) demonstrated that the protease is a component of the acrosome granule.

Bindin in Other Phyla

Bindinlike molecules have been described from two other invertebrates. Brandriff *et al.* (1978) isolated acrosome granules from the oyster *Crassostrea gigas*. The isolated granules resembled those of intact sperm in size and morphology and agglutinated oyster eggs. Gel electrophoresis separated the

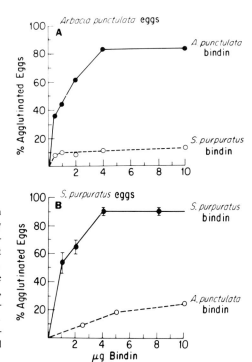

Figure 12. Agglutination of eggs from *A. punctulata* and *S. purpuratus* by bindin. (A) *A. punctulata* eggs are agglutinated by *A. punctulata* bindin, but only to a small extent by bindin from *S. purpuratus*. (B) *S. purpuratus* eggs are agglutinated by *S. purpuratus* bindin, but only limited agglutination is observed with bindin from *A. punctulata*. (Reproduced with permission of Rockefeller University Press from Glabe and Lennarz, 1979.)

isolated granules into two compnents of molecular weights 65,000 and 53,000. Unlike sea urchin bindin, these two components stain strongly with PAS, showing they are glycoproteins. Dry weight analysis reveals a protein composition of 85%.

Using the procedure developed by Brandriff et al (1978), Stephano Hornedo and Gould-Somero (personal communication) have recently isolated the acrosome region from the marine worm *Urechis caupo* (phylum Echiuroidea). The material is extremely insoluble. It does not appear to be species-specific in its surface interation with eggs because it also agglutinates sea urchin eggs and *Pelvetia* zygotes (Stephano Hornedo and Gould-Somero, personal communication). On acid-urea gels it migrates close to calf thymus histone, suggesting a low molecular weight. The purified protein appears to contain no carbohydrate (by gas chromatography analysis). Although 50% of the amino acid residues are lysine and arginine, the protein is not a histone.

Identification of a Bindin Receptor Glycoprotein from the Egg Vitelline Layer

Evidence for the Presence of Sperm Receptors on the Egg Surface

Bindin appears to be the species-specific molecule involved in the attachment of sea urchin sperm to the egg vitelline layer. It follows that sperm receptors exist on the surface of the egg. Their existence has been inferred from several lines of evidence outlined in Table III and discussed below.

Observation 1 (Table III) is concerned with the digestion of unfertilized eggs with trypsin, resulting in reduced fertilizability (Aketa et al., 1972; Schmell et al., 1977). Studies on the trypsinlike cortical granule protease released at fertilization (observation 2) extended the above results. Unfertilized eggs incubated in cortical granule protease bind sperm in greatly reduced numbers. Release of the cortical granules shortly after fertilization coincides with detachment of sperm from the vitelline layer as the layer transforms into the fertilization envelope. This detachment suggests that the protease removes specific protein receptors on the vitelline layer that interact with the bindin on the sperm surface. These conclusions are reinforced by the finding that sperm remain attached to the vitelline layer following fertilization in the presence of trypsin inhibitors, resulting in polyspermic eggs (Vacquier et al., 1972). This not only strengthens the conclusion that the cortical granule protease plays a role in removing these putative receptors but also suggests that in doing so it develops a block to polyspermy (Vacquier et al., 1973) by removing supernumerary sperm from the egg surface.

Observations 3 and 4 are both corollaries to the preceding discussion.

Table III

Evidence for Sperm Receptors of the Egg Vitelline Layer

---

1. Unfertilized eggs treated with trypsin show reduced fertilizability (Aketa *et al.*, 1972; Schmell *et al.*, 1977).
2. Unfertilized eggs incubated in cortical granule protease bind sperm in reduced numbers (Vacquier *et al.*, 1973; Carroll and Epel, 1975).
3. Unfertilized eggs treated with trypsin or cortical granule protease are not agglutinated by bindin (Vacquier and Moy, 1978).
4. Large glycoproteins can be isolated from egg vitelline layers that show species-specific inhibition of fertilization (Aketa, 1967, 1973, 1975; Schmell *et al.*, 1977; Tsuzuki, *et al.*, 1977; Glabve and Vacquier, 1978; Glabe and Lennarz, 1979, 1981).
5. Acrosome-reacted sperm exhibit species-specific binding (Summers and Hylander, 1975, 1976; Kinsey *et al.*, 1980).
6. Sperm binding exhibits saturation kinetics (Vacquier and Payne, 1973).
7. Sperm bind only to the external surface of isolated vitelline layers (Glabe and Vacquier, 1977b).
8. Bindin agglutinates eggs in a species-specific fashion (Glabe and Vacquier, 1977a; Vacquier and Moy, 1977; Glabe and Lennarz, 1979).

Unfertilized eggs that have been trypsinized or treated with cortical granule protease are not agglutinated by bindin (Vacquier and Moy, 1977, 1978), presumably because the receptor molecules on the egg surface have been removed. By the same token, the digest from eggs treated with cortical granule protease blocks bindin-dependent agglutination of intact eggs (Vacquier and Moy, 1977).

Observation 5, briefly mentioned in the previous section, involves the highly species-specific binding of sperm to eggs. Sperm will often undergo the acrosome reaction following exposure to egg jelly of a different species, but in almost every case, the same sperm will not bind to the vitelline layer of eggs of other species (Summers and Hylander, 1975, 1976; Kinsey *et al.*, 1980). Observation 6 deals with the kinetics of binding of sperm. There appears to be a maximum, species-specific number of sperm that can attach to an egg (Vacquier and Payne, 1973). A possible explanation for this phenomenon is that there are a limited number of receptors on the egg surface to which sperm can bind (although there are alternative explanations, such as steric hindrance by the binding sperm or degradation of receptors by enzymes released by sperm that are already attached).

Observation 7 suggests that there is an asymmetric arrangement of sperm receptor molecules on the vitelline layer, so that bindin will attach sperm only when they are in contact with the external surface of the vitelline layer (Figure 13; Glabe and Vacquier, 1977b). Observation 8, discussed in the preceding section, suggests that bindin must have its species-specific counterpart to complete the attachment step successfully (Glabe and Vacquier, 1977a; Vacquier and Moy, 1977).

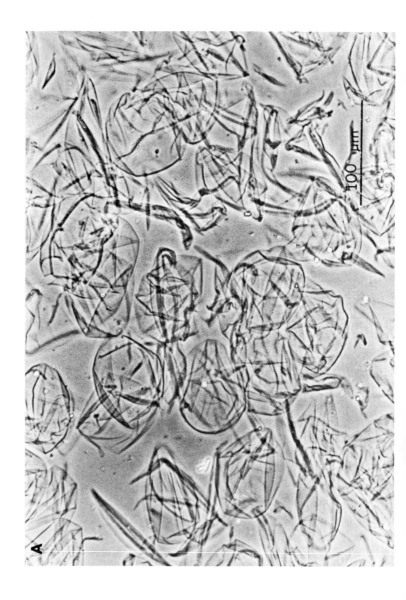

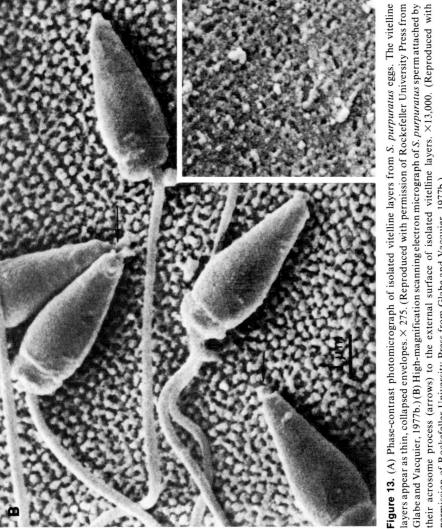

Figure 13. (A) Phase-contrast photomicrograph of isolated vitelline layers from *S. purpuratus* eggs. The vitelline layers appear as thin, collapsed envelopes. × 275. (Reproduced with permission of Rockefeller University Press from Glabe and Vacquier, 1977b.) (B) High-magnification scanning electron micrograph of *S. purpuratus* sperm attached by their acrosome process (arrows) to the external surface of isolated vitelline layers. ×13,000. (Reproduced with permission of Rockefeller University Press from Glabe and Vacquier, 1977b.)

Isolation of Bindin Receptors from the Vitelline Layer

To determine whether the protease-sensitive molecule(s) on the egg surface is a bindin receptor, Glabe and Vacquier (1978) isolated the material released from ^{125}I-labeled eggs following parthenogenetic activation with the ionophore A23187 in both the presence and the absence of protease inhibitors. A simple filter assay was used to determine whether this supernatant fraction contained the putative receptor to bindin. Binding of the putative receptor by bindin was saturable (Figure 14), showing that complex formation between bindin and an egg-surface-derived macromolecule occurred.

Because of previous evidence showing that sperm–egg binding is species-specific (Summers and Hylander, 1976; Kinsey *et al.*, 1980), the specificity of the receptor fraction was investigated using competition assays (Glabe and Vacquier, 1978). Cold receptor from *S. purpuratus* was found to be more effective than that of *S. franciscanus* in dissociating labeled bindin–receptor complexes from *S. purpuratus*. A preliminary biochemical characterization of the bindin receptor fraction showed that all the receptor activity was associated with a fraction of at least 5×10^6 molecular weight. The material was further fractionated by isoelectric focusing. This separated the fraction into two components, one of pI 2.25 (presumed to be egg jelly) and a second component of pI 4.02, containing an enrichment in binding affinity. This

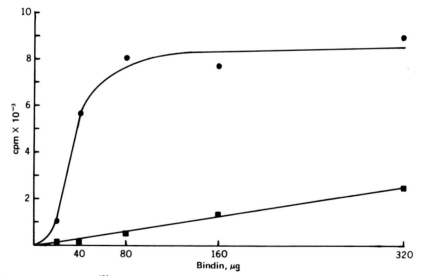

Figure 14. Binding of ^{125}I-labeled egg surface material released during activation to bindin. The crude receptor (●), obtained by activating ^{125}I-labeled eggs in soybean trypsin inhibitor, exhibits greater binding activity than does the degraded receptor (■) prepared in the absence of the inhibitor. (From Glabe and Vacquier, 1978.)

fraction was 4% sulfate and contained mannose, galactose, and no sialic acid, showing that it is not egg jelly, which is 17% sulfate and contains fucose and sialic acid (SeGall and Lennarz, 1979).

The nature of the egg surface bindin receptor material has been further investigated by Glabe and Lennarz (1979, 1981). They found, on examining the surface material released by Pronase digestion of unfertilized eggs, that it inhibited the bindin-dependent agglutination of eggs (Glabe and Lennarz, 1979). This was consistent with the earlier finding of Vacquier and Moy (1977; Glabe and Vacquier, 1977a). However, there was no species specificity observed: glycopeptide fractions from *A. punctulata* eggs were equally successful in inhibiting egg agglutination as those from *S. purpuratus* (Glabe and Lennarz, 1979).

Glabe and Lennarz (1981) biochemically characterized the egg surface Pronase digest. The material responsible for inhibition of egg agglutination also agglutinated bindin particles, making possible the affinity purification of the egg surface glycopeptide. Analysis of the activity thus obtained shows only the presence of fucose, xylose, and galactose.

Conclusions

The Sperm Surface. The 84K glycoprotein of the sea urchin sperm membrane is the first known membrane component that may have a role in the induction of the acrosome reaction. Similar components may exist on the surface of mammalian sperm, because of the many similarities in the physiological changes taking place during the acrosome reaction of sea urchin and mammalian sperm (Meizel, 1978). Further research on the role of 84K may help identify the ionic mechanisms responsible for initiation of this process. The many recent findings on the composition of the mammalian sperm surface (Feuchther and Eddy, 1980; Myles *et al.*, 1980; Primakoff *et al.*, 1980) may lead to the discovery of a mammalian counterpart to 84K.

Sperm–Egg Fusion. There is essentially no information on the molecular events of sperm–egg membrane fusion at fertilization. In the sea urchin the entire egg surface is apparently available for fusion. A consequence of fusion is that the egg membrane depolarizes, resulting in a transient rise in membrane potential to about $+10$ to $+20$ mV (Steinhardt *et al.*, 1971; Jaffe, 1976). This depolariztion prevents additional sperm from fusing with the egg (Jaffe, 1976).

Because sea urchin sperm bind to eggs by the bindin-coated acrosome process, the plasma membrane of the acrosome process is the portion of the sperm that fuses with the egg. This raises the possibility that the acrosome granule components may have a fusigenic role. The acrosin exposed during the acrosome reaction may modify bindin into a fusigenic protein, as is the case with the F protein of Sendai virus (Gething *et al.*, 1978). Also, there is evidence for the exposure of phospholipases during the acrosome reaction (Conway and Metz, 1976). These could function alone or in concert with an acrosin-modified bindin to mediate gamete fusion.

Sperm–Egg Binding. Sea urchin sperm bindin is the first protein to be isolated from any metazoan in fairly pure milligram quantities that mediates a specific intercellular adhesion. The isolation of the bindin receptor glyco-protein marks the first time the interacting surface components of both sperm and egg have been isolated from any organism. Because mammals also exhibit species-specific attachment of sperm to the egg zona pellucida (Yanagimachi, 1977), it is safe to assume that sperm bindin and egg surface bindin receptors also exist in higher organisms. Much work is urgently needed to understand the nature of bindin, the bindin receptor, and the interaction of these two gamete surface components. The information obtained from such endeavors will permit us to construct a truly molecular model of the events of animal fertilization.

ACKNOWLEDGMENTS

The authors wish to thank Dr. Stephen L. Wolfe for reviewing and editing the manuscript. We are also grateful to Drs. Nicholas L. Cross, Charles G. Glabe, Meredith Gould-Somero, William J. Lennarz, and Jose Stephano Hornedo for sharing their unpublished manuscripts and results with us. Supported by NIH HD 12986 to VDV. ACL is an NIH postdoctoral fellow.

References

Aketa, K., 1967, On the sperm–egg bonding as the initial step of fertilization in the sea urchin, *Embryologia* **9**:238–245.

Aketa, K., 1975, Physiological studies on the sperm surface component responsible for sperm-egg bonding in sea urchin fertilization. I. Effect of sperm-binding proteins on the fertilizing capacity of sperm, *Exp. Cell Res.* **80**:439–441.

Aketa, K., 1975, Physiological studies on the sperm surface component responsible for sperm-egg bonding in sea urchin fertilization. II. Effect of concanavalin A on the fertilizing capacity of sperm, *Exp. Cell Res.* **90**:56–62.

Aketa, K., Onitake, K., and Tsuzuki, H., 1972, Tryptic disruption of sperm-binding site of sea urchin egg surface, *Exp. Cell Res.* **71**:27–32.

Allen, G. J., and Bourne, F. J., 1978, Interaction of immunoglobulin fragments with the mammalian sperm acrosome, *J. Exp. Zool.* **203**:271–276.

Austin, C. R., 1966, *Fertilization*, Prentice–Hall, Englewood Cliffs, N. J.

Barros, C., and Yanagimachi, R., 1971, Induction of zona reaction in golden hamster eggs by cortical granule material, *Nature (London)* **233**:268–269.

Bellet, N. R., Vacquier, J. P., and Vacquier, V. D., 1977, Characterization and comparison of "bindin" isolated from sperm of two species of sea urchins, *Biochem. Biophys. Res. Commun.* **79:**159–165.

Bleil, J. D., and Wassarman, P. M., 1980a, Structure and function of the zona pellucida: Identification and characterization of the proteins of the mouse oocyte's zona pellucida, *Dev. Biol.* **76:**185–202.

Bleil, J. D., and Wassarman, P. M., 1980b, Mammalian sperm–egg interaction: Identification of a glycoprotein in mouse egg zonae pellucidae possessing receptor activity for sperm, *Cell* **20:**873–882.

Brandriff, B., Moy, G. W., and Vacquier, V. D., 1978, Isolation of sperm bindin from the oyster (*Crassostrea gigas*), *Gamete Res.* **1:**89–99.

Carroll, E. J., and Epel, D., 1975, Isolation and biological activity of the proteases released by sea urchin eggs following fertilization, *Dev. Biol.* **33:**22–32.

Chaffee, J. K., and Schachner, M., 1978, NS-6 (nervous system antigen-6): A new cell surface antigen of brain, kidney, and spermatozoa, *Dev. Biol.* **62:**173–184.

Chandler, J., and Heuser, J., 1980, The vitelline layer of the sea urchin egg and its modification during fertilization, *J. Cell Biol.* **84:**618–632.

Collins, F., 1976, A reevaluation of the fertilizin hypothesis of sperm agglutination and the description of a novel form of sperm adhesion, *Dev. Biol.* **49:**381–394.

Collins, F., and Epel, D., 1977, The role of calcium ions in the acrosome reaction of sea urchin sperm, *Exp. Cell Res.* **106:**211–222.

Colwin, L. H., and Colwin, A. L., 1967, Membrane fusion in relation to sperm–egg association, in: *Fertilization*, Volume 1 (C. B. Metz and A. Monroy, eds.), Academic Press, New York, pp. 295–367.

Conway, A. F., and Metz, C. B., 1976, Phospholipase activity of sea urchin sperm: Its possible involvement in membrane fusion, *J. Exp. Zool.* **198:**39–48.

Czihak, G., 1975, *The Sea Urchin Embryo: Biochemistry and Morphogenesis*, Springer-Verlag, New York.

Dan, J. C., 1952, Studies on the acrosome. I. Reaction to egg-water and other stimuli, *Biol. Bull.* **103:**543–61.

Dan, J. C., 1954, Studies on the acrosome. III. Effect of calcium deficiency, *Biol. Bull.* **107:**335–349.

Dan, J. C., 1956, The acrosome reaction, *Int. Rev. Cytol.* **5:**365–393.

Dan, J. C., 1967, Acrosome reaction and lysins, in: *Fertilization*, Volume 1 (C. B. Metz and A. Monroy, eds.), Academic Press, New York, pp. 237–293.

Decker, G. L., Joseph, D. B., and Lennarz, W. J., 1976, A study of factors involved in induction of the acrosomal reaction in sperm of the sea urchin, *Arbacia punctulata*, *Dev. Biol.* **53:**115–125.

Dunbar, B. S., Wardrip, N. J., and Hedrick, J. L., 1980, Isolation, physicochemical properties, and macromolecular composition of zona pellucidae from procine oocytes, *Biochemistry* **19:**356–365.

Epel, D., 1978, Mechanisms of activation of sperm and egg during fertilization of sea urchin gametes, *Curr. Top. Dev. Biol.* **12:**185–246.

Epel, D., and Vacquier, V. D., 1978, Membrane fusion events during invertebrate fertilization, *Cell Surface Rev.* **5:**1–63.

Feuchther, F. A., and Eddy, E. M., 1980, Monoclonal antibodies to mouse sperm surfaces, *J. Cell Biol.* **87:**147a.

Foerder, C. A., and Shapiro, B. M., 1977, Release of ovoperoxidase from sea urchin eggs hardens the fertilization membrane with tyrosine cross-links, *Proc. Natl. Acad. Sci. USA* **74:**4214–4218.

Fulton, B. P., and Whittingham, D. G., 1978, Activation of mammalian oocytes by intracellular injection of calcium, *Nature (London)* **273:**149–151.

Gabel, C. A., Eddy, E. M., and Shapiro, B. M., 1979, Regional differentiation of the sperm surface as studied with ^{125}I-diiodofluorescein isothiocyanate, an impermeant reagent that allows isolation of the labeled components, *J. Cell Biol.* **82:**742–754.

Garbers, D. L., and Kopf, G. S., 1980, The regulation of spermatozoa by cyclic nucleotides, *Adv. Cyclic Nucleotide Res.* **13:**251–306.

Gething, M. J., White, J. M., and Waterfield, N. D., 1978, Purification of the fusion protein of Sendai virus: Analysis of the NH₂-terminal sequence generated during precursor activation, *Proc. Natl. Acad. Sci. USA.* **75:**2737–2740.

Gilkey, J. C., Jaffe, L. S., Ridgway, L. S. B., and Reynolds, G. T., 1977, A free calcium wave traverses the activating egg of the medaka *Oryzias latipes, J. Cell Biol.* **76:**448–466.

Giudice, G., 1973, *Developmental Biology of the Sea Urchin Embryo,* Academic Press, New York.

Glabe, C. G., and Lennarz, W. J., 1979, Species-specific sperm adhesion in sea urchins: A quantitative investigation of bindin-mediated egg agglutination, *J. Cell Biol.* **83:**595–604.

Glabe, C. G., and Lennarz, W. J., 1981, Isolation and partial characterization of a high molecular weight egg surface glycoconjugate implicated in sperm adhesion, *J. Supramol. Struct.,* submitted.

Glabe C. G., and Vacquier, V. D., 1977a, Species-specific agglutination of eggs by bindin isolated from sea urchin sperm, *Nature (London)* **267:**836–838.

Glabe, C. G., and Vacquier, V. D., 1977b, Isolation and characterization of the vitelline layer of sea urchin eggs, *J. Cell Biol.* **75:**410–421.

Glabe, C. G., and Vacquier, V. D., 1978, Egg surface glycoprotein receptor for sea urchin sperm bindin, *Proc. Natl. Acad. Sci. USA* **75:**881–885.

Goldberg, G. H., Boyse, E. A., Bennett, D., Chied, N., and Carswell, E. A., 1971, Serological demonstration of H-Y (male) antigen on mouse sperm *Nature* **232:**478–480.

Gray, J. P., and Drummond, G. I., 1976, Guanylate cyclase of sea urchin sperm: subcellular localization, *Arch. Biochem. Biophys.* **172:**31–38.

Green, J. D., and Summers, R. G., 1980, Ultrastructural demonstration of trypsin-like protease in acrosome of sea urchin sperm, *Science* **209:**398–400.

Gwatkin, R. B. L., Williams, D. T., Hartmann, J. F., and Kniazuk, M., 1973, The zona reaction of hamster and mouse eggs: Production *in vitro* by a trypsin-like protease from cortical granules, *J. Reprod. Fertil.* **32:**259–265.

Hall, H. G., 1978, Hardening of the sea urchin fertilization envelope by peroxidase-catalyzed phenolic coupling of tryosines, *Cell* **15:**343–355.

Hanada, A., and Chang, M. C., 1972, Penetration of zona-free eggs by spermatozoa of different species, *Biol. Reprod.* **6:**300–309.

Hathaway, R. R., and Metz, C. B., 1962, Interactions between *Arbacia* sperm and ^{35}S-labeled fertilizin, *Biol. Bull.* **120:**360–369.

Isaka, S., Hotta, K., and Kurokawa, M., 1970, Jelly coat substances of sea urchin eggs, *Exp. Cell Res.* **59:**37–42.

Jaffee, L. A., 1976, Fast block to polyspermy in sea urchin eggs is electrically mediated, *Nature* **261:**68–71.

Kidd, P., 1978, The jelly and vitelline coats of the sea urchin egg: New ultrastructural features, *J. Ultrastruct. Res.* **64:**204–215.

Kinsey, W. H., Rubin, J. A., and Lennarz, W. J., 1980, Studies on the specificity of sperm binding in echinoderm fertilization, *Dev. Biol.* **74:**245–250.

Levine, A. E., and Walsh, K. A., 1979, Involvement of an acrosin-like enzyme in the acrosome reaction of sea urchin sperm, *Dev. Biol.* **72:**126–137.

Levine, A. E., and Walsh, K. A., 1980, Purification of an acrosin-like enzyme from sea urchin sperm, *J. Biol. Chem.* **255:**4814–4820.

Levine, A. E., Walsh, K. A., and Fodor, E. J. B., 1978, Evidence of an acrosin-like enzyme in the acrosome reaction of sea urchin sperm, *Dev. Biol.* **72:**126–137.

Lillie, F. R., 1915, Sperm agglutination and fertilization, *Biol. Bull.* **23**:18–33.

Lillie, F. R., 1919, *Problems of Fertilization*, University of Chicago Press, Chicago.

Loeb, J., 1916, *The Organism as a Whole*, University of Chicago Press, Chicago.

Longo, F. J., and Kunkle, M., 1978, Transformations of sperm nuclei upon insemination, *Curr. Top. Dev. Biol.* **12**:149–184.

Lopo, A. C., and Vacquier, V. D., 1980a, Radioiodination and characterization of the plasma membrane of sea urchin sperm, *Dev. Biol.* **76**:15–25.

Lopo, A. C., and Vacquier, V. D., 1980b, Antibody to a sperm surface glycoprotein inhibits the egg jelly-induced acrosome reaction of sea urchin sperm, *Dev. Biol.* **79**:325–333.

Lopo, A. C., and Vacquier, V. D., 1980c, Sperm-specific surface antigenicity common to seven animal phyla, *Nature (London)* **288**:397–399.

Lopo, A., Bean, C. P., and Epel, D., 1977, Studies on sperm–jelly interaction: Is there chemotaxis?, *Biol. Bull.* **153**:437.

Lui, C. W., and Meizel, S., 1979, Further evidence in support of a role for hamster sperm hydrolytic enzymes in the acrosome reaction, *J. Exp. Zool.* **207**:173–182.

Mar, H., 1980, Radial cortical fibers and pronuclear migration in fertilized and artificially activated eggs of *Lytechinus pictus*, *Dev. Biol.* **78**:1–13.

Meizel, S., 1972, Biochemical detection and activation of an inactive form of a trypsin-like enzyme in rabbit testes, *J. Reprod. Fertil.* **31**:459–462.

Meizel, S., 1978, The mammalian sperm acrosome reaction, a biochemical approach, in: *Development in Mammals*, Volume 3 (M. H. Johnson, ed.), North-Holland, New York, pp. 1–64.

Metz, C. B., 1967, Gamete surface components and their role in fertilization, in: *Fertilization*, Volume 1 (C. B. Metz and A. Monroy, eds.), Academic Press, New York, pp. 163–236.

Metz, C. B., 1978, Sperm and egg receptors involved in fertilization, *Curr. Top. Dev. Biol.* **12**:107–147.

Metz, C. B., and Monroy, A., (eds.), 1967, *Fertilization*, Academic Press, New York.

Miller, R. L., 1966, Chemotaxis during fertilization in the hydroid *Campanularia*, *J. Exp. Zool.* **162**:23–44.

Miller, R. L., 1975, Chemotaxis of the spermatozoa of *Ciona intestinalis*, *Nature (London)* **254**:244–245.

Miller, R. L., 1979a, Sperm chemotaxis in the hydromedusae, I. Species-specificity and sperm behavior, *Mar. Biol.* **53**:99–114.

Miller, R. L., 1979b, Sperm chemotaxis in the hydromedusae. II. Some chemical properties of the sperm attractants, *Mar. Biol.* **53**:115–124.

Miller, R. L., and Brokaw, C. J., 1970, Chemotactic turning behaviour of *Tubularia* spermatozoa, *J. Exp. Biol.* **52**:669–706.

Miller, R. L., and Tseng, C. Y., 1974, Properties and partial purification of the sperm attractant of *Tubularia*, *Am. Zool.* **14**:467–486.

Monroy, A., 1965, *Chemistry and Physiology of Fertilization*, Holt, Rinehart & Winston, New York.

Moy, G. W., and Vacquier, V. D., 1979, Immunoperoxidase localization of binding during the adhesion of sperm to sea urchin eggs, *Curr. Top. Dev. Biol.* **13**:31–44.

Müller, D. G., Gassmann, G., and Leining, K., 1979, Isolation of a spermatozoid-releasing and -attracting substance from female gametophytes of *Laminaria digitata*, *Nature* **279**:430–431.

Myles, D. G., Primakoff, P., and Bellve, A. R., 1980, Establishment and maintenance of cell surface domains of the guinea pig sperm, *J. Cell Biol.* **87**:99a.

Ohno, S., 1979, Major sex-determining genes, in: *Monographs on Endocrinology*, Volume 11 (F. Gross, A. Labhard, M. B. Lipsett, T. Mann, L. T. Samuels, and J. Sander, eds.), Springer-Verlag, New York, pp. 1–140.

Peterson, R. N., Russell, L., Bundman, D., and Freund, M., 1980, Sperm–egg interaction: Evidence for boar sperm plasma membrane receptors for procine zona pellucida, *Science* **207**:73–74.

Popa, G. T., 1927, The distribution of substances in the spermatozoon (*Arbacia* and *Nereis*), *Biol. Bull.* **52**:238–257.

Primakoff, P., Myles, D. G., and Bellve, A. R., 1980, Topographical organization of the mammalian sperm surface, *J. Cell Biol.* **87**:98a.

Runnstrom J., 1966, The vitelline membrane and cortical particles in sea urchin eggs and their function in maturation and fertilization, *Adv. Morphog.* **5**:221–325.

Russo, J., Metz, C. B., and Dunbar, B. S., 1975, Membrane damage to immunologically immobilized rabbit spermatozoa visualized by immunofluorescence and scanning electron microscopy, *Biol. Reprod.* **13**:136–141.

Schachner, M., Wortham, K. A., Carter, L. D., and Chaffee, J. K., 1975, NS-4 (nervous system antigen-4), a cell surface antigen of developing and adult mouse brain and sperm, *Dev. Biol.* **44**:313–325.

Schackmann, R. W., and Shapiro, B. M., 1981, A partial sequence of ionic changes associated with the acrosome reaction of *Strongylocentrotus purpuratus*, *Dev. Biol.* **81**:145–154.

Schackmann, R. W., Eddy, E. M., and Shapiro, B. M., 1978, The acrosome reaction of *Strongylocentrotus purpuratus* sperm: Ion requirements and movements, *Dev. Biol.* **65**:483–495.

Schatten, H., and Schatten, G., 1980, Surface activity at the egg plasma membrane during sperm incorporation and its cytochalasin B sensitivity, *Dev. Biol.* **78**:435–449.

Schmell, E. D., and Gulyas, B. J., 1980, Ovoperoxidase activation in ionophore-treated mouse eggs. II. Evidence for the enzyme's role in hardening the zona pellucida, *Gamete Res.* **3**:279–290.

Schmell, E., Earles, B. J., Breaux, C., and Lennarz, W. J., 1977, Identification of a sperm receptor on the surface of the eggs of the sea urchin *Arbacia punctulata*, *J. Cell. Biol.* **72**:35–46.

SeGall, G. K., and Lennarz, W. J., 1979, Chemical characterization of the component of the jelly coat from sea urchin eggs responsible for induction of the acrosome reaction, *Dev. Biol.* **71**:33–48.

Silvers, W. K., and Wachtel, S. S., 1977, H-Y antigen: Behavior and function, *Science* **195**:956–960.

Solter, D., and Schachner, M., 1976, Brain and cell surface antigens (NS-4) on preimplantation mouse embryos, *Dev. Biol.* **52**:98–104.

Steinhardt, R. A., Lundin, L., and Mazia, D., 1971, Bioelectric responses of echinoderm egg to fertilization, *Proc. Natl. Acad. Sci.* **68**:2426–2430.

Summers, R. G., and Hylander, B. L., 1975, Species-specificity of acrosome reaction and primary gamete binding in echinoids, *Exp. Cell Res.* **96**:63–68.

Summers, R. G., and Hylander, B. L., 1976, Primary gamete binding: Quantitative determination of its specificity in echinoid fertilization, *Exp. Cell Res.* **100**:190–194.

Summers, R. G., Hylander, B. L., Colwin, L. H., and Colwin, A. L., 1975, The functional anatomy of the echinoderm spermatozoon and its interaction with the egg at fertilization, *Am. Zool.* **15**:523–551.

Summers, R. G., Talbot, P., Keough, E. M., Hylander, B. L., and Franklin, L. E., 1976, Ionophore A23187 induces acrosome reactions in sea urchin and guinea pig spermatozoa, *J. Exp. Zool.* **196**:381–386.

Talbot, P., Summers, R. G., Hylander, B. L., Keough, E. M., and Franklin, L. E., 1976, The role of calcium in the acrosome reaction: An analysis using ionophore A23187, *J. Exp. Zool.* **198**:383–392.

Tilney, L. G., 1976a, The polymerization of actin. II. How nonfilamentous actin becomes nonrandomly distributed in sperm: Evidence for the association of this actin with membrane, *J. Cell Biol.* **69**:51-72.

Tilney, L. G., 1976b, The polymerization of actin. III. Aggregates of nonfilamentous actin and its associated proteins: A storage form of action, *J. Cell Biol.* **69**:73-89.

Tilney, L. G., 1978, The polymerization of actin, IV. A new organelle, the actomere, that initiates the assembly of actin filaments in *Thyone* sperm, *J. Cell Biol.* **71**:46.

Tilney, C. G., and Mooseker, M. S., 1976, Actin filament-membrane attachment: Are membrane proteins involved? *J. Cell Biol.* **71**:402-416.

Tilney, L. G., Hatano, S., Ishikawa, H., and Mooseker, M. S., 1973, The polymerization of actin: Its role in the generation of the acrosomal process of certain echinoderm sperm, *J. Cell Biol.* **59**:109-126.

Tilney, L. G., Kiehart, D. P., Sardet, C., and Tilney, M., 1978, Polymerization of actin. IV. Role of Ca^{+2} and H^+ in the assembly of actin and in membrane fusion in the acrosomal reaction of echinoderm sperm, *J. Cell Biol.* **77**:536-550.

Tilney, L. G., Clain, J. C., and Tilney, M. S., 1979, Membrane events in the acrosomal reaction of *Limulus* sperm, *J. Cell biol.* **81**:229-253.

Tsuzuki, H., and Aketa, K., 1969, A study on the possible significance of carbohydrate moiety in the sperm-binding protein from sea urchin egg, *Exp. Cell Res.* **55**:43-45.

Tsuzuki, H., Yoshida, M., Onitake, K., and Aketa, K., 1977, Purification of the sperm-binding factor from the egg of the sea urchin, *Hemicentrotus pulcherrimus*, *Biochem. Biophys. Res. Commun.* **76**: 502-508.

Tyler, A., 1949, Properties of fertilizin and related substances of eggs and sperm of marine animals, *Am. Nat.* **83**:195-219.

Uno, Y., and Hoshi, M., 1978, Separation of the sperm agglutinin and the acrosome-reaction inducing substance in egg jelly of starfish, *Science* **200**:58-59.

Vacquier, V. D., 1979a, The fertilizing capacity of sea urchin sperm rapidly decreases after induction of the acrosome reaction, *Dev. Growth Differ.* **21**:61-69.

Vacquier, V. D., 1979b, The interactions of sea urchin gametes during fertilization, *Am. Zool.* **19**:839-849.

Vacquier, V. D., 1980, The adhesion of sperm to sea urchin eggs, in: *The Cell Surface, Mediator of Developmental Processes* (N. K. Wessells, ed.), 38th Symposium of the Society for Developmental Biology.

Vacquier, V. D., and Moy, G. W., 1977, Isolation of bindin: The protein responsible for adhesion of sperm to sea urchin eggs, *Proc. Natl. Acad. Sci. USA* **74**:2456-2460.

Vacquier, V. D., and Moy, G. W., 1978, Macromolecules mediating sperm-egg recognition and adhesion during sea urchin fertilization, in: *Cell Reproduction* (E. R. Dirksen, D. M. Prescott, and C. F. Fox, eds.), Academic Press, New York, pp. 389-397.

Vacquier, V. D., and Payne, J. E., 1973, Methods for quantitating sea urchin sperm-egg binding, *Exp. Cell Res.* **82**;227-235.

Vacquier, V. D., Tegner, M. J., and Epel, D., 1972, Protease activity established the block against polyspermy in sea urchin eggs, *Nature (London)* **240**:352-353.

Vacquier, V. D., Tegner, M. J., and Epel, D., 1973, Protease released from sea urchin eggs at fertilization alters the vitelline layer and aids in preventing polyspermy, *Exp. Cell Res.* **80**:111-119.

Vacquier, V. D., Brandriff, B., and Glabe, C. G., 1979, The effect of soluble egg jelly on the fertilizability of acid-dejellied sea urchin eggs, *Dev. Growth Differ.* **21**:47-60.

Wachtel, S. S., 1977a, H-Y antigen: Genetics and serology, *Immunol. Rev.* **33**:3-58.

Wachtel, S. S., 1977b, H-Y antigen and the genetics of sex determination, *Science* **198**:797-799.

Yanagimachi, R., 1972, Fertilization of guinea pig eggs *in vitro*, *Anat. Rec.* **174**:9-20.

Yanagimachi, R., 1977, Specificity of sperm-egg interaction, in: *Immunobiology of Gametes* (M.

H. Johnson and M. Edidin, eds.), Cambridge University Press, London, pp. 255–296.

Yanagimachi, R., 1978, Spern–egg association in mammals, *Curr. Top. Dev. Biol.* **12:**83–106.

Yanagimachi, R., and Usui, N., 1974, Calcium dependence of the acrosome reaction and activation of guinea pig spermatozoa, *Exp. Cell Res.* **89:**161–174.

Zucker, R. S., Steinhardt, R. A., and Winkler, M. M., 1978, Intracellular calcium release and the mechanisms of parthenogenetic activation of the sea urchin egg, *Dev. Biol.* **65:**285–295.

8

AWAKENING OF THE INVERTEBRATE EGG AT FERTILIZATION

BENNETT M. SHAPIRO

The previous chapter dealt with mechanisms by which the invertebrate sperm responds to the egg, first undergoing the acrosome reaction and then binding to it before gamete membrane fusion. The fusion of sperm and egg is catastrophic for both the organism and the species. A new individual is formed with a reassortment of meiotic products that constitutes a new roll of the evolutionary dice. The mechanism of formation of the zygote has received increasing attention over the past decade with the application of modern techniques in molecular and cellular biology. In this chapter I will focus on some recent insights concerning several phenomena associated with activation of the sea urchin egg after fertilization. Work in this field occurs in the context of an excellent scientific literature that dates back well over a century; I shall try to point out some of the classical antecedents of the modern study of fertilization mechanisms.

Sperm–Egg Fusion and the Rapid Block to Polyspermy

The fusion of sperm and egg was first analyzed by Fol (1877), who noted that a filament seemed to attach the sperm to the egg before sperm penetration (Figure 1). The relationship of this filament to sperm entry was clarified by the elegant morphological analyses of the Colwins (e.g., 1967), who showed that the intergametic liason was effected by an acrosomal process that extended from the tip of the sperm to initiate contact with the egg. This interaction

BENNETT M. SHAPIRO • Department of Biochemistry, University of Washington, Seattle, Washington 98195

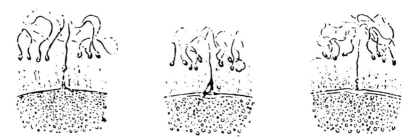

Figure 1. Attachment of sperm to egg by the acrosomal filament, a phenomenon first noticed by Fol (1877) and later shown to reflect the extension of an acrosomal process (Colwin and Colwin, 1967). (Figure from Fol, 1877.)

between the tip of the acrosome and the egg plasma membrane occurs in many marine invertebrates. The acrosomal process is formed by the assembly or uncoiling of an actin-containing filament (e.g., Tilney *et al.*, 1973, 1978, 1979), which then initiates contact with the egg plasma membrane. This contact elicits responses in the egg that reduce the probability of entry of the subsequent sperm; collectively these processes are called the blocks to polyspermy. As a phenomenon the block to polyspermy was best characterized 25 years ago by Rothschild (1956) as an event composed of two separate processes (Figure 2): a transient, incomplete block to polyspermy in

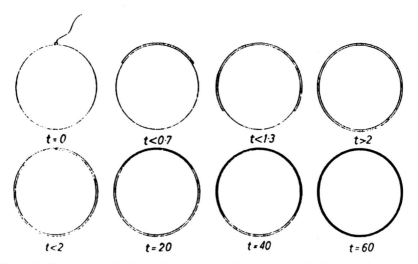

Figure 2. The existence of both a rapid and a delayed component to the block to polyspermy as discussed in Rothschild (1956). The assignment of two phases was based principally on the kinetics of interaction of sperm with eggs. (Figure from Rothschild, 1956.)

the first few seconds, and a slower, complete block accomplished within minutes of fertilization. The delayed, definitive block to polyspermy is effected by alterations in the fertilization membrane that occur during the cortical reaction, as discussed below. Although the existence of a rapid block to polyspermy has been questioned on occasion (e.g., Byrd and Collins, 1975), it appears not only to exist but to have a physiological mechanism based upon the electrical response of the egg to fertilization (Jaffe, 1976). The membrane potential of the egg depolarizes at fertilization (e.g., Steinhardt *et al.*, 1971; Jaffe, 1976), often simultaneously with the occurrence of the rapid block to polyspermy. Moreover, if the egg is subjected to a voltage clamp at a positive membrane potential, fertilization is impaired. Conversely, if depolarization is blocked by an appropriate voltage clamp, polyspermy occurs (Jaffe, 1976). Thus, the membrane potential of the egg seems to regulate some aspect of sperm–egg receptivity, although the involved step has not yet been elucidated.

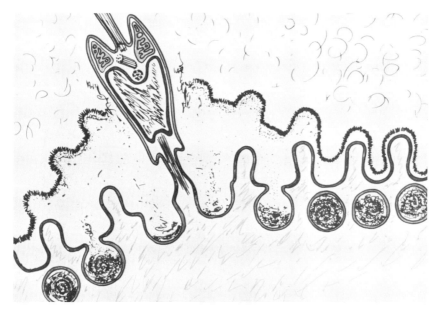

Figure 3. A cartoon of sperm–egg fusion in echinoderms. In this drawing, but not necessarily in reality, fusion is initiated between the acrosomal process of the sperm and the tip of an egg microvillus. The surrounding cortical vesicles have begun to release their contents, which participate in the elevation of the vitelline layer and in its conversion into a fertilization membrane. The cortical vesicles undergo exocytosis in a wave from the point of attachment of the fertilizing sperm, more than doubling the surface area of the egg plasma membrane. Sperm components seem to be internalized by a microfilament-mediated process that pulls the sperm in despite the forceful rearrangement of the egg surface in the cortical reaction.

Insertion and Localization of Sperm Components in the Egg

What happens to the sperm after it fuses with the egg? As shown in Figure 3, sperm–egg membrane fusion leads to secretion of some thousands of cortical vesicles that underlie the plasma membrane, resulting in the elevation of the fertilization membrane. Starting at the apical end of the acrosome, the

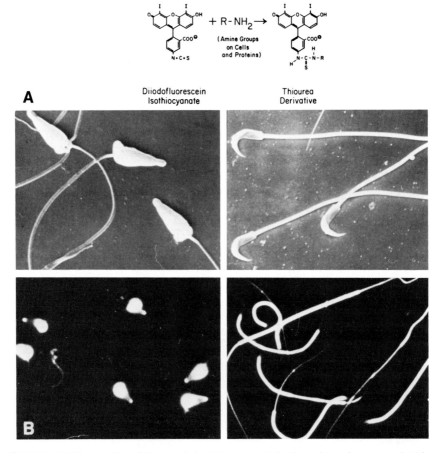

Figure 4. (A) The reaction of fluorescein isothiocyanate derivatives with amine groups. In this case the fluorescent and potentially radioactive diiodofluorescein isothiocyanate is shown. The amine groups can be constituents of proteins or phospholipids in the cell membrane; representatives of each class seem to be modified in labeled sperm. (B) Scanning electron micrographs (upper photos) and fluorescence micrographs (lower photos) of sea urchin (left) and hamster (right) sperm. In the fluorescence micrographs the sperm were labeled with fluorescein isothiocyanate; the most intense labeling is found over the midpiece in both species. In the case of the sea urchin the midpiece is a small region at the base of the head; in mammalian sperm the midpiece is elongated in the initial region of the tail.

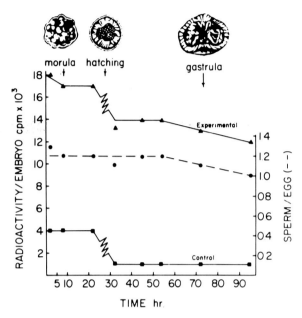

Figure 5. Persistence of sperm-derived radioactivity throughout early development. Sea urchin (*S. purpuratus*) sperm were labeled with [125]IFC, washed, and then used to fertilize eggs. Embryos recovered at different times after fertilization were washed and their radioactivity determined. Control embryos were first fertilized with nonradioactive sperm, after which radioactive sperm were added in an amount equivalent to the experimental embryos; the radioactivity was then similarly determined at various times during early development. A decrease in radioactivity at the time of hatching probably reflects the loss of sperm components that are adventitiously bound to the fertilization membrane. Note that the difference between experimental and control remains constant throughout development to the late gastrula stage. When the specific radioactivity of the sperm was used to determine the number of sperm equivalents per embryo, the result was the expected one sperm per egg. (Data from Gabel *et al.*, 1979b.)

echinoderm sperm plasma membrane fuses with that of the egg, presumably forming a mosaic membrane, as well as establishing a continuity between sperm and egg cytoplasms. In order to study the fate of the sperm surface material after membrane fusion, we have covalently labeled the sperm with fluorescent and radioactive isothiocyanate derivatives as shown in Figure 4. Fluorescein isothiocyanate, a well-studied reagent for labeling cell surfaces reacts with exposed amino groups. We have made a radioactive derivative, [125]Idiiodofluorescein isothiocyanate, that reacts with the surface of erythrocytes (Gabel and Shapiro, 1978) and sperm (Gabel *et al.*, 1979a). This reagent serves as a convenient tag of sperm components throughout the developmental sequence. Surprisingly, labeled sperm components persist in the developing embryo (Figure 5) even as late as the pluteus larval stage (Gabel *et al.*, 1979b). We would have expected sperm components to undergo

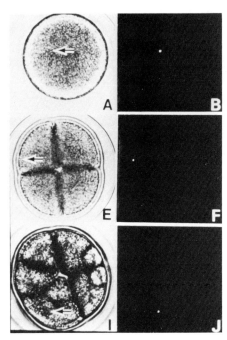

Figure 6. Sperm-derived fluorescence remains as a patch throughout early development of the sea urchin, *S. purpuratus.* Phase-contrast micrographs (A, C, E, G, I, K) and the corresponding fluorescence micrographs (B, D, F, H, J, L) are shown for 1-, 2-, 4-, 8-, and 16-cell embryos, as

turnover at a finite rate if they behaved like components of somatic cells; however, the radioactivity of the labeled surface components persisted in macromolecular form throughout the multiple cell divisions occurring over a 4-day period (Figure 5). The persistence is more striking when the location of the labeled material in the embryo is studied by fluorescence microscopy. As shown in Figure 6, labeled sperm components persist as a patch throughout early development. One blastomere serves as the repository of the sperm components, which seem to remain localized even up to the pluteus larval stage in those experiments where we have obtained optimal visualization of the patch (Gundersen, unpublished data). The patch has no unusual association with the animal–vegetal axis (Gabel *et al.*, 1979b), a developmental gradient laid down during oogenesis. We are interested in carefully analyzing later embryos to see whether any relationship exists between the patch and the dorsal–ventral axis, a developmental gradient that may be related to the point of sperm entry. The patch is not only localized in sea urchins, but also remains in one blastomere of mouse embryos throughout early embryogenesis (Gabel *et al.*, 1979b). Thus, as early as the first cell division the two blastomeres of the embryo may be distinguished; one of them

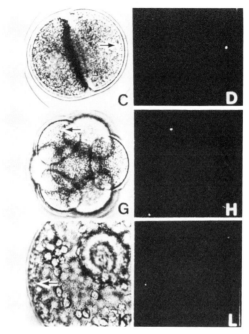

well as for gastrula, respectively. The arrows in the phase-contrast micrographs show the location of the fluorescent patch from the corresponding fluorescence micrograph. Sperm were labeled with FITC and washed before fertilization; the data were obtained and taken from experiments similar to those reported in Gabel *et al.* (1979b).

contains a complement of paternal cytoplasmic components. In other words, both sea urchin and mammalian embryos are differentiated in their molecular composition, a finding of unknown significance for their further development. In this regard, the location of the components in the embryo is of interest: although labeling in the sperm is predominantly on the surface, the labeled materials are found just beneath the surface in the embryo (Gundersen *et al.*, 1980).

Being able to trace sperm components after fertilization affords us an opportunity to ask questions about the mechanism of internalization of the sperm. A clue to the workings of this process came from studies with cytochalasins, which do not block the cortical reaction (Eddy and Shapiro, 1976) of fertilization and yet inhibit incorporation of the sperm pronucleus (Gould-Somero *et al.*, 1977; Longo, 1978; Byrd *et al.*, 1977). We repeated these experiments with sperm and eggs of the sea urchin, *Strongylocentrotus purpuratus*, but examined the fate of both fluorescent sperm surface components and pronuclei after fertilization. About half of the eggs that are fertilized in the presence of cytochalasin B or D have no sperm pronucleus or

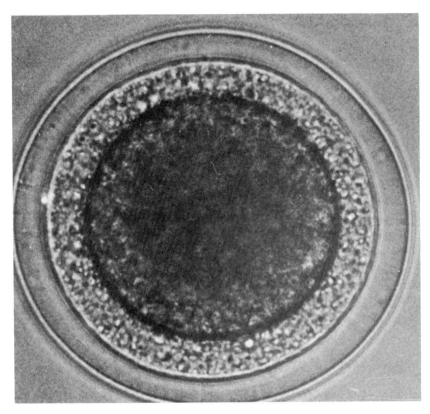

Figure 7. The fluorescent sperm patch in cytochalasin-treated eggs. Eggs of *S. purpuratus* were incubated with 10 μg/ml cytochalasin B for 5 min prior to fertilization. The sperm, fluorescently labeled with FITC, transfers fluorescent components to the egg, but they remain just at the point of focus of the egg surface, inside the fertilization membrane, instead of becoming internalized as seen in controls. Note the distortion of the cortex in the cytochalasin-treated egg.

patches in them. The other half of the eggs have the fluorescent patch from the sperm located just at the surface of the egg, having apparently arrested at the plasma membrane (Figure 7). The patch rests inside the fertilization membrane, but has not moved into the deeper cortical location characteristic of unperturbed fertilization. The pronucleus is also found just at the level of the plasma membrane (Figure 8A) in about half of the embryos treated with cytochalasin B or D. When the cytochalasin is washed away from the fertilized eggs, the fluorescent patch migrates to a position inside of the egg, in the cortical region; the pronucleus also becomes internalized and begins to decondense (Figure 8B; Gundersen *et al.*, 1980). The progression of the patch from a surface site to an internal site may be conveniently monitored by image-intensified fluorescent microscopy, giving a kinetic measurement of internalization. As internalization of sperm components is inhibited by cytochalasin at concentrations similar to those that block cleavage, its effect on sperm internalization is most likely due to a disruption of an actin-dependent cytoskeletal process that we propose to be involved in the incorporation process.

The Cortical Reaction and Extracellular Peroxidative Reactions

As shown in Figure 3, sperm–egg fusion is accompanied by a secretory response, the cortical reaction, in which the release of the contents of the cortical vesicles changes the properties of the vitelline layer, converting it into a fertilization membrane. The secretion process, shown by scanning electron microscopy in Figure 9, proceeds in a wave from the point of attachment of the fertilizing sperm; the inserted cortical granule membranes more than double the surface area of the egg. The secretory product contains protease activity that functions not only to promote the elevation of the vitelline layer, but also to remove sperm receptors, thereby serving as one of the components of the delayed block to polyspermy (Vacquier et al., 1972; Schuel et al., 1973). Preliminary purification attempts have suggested that two activities reside in distinct proteolytic enzymes (Carroll and Epel, 1975). However, a homogeneous serine protease has been purified and identified as the cortical vesicle protease; it is inactive in eggs but activated after fertilization (Fodor et al., 1975). In addition to elevating the fertilization membrane and removing sperm receptors, there may be additional roles for the protease(s), as a limited proteolytic cleavage of several egg surface components occurs at fertilization or after artificial activation of eggs (Shapiro, 1975). The role, if any, of this limited proteolysis in development has not been identified.

Elevation of the fertilization membrane occurs in a well-defined sequence of steps (Veron et al., 1977), resulting in a hard glycoprotein coat that is resistant to most forms of denaturation. Although some proteins may be extracted from the assembled structure (Carroll and Baginski, 1978), it is only fully solubilized when polypeptide bonds are broken. The assembly sequence proceeds from a soft fertilization membrane that readily collapses down on the surface of the egg (Figure 10A) and contains domelike casts of the microvilli (called "igloos") (Figure 10C) to a final hardened structure that resists denaturation or the drying resulting from sample preparation for microscopy (Figure 10B), the casts having been converted to pyramidal, tentlike forms (Figure 10D). This assembly sequence is subject to inhibition at several stages (Veron et al., 1977). For example, as shown in Figure 10E, a soft fertilization membrane with domelike casts is obtained in the presence of glycine ethyl ester. The final hardened structure (Figure 10F) with tentlike projections is raised from the plasma membrane, whose microvilli are

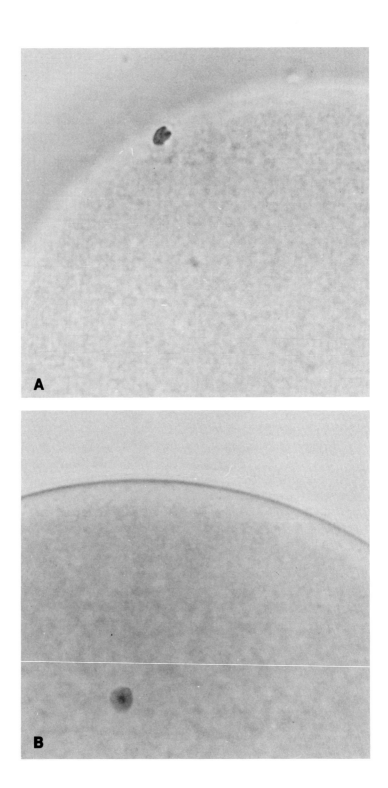

elongated, probably in order to incorporate the additional membrane introduced by cortical vesicle exocytosis.

The hardening reaction is effected by the formation of dityrosine cross-links between adjacent polypeptide chains of the assembled soft fertilization membrane (Foerder and Shapiro, 1977). The egg secretes an ovoperoxidase from the cortical granules to catalyze the cross-linking, using as the oxidative substrate hydrogen peroxide made at the time of fertilization from molecular oxygen (Foerder et al., 1978). Several pieces of evidence support this hypothesis (Foerder and Shapiro, 1977; Hall, 1978). The enzyme, ovoperoxidase, is released from eggs at the time of fertilization; it resides in the cortical granules before fertilization and afterwards is incorporated into the assembled fertilization membrane (Figure 11). Inhibitors of the hardening reaction that were known from classical embryology all inhibit the ovoperoxidase. Conversely, known peroxidase inhibitors are potent inhibitors of hardening. Dityrosine synthesis is a known property of peroxidases, and dityrosine residues are found in hardened fertilization membranes at one per 50,000–100,000 daltons of protein, an appropriate amount to account for the cross-linking (Foerder and Shapiro, 1977).

The peroxidase inhibitors have afforded us the ability to study the chemistry of fertilization membrane assembly. Thus, by using 3-amino-1,2,4-triazole to inhibit ovoperoxidase activity, the fertilization membranes remain soft and eggs may be removed from them at any time (Showman and Foerder, 1979). We have exploited this property to isolate soft fertilization membranes as shown in Figure 12 (Kay et al., 1980). Although they are stable in seawater, these soft fertilization membranes fall apart in solutions of low ionic strength. This disappearance of the soft fertilization membrane is termed *wraithing* and may be measured by several procedures: a decrease in light scattering, a loss of refractivity by phase microscopy, or by the release of specific proteins as determined by gel electrophoresis. An example of the light-scattering change seen in the wraithing process is shown in Figure 13. In seawater the soft fertilization membranes are stable and maintain their refractivity; however, in dilute buffers the light scattering of the preparations decreases. This phenomenon can be reversed or protected by specific cations. The cations that are effective in blocking the wraithing process, or in reversing it at the concentrations present in normal seawater, include: Mg^{2+} (Figure 13), Ca^{2+}, and Na^+. The soft fertilization membrane is thus a noncovalently assembled structure that is stabilized by specific cations; when these cations are removed,

---

Figure 8. Pronuclear location in cytochalasin-treated sea urchin eggs. When the pronuclear location was assessed in eggs fertilized in the presence of cytochalasin B, the sperm pronuclei remain condensed just at the egg surface (A). This is in contrast to that occurring in normal fertilization, or when cytochalasin is washed away, when the pronucleus enters and decondenses (B).

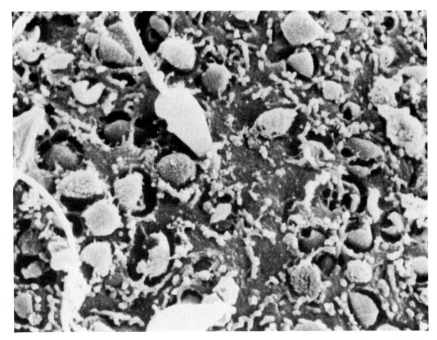

Figure 9. Scanning electron micrographs of the surface of *S. purpuratus* eggs from which the fertilization membrane has been removed. The sperm is seen fusing with the plasma membrane, and the exocytotic release of the contents of surrounding cortical vesicles may be observed. (Data from Eddy and Shapiro, 1976.)

it falls apart. We view the wraithing process as an experimental reversal of fertilization membrane assembly and think that the ionic composition of seawater modulates the coordinated assembly of that structure (Kay *et al.*, 1980).

Once assembled, the soft fertilization membrane can be hardened, as shown *in vivo* (Foerder and Shapiro, 1977) and also *in vitro* (Figure 14). The soft fertilization membrane is composed of 8–10 polypeptides, one of which (of 50,000 daltons) is the ovoperoxidase. It may be hardened *in vitro* by the addition of hydrogen peroxide. As shown in Figure 14, addition of hydrogen peroxide causes several high-molecular-weight peptides to disappear from the gel: protein is instead found on top of the stacking gel, a characteristic of

Figure 10. Stages in assembly of the fertilization membrane of *S. purpuratus*. As initially elevated, the fertilization membrane is soft and wrinkles under the conditions of drying (A) used in microscopy; it contains casts of the tips of the egg plasma membrane microvilli (C). However, within a few minutes the fertilization membrane becomes hard (B) and the casts are changed from a domelike configuration to a pyramidal one (D). The pyramidal forms may be seen on end as tentlike structures, by transmission electron microscopy (F). In the presence of inhibitors of the hardening reaction, like glycine ethyl ester, the hardening does not occur and often the transition from domelike to tentlike casts is blocked (E). (Data from Vernon *et al.*, 1977.)

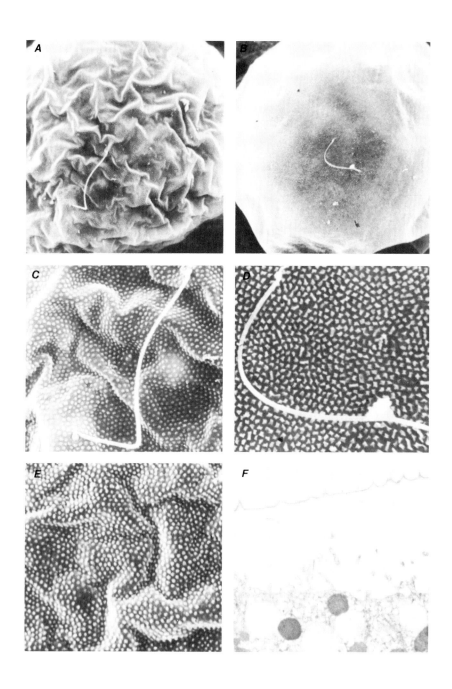

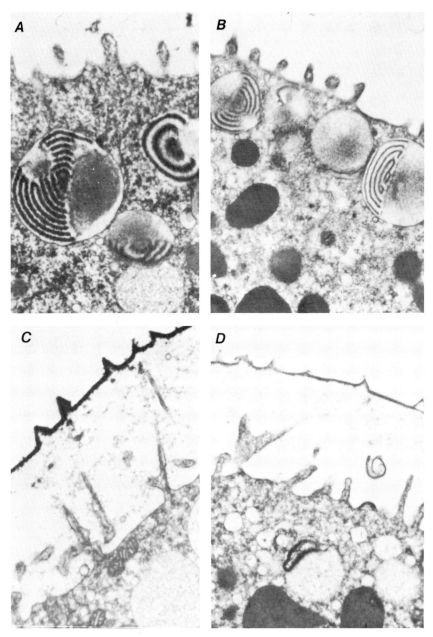

Figure 11. Location of the ovoperoxidase before and after fertilization. (A) Stained with diaminobenzidine and hydrogen peroxide, the peroxidase is localized in the lamellae of the cortical granules. (B) In the presence of the peroxidase inhibitor aminotriazole, these lamellae do not stain. (C) After fertilization, the ovoperoxidase is found in the assembled hard fertilization membrane. (D) A control in the presence of aminotriazole shows no staining.

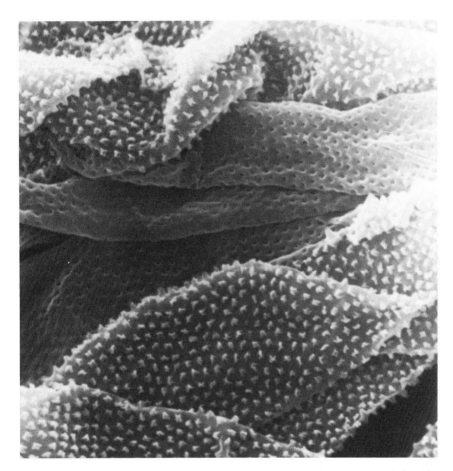

Figure 12. A soft fertilization membrane of *S. purpuratus* eggs. This structure was isolated by fertilizing eggs in the presence of aminotriazole and passing the eggs through Nytex, to remove the soft fertilization membranes, as described by Showman and Foerder (1979). Note that the fertilization membrane prepared under these conditions has the tentlike forms, although it is clearly wrinkled and not hardened by several criteria.

hardened fertilization membrane (Shapiro, 1975). *In vitro* hardening is independent of exogenously added ovoperoxidase, suggesting that the endogenous ovoperoxidase of the fertilization membrane is capable of catalyzing the cross-linking; thus, it must be juxtaposed to the residues that will be cross-linked. However, the ovoperoxidase itself is not cross-linked, as shown by its entry into the gel even after the hardening reaction. When the hardening reaction is performed in the presence of trace amounts of ^{125}I, radioactivity is rapidly incorporated into protein. After a 30-sec incubation, certain protein bands become highly radioactive (Figure 14, gel 30 s) and are

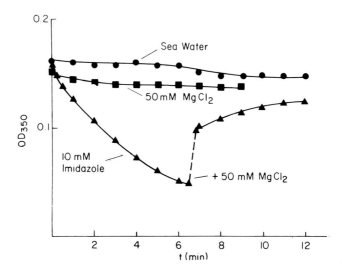

Figure 13. Light-scattering changes accompanying the dilution of soft fertilization membranes into media of low ionic strength. Upon dilution into 10 mM imidazole, the light scattering at 350 nm decreases, a reaction that is inhibited in seawater or by elevated concentrations of bivalent cations (here 50 mM MgCl$_2$). Readdition of bivalent cation causes a restoration of the light-scattering properties.

finally excluded (Figure 14, gel 18 m); the other proteins become only moderately radioactive at both time periods. As iodine is a substrate for peroxidative reactions, and the ovoperoxidase catalyzes iodination of the fertilization membrane *in vivo* (Hall, 1978; Klebanoff *et al.*, 1979), we can use this reaction to identify the proteins that are most susceptible to peroxidatic attack. As expected, these are the proteins that are excluded from the gel during the cross-linking reaction. Taken together these data suggest that cortical vesicle proteins join components of the vitelline layer to assemble a soft fertilization membrane in a reaction modulated by ions in the seawater. This structure is cross-linked by the appropriately positioned ovoperoxidase using the hydrogen peroxide synthesized by the egg.

The synthesis of hydrogen peroxide is an interesting phenomenon that recalls the observations of Warburg (1908) on activation of metabolism at fertilization. Hydrogen peroxide synthesis occurs in a burst after fertilization (Foerder *et al.*, 1978) as shown in Figure 15, and this burst of hydrogen peroxide synthesis accounts for two-thirds of the oxygen uptake during the first 15 min after fertilization; it occurs concomitantly with the burst of oxygen uptake. Hydrogen peroxide is toxic to sperm as are peroxidatic reactions (see discussion in Foerder *et al.*, 1978), and in addition to hardening of the fertilization membrane this system may effect an additional block to polyspermy.

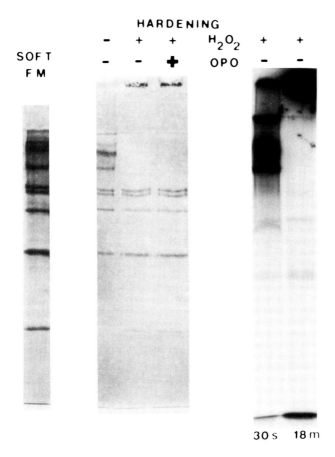

Figure 14. SDS–polyacrylamide gel electrophoresis of soft fertilization membrane before and after hardening. On the left the protein composition of soft fertilization membranes is shown. The marked band of lowest molecular weight is the ovoperoxidase. In the center are shown the effects of addition of either hydrogen peroxide alone or hydrogen peroxide and ovoperoxidase to soft fertilization membranes. Note that the three bands of high molecular weight disappear upon addition of hydrogen peroxide and can now be seen accumulating on top of the stacking gel. The addition of ovoperoxidase is unnecessary for this reaction, which is thus apparently catalyzed by the endogenous ovoperoxidase. The two gels on the right show the effect of adding a tracer amount of ^{125}I to fertilization membranes during the hardening reaction. As previously shown (Klebanoff *et al.*, 1979), the peroxidase is capable of iodinating proteins. In this case the proteins that are iodinated after short incubation (30 s) are the ones that are later cross-linked and excluded from the gel (18 m). Thus, the proteins that are cross-linked are optimal peroxidative targets; the other proteins in the gel are iodinated to only a small extent.

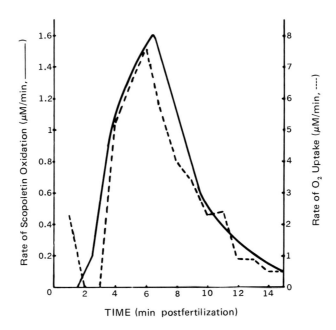

Figure 15. Oxygen uptake and hydrogen peroxide production at fertilization. Oxygen uptake increases in a burst after fertilization as first described by Warburg (1908). This burst occurs concomitantly with increased hydrogen peroxide synthesis, here detected by the peroxidase-catalyzed oxidation of scopoletin (see Foerder *et al.*, 1978).

The egg has developed a complex series of oxidative reactions that it carries on extracellularly in order to cross-link its fertilization membrane and perhaps to kill extra sperm in its vicinitiy. This system is reminiscent of one used by the polmorphonucleur leukocyte (PMN) during phagocytosis (Klebanoff *et al.*, 1979). As shown in Table I, an oxidase makes activated oxygen species in both cases and a peroxidase uses these activated oxygen species to effect some redox reaction. In phagocytosis the oxidase accounts for the respiratory burst, the reductant for oxygen being either NADH or NADPH. The reductant has not yet been identified in fertilization, although increased hexose monophosphate shunt activity in fertilization suggests that NADPH may be employed. In both systems hydrogen peroxide is made; the PMN also makes superoxide anion. The peroxidative reaction of fertilization uses an ovoperoxidase and the PMN uses a myeloperoxidase. In both systems enzymes located in cytoplasmic granules are released after specific stimuli. Chemiluminescence accompanies both peroxidative reactions, and both systems catalyze model reactions like iodination, deiodination, and estradiol binding. The similarities in these two systems that function in widely

Table I
Similarities between Fertilization and Phagocytosis

$$O_2 \xrightarrow{\text{oxidase}} \text{activated oxygen} \xrightarrow{\text{peroxidase}} \text{chemical modification}$$

	Fertilization	Phagocytosis
Oxidase		
Respiratory burst	+	+
NAD(P)H	?	+
Increase hexose monophosphate shunt	+	+
H_2O_2	+	+
Superoxide production	?	+
Peroxidase	(ovoperoxidase)	(myeloperoxidase)
Located in cytoplasmic granule	+	+
Released upon specific stimuli	+	+
Chemiluminescence	+	+
Iodination	+	+
Spermicidal	?	+
Deiodination	+	+
Estradiol binding	+	+
Dityrosine synthesis	+	?

separated cells from different animal phyla are striking and demonstrate yet another fascinating example of the economy of the evolutionary process.

Activation of Egg Metabolism

The past few years have seen an increase in the study of the regulation of egg activation by ions and other small molecules. Table II summarizes some of our current ideas about the roles of ions in the activation process. The fertilization action potential is the first ionic event and generally is dependent upon an increased sodium permeability. This, as noted earlier, is correlated with a decreased receptivity of the egg to sperm. This process is followed by a transient increase in intracellular free Ca^{2+} levels that occurs soon after fertilization and appears to be the mediator of exocytosis of the cortical reaction (e.g., Ridgeway et al., 1977; Steinhardt et al., 1977). Although the Ca^{2+} release has not been well defined, some evidence suggests that a microsomal fraction of eggs is capable of Ca^{2+} uptake and release, perhaps analogous to the sarcoplasmic reticulum of muscle. Many aspects of metabolic activation of the egg occur slightly later than the Ca^{2+}-dependent effects and appear to be mediated by an increase in intracellular pH. These

Table II

Ions and Activation

Ionic flux	Physiological response
Action potential	Decreased receptivity to sperm
Na permeability	(rapid block to polyspermy)
Ca^{2+} increase—transient	Cortical reaction
? Ooplasmic reticulum	Vesicle exocytosis
	Fertilization membrane elevation
	Peroxidative system
	(O_2 uptake, H_2O_2 production,
	dityrosine)
pH increase	Metabolic activation
Na^+ requirement—	Protein synthesis
exchange vs. activation	DNA synthesis
? Protein phosphorylation	Chromosome cycle

include the activation of protein and DNA synthesis as well as initiation of chromosome replication (e.g., Steinhardt and Mazia, 1973). The intracellular pH increase requires extracellular sodium (Chambers, 1975, 1976; Epel *et al.*, 1974) either for a Na^+-H^+ antiport system or as a regulator of acid release (e.g., see Epel, 1978, for review). Metabolic activation is accompanied by changes in the capacity of the egg to catalyze phosphorylation of endogenous proteins. Such a change has the capacity to couple the ionic fluxes to metabolic activation, although this relationship has not yet been established (Keller *et al.*, 1980). Thus, the biochemistry of the early events of fertilization seems to be intimately associated with altered ionic fluxes, and the relationship between the different fluxes is just beginning to be worked out. The mechanism by which increased pH mediates an increase in protein synthesis or DNA synthesis is still not clear for example, nor is the mechanism by which Ca^{2+} mediates exocytosis in this (or, for that matter, in any other) system. Clarifying these interrelationships constitutes a most exciting aspect of the current research on fertilization mechanisms.

Conclusions

I have tried to outline some of the current directions of research concerning the activation of the invertebrate egg. I have concentrated on results from my laboratory but have also attempted to indicate some important directions taken by other workers in this rapidly moving area. Some of the observations being actively pursued today trace their roots back to the last century, and others involve phenomena that have only been discovered within the past few years. Although we are just beginning to understand the molecular aspects of the regulation of cellular events in fertilization, the problem is beginning to take form. We seem to be in an equivalent position to that of students of metabolism about 100 years ago. Some of the reactions are understood in the the broadest general form, but the links between them and the significance of the pathways are still very hazy. With the vigorous research that is presently taking place in this area, the details should continue to emerge. This type of understanding is absolutely essential for any rational consideration of means to either improve or decrease reproductive efficiency. We have not yet begun to exploit the modern molecular and cellular biology of fertilzation either to treat reproductive failure or to design more effective contraceptive agents. I am sure that as our knowledge of these processes continues to grow, we shall discover more similarities between fundamental fertilization processes in mice, man, cattle, and sea urchins, and this knowledge will aid us enormously in responding to problems in human and animal reproduction.

ACKNOWLEDGMENTS

I am indebted to Erica Kay and Gregg Gundersen for their comments on the manuscript. The work was supported by National Science Foundation Grant PCM 77 20472 and United States Publc Health Services Grant GM 23910.

References

Byrd, E. W., Jr., and Collins, F. D., 1975, Absence of a fast block to polyspermy in eggs of sea urchin *Strongylocentrotus purpuratus*, *Nature (London)* **257**:675–677.

Byrd, W., Perry, G., and Weidener, E., 1977, Role of the egg cortex and actin in fertilization of the sea urchin egg, *J. Cell Biol.* **75**:267a.

Carroll, E. J., Jr., and Baginski, R. M., 1978, Sea urchin fertilization envelope: Isolation, extraction and characterization of a major protein fraction from *Strongylocentrotus purpuratus* embryos, *Biochemistry* **17**:2605–2612.

Carroll, E. J., Jr., and Epel, D., 1975, Isolation and biological activity of the proteases released by sea urchin eggs following fertilization, *Dev. Biol.* **44**:22–32.

Chambers, E. L., 1975, Na$^+$ is required for nuclear and cytoplasmic activation of sea urchin eggs by sperm and divalent ionophores, *J. Cell Biol.* **67**:60a.

Chambers, E. L., 1976, Na$^+$ is essential for activation of the inseminated sea urchin egg, *J. Exp. Zool.* **197**:149–154.

Colwin, L. H., and Colwin, A. L., 1967, Membrane fusion in relation to sperm egg association, in *Fertilization: Comparative Morphology, Biochemistry and Immunology*, Volume 1 (C. Metz and A. Monroy, eds.), Academic Press, New York, pp. 295–367.

Eddy, E. M., and Shapiro, B. M., 1976, Changes in the topography of the sea urchin egg after fertilization, *J. Cell Biol.* **71**:35–48.

Epel, D., 1978, Mechanisms of activation of sperm and egg during fertilization of sea urchin gametes, *Curr. Top. Dev. Biol.* **12**:185–246.

Epel, D., Steinhardt, R., Humphreys, T., and Mazia, D., 1974, An analysis of the partial metabolic derepression of sea urchin eggs by ammonia: The existence of independent pathways, *Dev. Biol.* **40**:245–255.

Fodor, E. J. B., Ako, H., and Walsh, K. A., 1975, Isolation of a protease from sea urchin eggs before and after fertilization, *Biochemistry* **14**:4923–4927.

Foerder, C. A., and Shapiro, B. M., 1977, Release of ovoperoxidase from sea urchin eggs hardens the fertilization membrane with tyrosine crosslinks, *Proc. Natl. Acad. Sci. USA* **74**:4214–4218.

Foerder, C. A., Klebanoff, S. J., and Shapiro, B. M., 1978, Hydrogen peroxide production, chemiluminescence, and the respiratory burst of fertilization: Interrelated events in early sea urchin development, *Proc. Natl. Acad. Sci. USA* **75**:3183–3187.

Fol, H., 1877, Sur le commencement de l'hémogénie chez divers animaux, *Arch. Zool. Exp. Gen. Ser. I* **6**:145–169.

Gabel, C. A., and Shapiro, B. M., 1978, ^{125}I-diiodofluorescein isothiocyanate: Its synthesis and use as a reagent for labeling proteins and cells to high specific radioactivity, *Anal. Biochem.* **86**:396–406.

Gabel, C. A., Eddy, E. M., and Shapiro, B. M., 1979a, Regional differentiation of the sperm surface as studied with ^{125}I-diiodofluorescein isothiocyanate, an impermeant reagent that allows isolation of the labeled components, *J. Cell Biol.* **82**:742–754.

Gabel, C. A., Eddy, E. M., and Shapiro, B. M., 1979b, After fertilization, sperm surface components remain as a patch in sea urchin and mouse embryos, *Cell* **18**:207–215.

Gould-Somero, M., Holland, L., and Paul, M., 1977, Cytochalasin B inhibits sperm penetration into eggs of *Urechis caupo*, *Dev. Biol.* **58**:11–22.

Gundersen, G., Gabel, C., and Shapiro, B., 1980, An intermediate state in fertilization, *J. Cell Biol.* **87**:143a.

Hall, H. G., 1978, Hardening of the sea urchin envelope by peroxidase catalyzed phenolic coupling of tyrosines, *Cell* **15**:343–355.

Jaffe, L. A., 1976, Fast block to polyspermy in sea urchin eggs is electrically mediated, *Nature (London)* **261**:68–71.

Kay, E., Turner, E., Weidman, P., and Shapiro, B., 1980, Assembly of the fertilization membrane of *Strongylocentrotus purpuratus*, *J. Cell Biol.* **87**:143a.

Keller, C. J., Gundersen, G. G., and Shapiro, B. M., 1980, Altered *in vitro* phosphorylation of specific proteins accompanies fertilization of *Strongylocentrotus purpuratus* eggs, *Dev. Biol.* **74**:86–101.

Klebanoff, S. J., Foerder, C. A., Eddy, E. M., and Shapiro, B. M., 1979, Metabolic similarities between fertilization and phagocytosis: Conservation of a peroxidatic mechanism, *J. Exp. Med.* **149**:938–953.

Longo, G., 1978, Effects of cytochalasin on sperm–egg interactions, *Dev. Biol.* **67**:249–265.

Ridgeway, E. B., Gilkey, J. C., and Jaffe, L. F., 1977, Free calcium increases explosively in activating medaka eggs, *Proc. Natl. Acad. Sci. USA* **74**:623–627.

Rothschild, L., 1956, *Fertilization*, Methuen, London.

Schuel, J., Wilson, W. L., Chen, K., and Lorand, L., 1973, A trypsin-like proteinase localized in cortical granules isolated from unfertilized sea urchin eggs by zona centrifugation: Role of the enzyme in fertilization, *Dev. Biol.* **34**:175–180.

Shapiro, B. M., 1975, Limited proteolysis of some egg surface components is an early event following fertilization of the sea urchin *Strongylocentrotus purpuratus*, *Dev. Biol.* **46**:88–102.

Showman, R. M., and Foerder, C. A., 1979, Removal of the fertilization membrane of sea urchin embryos employing aminotriazole, *Exp. Cell Res.* **120**:253–255.

Steinhardt, R. A., and Mazia, D., 1973, Development of a K^+-conductance and membrane potentials in unfertilized sea urchin eggs after exposure to NH_4OH, *Nature (London)* **241**:400–401.

Steinhardt, R. A., Lundin, L., and Mazia, D., 1971, Bioelectric responses of the echinoderm egg to fertilization, *Proc. Natl. Acad. Sci. USA* **68**:2426–2430.

Steinhardt, R., Zucker, R., and Schatten, G., 1977, Intracellular calcium release at fertilization in the sea urchin egg, *Dev. Biol.* **58**:185–196.

Tilney, L. G., Hatano, S., Ishikawa, H., and Mooseker, M. S., 1973, The polymerization of actin: Its role in the generation of the acrosomal process of certain echinoderm sperm, *J. Cell Biol.* **59**:109–126.

Tilney, L. G., Kiehart, D. P., Sardet, C., and Tilney, M., 1978, Polymerization of actin. IV. Role of Ca^{2+} and H^+ in the assembly of actin and in membrane fusion in the acrosomal reaction of echinoderm sperm, *J. Cell Biol.* **77**:536–550.

Tilney, L. G., Clain, J. G., and Tilney, M. S., 1979, Membrane events in the acrosomal reaction of *Limulus* sperm, *J. Cell Biol.* **81**:229–253.

Vacquier, V. D., Epel, D., and Douglas, L. A., 1972, Sea urchin eggs release protease activity at fertilization, *Nature* (*London*) **237**:34–36.

Veron, M., Foerder, C., Eddy, E. M., and Shapiro, B. M., 1977, Sequential biochemical and morphological events during assembly of the fertilization membrane of the sea urchin, *Cell* **10**:231–328.

Warburg, O., 1908, Beobachtungen über die Oxidationsprozesse in Seeigelei, *Z. Physiol. Chem.* **57**:1–16.

9

CHROMOSOME ABERRATIONS AND MAMMALIAN REPRODUCTION

MITCHELL S. GOLBUS

Chromosome heteroploidy is responsible for a substantial segment of observed birth defects and reproductive inefficiency. Sterility, reduced fertility, embryonic or fetal death, stillbirths, and/or congenital malformation may result from an aberration in chromosome number. Sandler and Hecht (1973) argue that the maximum nonlethal excess of autosomal DNA in humans is 5–6% and that deletion of more than 2–3% of the haploid autosomal complement is incompatible with life.

The potential of using techniques of ova collection, *in vitro* fertilization, and embryo transfer to alleviate certain types of human infertility has generated concern regarding the risks of embryo/fetal abnormalities being induced by these procedures. To consider such a risk appropriately one must have a firm understanding of the role of chromosomal aneuploidy in mammalian reproduction. Each year in the United States *in vivo* fertilization produces 15,000 neonates with chromosome abnormalities, and there are 200,000 spontaneous abortions of chromosomally abnormal fetuses.

The 1950s witnessed four technical developments that permitted mammalian chromosomes to be studied more readily. These were (1) the hypotonic treatment of cells to spread the chromosomes before fixation, (2) the use of mitosis-arresting agents to allow accumulation of cells at a mitotic stage suitable for chromosome study, (3) the improvement of tissue culture techniques, and (4) the discovery that certain substances would induce lymphocytes to undergo mitosis. These developments rapidly led to the

MITCHELL S. GOLBUS • Departments of Obstetrics, Gynecology, and Reproductive Sciences and of Pediatrics, University of California Medical Center, San Francisco, California 94143.

establishment of the correct karyotypes for numerous mammalian species and to an understanding that speciation was, to a significant extent, dependent upon chromosomal evolution. The other significant technical development in cytogenetics was the introduction in the 1970s of banding techniques that allowed specific identification of each chromosome in the karyotype.

The utilization of these technical advances has led to a greater understanding of the influence of chromosomal aneuploidy on mammalian reproduction. The available data will be considered for various developmental stages with reference to humans, mice, and other mammals. The incidence of chromosomal aneuploidy will be presented first, so that considerations of the role of *in vitro* fertilization and of the applicability of subprimate data to the human situation may follow.

The Newborn

The incidence of human heteroploidy varies with the population selected for study. The incidence may be as high as one-third of children studied because of a suspected cytogenetic abnormality (Mulcahy and Jenkyn, 1972), but falls to 5.05% of neonatal deaths and 5.75% of stillbirths (Sutherland *et al.*, 1978). A number of surveys have been performed on unselected newborns with a total of 326 major chromosomal aberrations found among 54,749 neonates, an incidence of 0.59% (Jacobs, 1977).

Similar data are not available for other mammalian species. Clinical recognition of intersexuality and pseudohermaphroditism has led to the demonstration of sex chromosome aberrations in the mouse, pig, cow, sheep, goat, and horse (Fechheimer, 1971; McFeely, 1975). Although sporadic cases of mouse aneuploidy have been reported, a survey of 756 newborn mice found no examples of aneuploidy (Goodlin, 1965). However, the limited size of this study population still permits (at the 5% confidence level) an incidence of approximately 1:200. The data are not available to allow any definitive statement regarding the incidence of cytogenetic abnormalities in any newborn mammalian population other than humans.

Postimplantation Embryos

There are three sources of data on the incidence of chromosome abnormalities in the postimplantation human embryo and fetus. The largest amount of data has been gathered on the early midtrimester fetus from amniocentesis programs. A number of points of information pertinent to this discussion have come from these data. Patients having an amniocentesis because of a fetus at risk for a metabolic defect represent an unbiased group from a cytogenetic point of view. Reports on 648 such patients have included ten fetuses found to be aneuploid (1.5%) at 14 weeks of fetal development. Comparison of this figure to the 0.59% newborn incidence indicates that 60% of fetuses known to be aneuploid at 14 weeks will die before delivery. A small but pertinent study was conducted by surveying those cases in which an aneuploid fetus was identified by amniotic fluid cell karyotyping but the parents opted to not have a selective abortion. Twenty-four per cent of trisomy 21 fetuses and 57% of trisomy 13 or 18 fetuses died before delivery. This phenomenon is further verified by examining the maternal age-specific risks of having a chromosomally abnormal fetus at the time of amniocentesis and at delivery (Figure 1). Although the maternal age effect on aneuploidy can be seen in both curves, it is clear that many aneuploid fetuses will not be liveborn. The ratio of aneuploid liveborn to aneuploid fetuses remains steady at approximately 40% over the ages examined, suggesting that there is no age effect among older mothers on the ability of *in utero* selection factors.

A further lesson about fetal aneuploidy has been learned from patients undergoing amniocentesis because of a prior child with trisomy 21. It has been argued that such couples are at an increased risk of having a second affected offspring. However, analysis of the prenatal diagnosis program data on recurrent trisomy 21 indicates a recurrence risk approximately equal to the age-specific risk for women of all ages. Thus, women with a prior trisomic child are not really at an increased risk in subsequent gestations.

The second source of information regarding human fetal aneuploidy has been karyotypes of spontaneously aborted first-trimester fetuses. A number of such cytogenetic surveys have been published and, as seen in Table I, it is generally agreed that about 50% of unselected clinically recognized spontaneous abortions are chromosomally aberrant. Of these, some 50% are trisomic, 20% are 45,X, 15% are triploid and the remainder tetraploid or structurally abnormal. A study of the incidence and distribution of cytogenetic abnormalities as a function of race found no significant differences among the different racial groups (Hassold *et al.*, 1978).

There have been 108 couples who have had karyotypes on two consecutive abortuses (Table II) (Alberman *et al.*, 1975; Boue *et al.*, 1975; Lauritsen, 1976; Hassold, 1978; Kajii and Ferrier, 1978). As expected, approximately 50% of the first abortuses and 50% of the second abortuses had abnormal chromosome constitutions. However, the karyotypes of the first and second abortuses of each couple were found to be highly correlated. Seventy-six per cent (42/55) of couples whose first abortus was chromosomally normal had a chromosomally normal second abortus, and, similarly, seventy-five per cent (40/53) of couples whose first abortus was chromosomally abnormal had a chromosomally abnormal second abortus. Furthermore, the forty pairs of abnormal abortuses had the same class of chromosome aberrations in each of twenty-nine pairs. This indicates the presence of

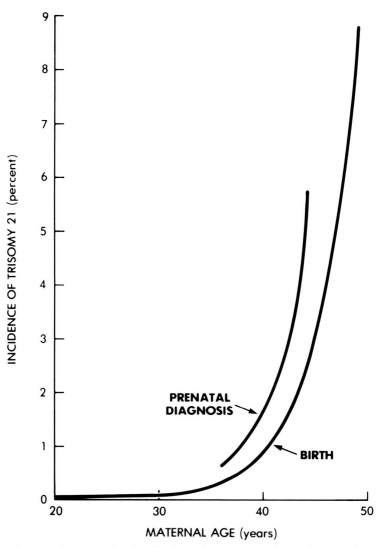

Figure.1 Maternal age-specific risks of having a chromosomally abnormal fetus at the time of amniocentesis and at delivery. Birth data are means of Massachusetts, New York, and Sweden statistics (Hook and Fabia, 1978). Prenatal diagnosis data are from San Francisco (Golbus *et al.*, 1979).

significant genetic and/or environmental factors controlling the conception and spontaneous abortion of chromosomally abnormal fetuses.

Trisomic spontaneous abortion material, as well as neonates with trisomy 21, have been used to demonstrate the origin of the additional chromosome based on observations of chromosome heteromorphisms (Lauritsen and Friedrich, 1976; Jacobs and Morton, 1977). In spite of serious

Table I

Results of Five Cytogenetic Surveys of Spontaneous Abortions[a]

Total abortuses karyotyped	3080			
Normal karyotypes	1541	(50%)		
Abnormal karyotypes	1539	(50%)		
Trisomic			810	(26%)
45,X			287	(9%)
Triploid			260	(8%)
Tetraploid			92	(3%)
Structural abnormalities			61	(2%)
Mosaics			25	(1%)
Other			4	—

[a] Adapted from Hassold et al. (1978).

methodologic biases in these studies it is clear that the majority of trisomies are due to nondisjunction at the first maternal meiotic division. The finding that 5–10% of trisomic spontaneous abortions are mosaics suggests that mitotic nondisjunction also may play a significant role in the production of trisomic fetuses (Warburton et al., 1978).

The incidence of chromosome abnormalities among first-trimester spontaneous abortions allows an estimate of the incidence of aneuploid human conceptions. Approximately 15% of clinically recognized pregnancies result in spontaneous abortions, and if 50% of these are chromosomally abnormal, then approximately 7.5% of recognized conceptions must be aneuploid. At another extreme, Boué et al. (1975) argue that meiotic nondisjunction occurs with equal probability for each chromosome and that the incidence of trisomy 16 and monosomy X among spontaneous abortions can be used to estimate the aneuploid load of conceptions. Allowing that 1000 recognized pregnancies would produce 150 spontaneous abortions of which 15 would be trisomy 16 and 15 would be monosomy X, this leads to the conclusion that 345 trisomies and 345 monosomies were conceived (23 sets of chromosomes × 15). Thus at conception there would have been 690 monosomies and trisomic embryos, 22 polyploids and miscellaneous chromosome abnormalities, 75 embryos destined to become euploid abortuses, 5

Table II

Correlation between Karyotypes of Two Consecutive Abortuses in 108 Couples

	Second abortus	
First abortus	Normal	Abnormal
Normal	42	13
Abnormal	13	40

Table III

Selection Against Fetuses with Chromosome Abnormalities[a]

	Frequency of abnormality			
	Among spontaneous abortions	Among recognized pregnancies[b]	Among liveborns	Recognized pregnancies resulting in spontaneous abortion (%)
Trisomy 13	3.94	0.59	0.13	78
Trisomy 16	11.84	1.78	0.0	100
Trisomy 17–18	1.32	0.20	0.01	95
Trisomy 21	1.46	0.22	0.11	50
45,X	9.34	1.40	0.004	99.7
Triploidy	12.22	1.83	0.0	100

[a] Adapted from Stein et al. (1975).
[b] Assumes 15% of recognized pregnancies end in spontaneous abortion.

destined to become aneuploid liveborn, and 845 destined to become euploid liveborns. This is an aneuploidy rate of 43.8% (717/1637). The most tenuous assumption in this argument is that meiotic nondisjunction occurs with equal probability for each chromosome.

The fact that only 0.59% of newborns are chromosomally abnormal indicates that the spontaneous abortion mechanism selectively removes 92% of the aneuploid conceptions. Table III shows the relative efficiency of this selection mechanism for various chromosome abnormalities (Stein et al., 1975). The concept of increasing this selectivity by stressing the early gestation has been termed *terathanasia* by Warkaney (1978).

More recently, a number of cytogenetic surveys have been conducted on induced abortuses (Kajii, 1973; Kajii et al., 1978; Yamamoto and Watanabe, 1979). This is, to date, the earliest estimate of aneuploidy in human conceptions, but it is also limited to clinically recognizable pregnancies. Table IV shows that 2.6% of first-trimester induced abortions were chromosomally

Table IV

Chromosome Abnormalities in Induced Abortions

Author	Incidence of abnormality	Mean developmental age (days)	Mean maternal age (years)
Sasaki	16/1297	39	26.6
Tonomura	11/609	36	27.1
Yasuda	5/188	37	29.0
Ford	0/307	51	27.7
Kajii	23/728	49	28.4
Hahnemann	6/172	73	26.5
Yamamoto	80/1250	45	28.0
Klinger	9/1233	—	24.7
Total	150/5784 (2.6%)		

abnormal. That this represents a low estimate is seen in that the early studies devoted themselves to complete specimens containing both membranes and an embryo and found a 1.1% incidence of chromosome abnormality, while more recent studies, which have included incomplete anembryonic specimens, found a 5.0% incidence of chromosome anomaly. The rate of karyotype abnormality also is a function of the developmental age of the embryo (Table V), and these data suggest an abnormality rate of approximately 10% in the early postimplantation human embryo.

Midgestation mouse fetuses of a number of strains have been examined for karyotype anomalies (Yamamoto *et al.*, 1973; Basler *et al.,* 1976; Fabricant and Schneider, 1978). Eight of 494 (1.62%) fetuses of 2- to 5-month-old females and 24 of 270 (8.89%) fetuses of 11- to 16-month-old females were chromosomally abnormal. There were no differences between gestations achieved by natural ovulation and those achieved by superovulation. These are incidences similar to those found by amniocentesis in humans at a somewhat later developmental stage. The maternal age effect on trisomy appears to exist for mouse fetuses as it does for human fetuses and neonates. Postimplantation incidences of chromosome abnormality for the 9-day-old hamster embryo (2/150, 1.3%), the 10- to 16-day-old rabbit embryo (1/104, 0.96%), and the 11-day-old rat embryo (6/410, 1.5%) are compatible with the data on humans and mice (Table VI).

Preimplantation Embryos

There are no human studies bearing directly on the question of pre- and periimplantation embryos, but there is the much-quoted work of Hertig *et al.*, (1959). Thirty-four early embryos were found in reproductive organs removed surgically. Ten of these embryos were morphologically abnormal, including four of the eight preimplantation embryos. Although no statement regarding chromosome anomalies is possible, it is clear that a minimum of 29.4% (10/34) of these early embryos were unsuccessful gestations.

The mouse has served as a common model for preimplantation chromosome studies. Virtually all of the investigations have employed superovulation techniques; however, there are insufficient studies to demonstrate that these hormones do not influence the chromosome constitution of

Table V
Chromosome Abnormalities in Induced Abortions by Developmental Age[a]

Developmental age (weeks)	Number of karyotypes	Chromosome abnormalities
3–4	108	10 (9.3%)
5–10	1558	90 (5.8%)
>10	259	2 (0.8%)

[a]Combined data of Kajii *et al.* (1978) and Yamamoto and Watanabe (1979).

Table VI
Chromosomal Abnormalities in Postimplantation Mammalian Species

Species	Developmental stage	Maternal age	Embryos karyotyped	Chromosome abnormalities
Mouse	Midgestation	Young	494	8 (1.6%)
		Old	270	24 (8.9%)
Rat	11 days	Young	410	6 (1.5%)
Syrian hamster	9 days	Young	150	2 (1.3%)
Rabbit	10–16 days	Young	104	1 (1.0%)
Human	3–10 weeks (induced abortions)	Young	1,668	100 (6.0%)
	>10 weeks (induced abortions)	Young	259	2 (0.8%)
	14–16 weeks (amniocentesis)	Young	648	10 (1.5%)
	14–16 weeks (amniocentesis)	Old (>40)	5,718	212 (3.7%)
	Neonates	Young	54,749	326 (0.6%)

the embryo. Takagi and Sasaki (1976) found that superovulation had no effect on the incidence of trisomy in Day $6\frac{1}{2}$ embryos, but they found so great an incidence of polyploidy as to call the entire study into question. Rohrborn (1972) found no difference in trisomy incidence in metaphase II oocytes obtained with and without superovulation. Maudlin and Fraser (1977) did not find a PMS (pregnant mare serum) dose-related incidence of triploidy in superovulated embryos, but no naturally ovulated control group was available for comparison. There is a series of studies suggesting that the incidence of triploidy in embryos from natural ovulations is approximately 1% (Beatty and Fischberg, 1951; Beatty, 1957; Evans quoted by Fraser *et al.*, 1976) and that that in embryos from superovulation is 0.3% (Vickers, 1969), 2.7% (Fraser *et al.*, 1976), 4.9% (Maudlin and Fraser, 1977), and 5.5% (Gosden, 1973). Comparative data with regard to strain and methodology are not available. The data that are available allow an estimate of aneuploidy in the mouse embryo of 4.30% (18/419) in superovulated morulae/blastocysts (Vickers, 1969; Gosden, 1973), 4.51% (39/864) in naturally ovulated blastocysts (Beatty and Fischberg, 1951), and 2.7% (46/1710) at the first cleavage division of embryos obtained by superovulation (Rohrborn *et al.*, 1971; Donahue, 1972; Kaufman, 1973; Luthardt, 1976; Maudlin and Fraser, 1977, 1978a,b). These estimates were obtained by doubling the number of trisomies, ignoring the monosomies that may have been methodologically caused, and adding the other forms of heteroploidy. There is insufficient data to examine strain variation except to state that the "silver" strain appears to have an increased polyploidy rate. The hyperdiploidy rate rises as a function of increasing maternal age from 1.17% to 4.79% at the first cleavage division (Maudlin and Fraser, 1978b) and from 0.91% to 6.90% in morulae/blastocysts (Gosden, 1973).

The rabbit blastocyst has been the object of many cytogenetic surveys (Shaver and Carr, 1967 and 1969; Shaver, 1970, 1975; Hofsaess and Meacham, 1971; Martin and Shaver, 1972; Widmeyer and Shaver, 1972;

Table VII
Chromosome Aberrations in Rabbit Blastocysts

	Number karyotyped	Chromosomal aberrations
Natural ovulation	240	3 (1.25%)
HCG only	328	13 (3.96%)
Superovulation	339	17 (5.01%)

Fechheimer and Beatty, 1974; Fujimoto *et al.*, 1974). The incidences of aneuploidy have been 1.25% (3/240) among blastocysts obtained by natural ovulation, 3.96% (13/328) where only human chorionic gonadotropin was utilized to synchronize ovulation, and 5.01% (17/339) among superovulated blastocysts (Table VII). The difference between naturally ovulated blastocysts and those obtained by hormonal intervention is statistically significant ($p < 0.01$), while the difference between the two hormonal methods is not significant.

There have been only sporadic reports of chromosome studies of other mammalian preimplantation embryos (Table VIII). Yamamoto and Ingalls (1972) found that only 1/135 (0.74%) naturally ovulated four- to eight-cell embryos of Syrian hamsters was aneuploid, while Binkert and Schmid (1977) noted a 12/226 (5.3%) aberration rate among naturally ovulated four- to eight-cell embryos of Chinese hamsters. One hundred and one naturally ovulated pig blastocysts have been cytogenetically examined with thirteen (12.8%) of them proving to be aneuploid; however, all but one of these were polyploid (McFeely, 1967; Moon *et al.*, 1975). Long and Williams (1980) found that 5/84 (5.95%) naturally ovulated two- to eight-cell domestic sheep embryos were chromosomally abnormal.

This summary of the available data on chromosomal aneuploidy in preimplantation mammalian embryos (Table VIII) indicates the extreme variability of the results. Note that data on the postimplantation embryo were

Table VIII
Chromosomal Abnormalities in Preimplantation Mammalian Embryos

Species	Developmental stage	Ovulation method	Embryos karyotyped	Chromosome abnormalities
Mouse	One- to two-cell	Superovulated	1710	46 (2.7%)
	Morula/blastocyst	Superovulated	419	18 (4.3%)
Rabbit	Blastocyst	Natural	240	3 (1.2%)
	Blastocyst	Hormonal	667	30 (4.5%)
Syrian hamster	Four- to eight-cell	Natural	135	1 (0.7%)
Chinese hamster	Four- to eight-cell	Natural	226	12 (5.3%)
Pig	Blastocyst	Natural	101	13 (12.9%)
Sheep	Two- to eight-cell	Natural	84	5 (6.0%)

much less variable (Table VI). In the presence of so little information available regarding the human, it is impossible to argue that any one of these species is the best model for the human situation.

Germ Cells

Two karyotype studies of human sperm in testicular biopsy specimens found, respectively, 73/487 (14.9%) and 10/48 (20.83%) incidences of hyperploidy (Beatty et al., 1975; Polani and Jagiello, 1976). A third investigation utilized quinacrine fluorescence to estimate that 1.3% of sperm have two Y bodies and Giemsa-11 staining to estimate that 2% of sperm have two chromosomes 9 (Pawlowitzki and Pearson, 1972). The authors then concluded that this intimated a 38% incidence of chromosomal abnormalities in ejaculated sperm. This seems quite high compared to investigations in male mice of various strains where only 23 of 6733 (0.34%) of metaphase II sperm were hyperploid (Hulten and Linsten, 1970; Skakkebaek et al., 1973). The newly developed technique of analyzing human sperm that have penetrated zona-free hamster eggs should allow the accumulation of further data; however, there may be selection involved in which sperm are capable of egg penetration.

Not surprisingly, no cytogenetic studies of human oocytes have been performed to date. The syrian hamster, Chinese hamster, sheep, and cow oocytes examined have had no hyperploidy (Jagiello et al., 1974; Basler, 1978; Hansmann and Probeck, 1979), whereas the few pig oocytes studied had an 11.1% incidence of hyperploidy (McGaughey and Polge, 1971).

The mouse oocyte has been the most extensively studied model. Different strains, females of different ages, and different oocyte maturation methods have been employed, leading to an array of confusing results. In vitro maturation of oocytes from young females produces almost no (1/1804) hyperploid metaphase II spreads (Karp and Smith, 1975; Martin et al., 1976; Polani and Jagiello, 1976; Uchida and Freeman, 1977), while oocytes from older females produced enough more (6/1822) to represent a significant increase in aneuploidy (Martin et al., 1976; Polani and Jagiello, 1976; Speed, 1977; Uchida and Freeman, 1977). It is difficult to interpret biologically the data of Martin et al., (1976), who found no hyperploidy in oocytes of younger or older females but a 5.2% hyperploidy rate among those of "middle-aged" mice. Naturally ovulated oocytes were examined by Rohrborn (1972), who found 3/128 (2.3%) to be hyperploid. He compared this with superovulated oocytes of the same strain (C3H), which had a 2.4% (8/335) incidence of hyperploidy. The total reported experience with superovulated oocytes of young females of various strains demonstrated a 3.0% (14/466) incidence of hyperploidy (Rohrborn, 1972; Basler et al., 1976), while oocytes of older females had a 4.3% (14/328) incidence (Chebotar, 1978). Comparison of aneuploidy rates shows no significant difference ($x^2 = 1.87, 0.10 < p < 0.25$).

Table IX
Hyperploidy in Swiss–Webster Oocytes at Metaphase II

	Number	Hyperploid
6–8 weeks old		
In vitro	450	11 (2.44%)
Natural	350	4 (1.14%)
Superovulated	350	4 (1.14%)
13–15 months old		
In vitro	225	8 (3.56%)
Natural	175	3 (1.71%)
Superovulated	225	7 (3.11%)

The absolute nature of percentages should not obscure the uncertainty engendered by quoting studies done over a six-year period by eight different laboratories utilizing eight different strains of mice of varying ages and three different methods of oocyte maturation. Our laboratory has been interested in understanding the influence of maturation method, strain, and maternal age on oocyte aneuploidy. Examination of 6- to 8-week-old Swiss–Webster mice (Table IX) indicated no difference between naturally ovulated and super-ovulated oocytes, while *in vitro* maturation caused a statistically significant rise in aneuploidy ($\chi^2 = 5.8$, $p < 0.02$). Oocytes of 12- to 15-month-old Swiss–Webster mice did not have a significantly higher aneuploidy rate when comparing those matured by superovulation or *in vitro* with those obtained by natural ovulation. There was a maternal age-related increase only for the superovulated oocytes ($\chi^2 \div 5.76$, $p < 0.01$) and not for the *in vitro* or naturally matured oocytes.

The data from the CBA mice were remarkably similar (Table X). There was no difference between natural ovulation and superovulation in oocytes of young mice, while *in vitro* maturation caused a significant rise in hyperploidy. Also similar to the Swiss–Webster findings, oocytes of older females did not have a significantly higher aneuploidy rate when matured by superovulation

Table X
Hyperploidy in CBA Oocytes at Metaphase II

	Number	Hyperploid
6–8 weeks old		
In vitro	275	17 (6.19%)
Natural	275	2 (0.73%)
Superovulated	275	2 (0.73%)
9–10 months old		
In vitro	200	6 (3.00%)
Natural	200	2 (1.00%)
Superovulated	200	4 (2.00%)

or *in vitro* as compared to natural ovulation. A maternal age-related increase in aneuploidy was not found for any mode of maturation.

These data can be analyzed for a number of factors. Regarding the mode of maturation, there was no difference between superovulated and naturally ovulated oocytes of either strain at any age. *In vitro* maturation caused hyperdiploidy only for oocytes of younger females in both strains, with the more marked effect on CBA oocytes ($\chi^2 = 6.42, p < 0.02$). It is noteworthy that we had a higher *in vitro* aneuploidy incidence than that seen by other authors. Our system allowed 80% of ova to proceed to metaphase II while most other reports had only a 50% success rate. Our culture system may have allowed more marginal oocytes to mature. Regarding strain differences, aside from the *in vitro* matured oocytes of young mice mentioned above, there were no differences. Regarding a maternal age effect, of the six possible comparisons an aneuploidy increase was seen only for superovulated oocytes of Swiss–Webster mice and does not appear to be a general effect. Since a maternal age effect does appear to exist in the preimplantation mouse embryo, this raises the question of whether there could be a maternal age effect on the second meiotic division, on fertilization, or on early selection.

Previous data had indicated that oocytes of older females are more sensitive to meiosis alteration and the induction of aneuploidy by radiation (Uchida and Freeman, 1977). Although our *in vitro* maturation system appears to be a stress situation for the oocytes it is noteworthy that oocytes of older females were not more influenced by this stress. Therefore, we utilized a "temperature stress" mechanism described by Karp and Smith (1975). Table XI demonstrates that although we could markedly increase the hyperidploidy rate, there was no greater increase among oocytes of older mice.

In view of the evidence that maternal age, radiation, oocyte maturation method, and temperature may cause an increase in the incidence of oocyte/embryo chromosomal aberrations, consideration must be given as to whether *in vitro* fertilization might increase the aneuploidy rate. It is known that *in vitro* fertilization in the mouse and hamster does increase the incidence of polyploidy in the embryo (Barros *et al.*, 1972; Fraser *et al.*, 1976). The incidence of mouse embryo polyploidy resulting from *in vitro* fertilization

Table XI
Effect of Temperature Stress on Oocyte Hyperploidy

	Number	Hyperploid
6–8 weeks old		
Control	450	11 (2.44%)
Stressed	125	24 (19.20%)
13–15 months old		
Control	225	8 (3.56%)
Stressed	90	9 (10.0%)

may be a function of sperm and ova genotype (Maudlin and Fraser, 1978a), sperm concentration (Fraser and Maudlin, 1978), and the dose of PMS used to obtain the oocytes (Maudlin and Fraser, 1977). It is clear each of these factors will have to be monitored in considering human *in vitro* fertilization.

Conclusions

What conclusion can be drawn regarding the appropriate mammalian model for the human situation? The similarities among mammals in postimplantation incidences of heteroploidy and their ability to selectively reabsorb or abort abnormal embryos is reassuring; however, the differences, such as the fact that superovulation increases the incidence of chromosomal abnormalities in the rabbit but not in the mouse and the variability of preimplantation incidences of heteroploidy, make one conclude that we do not yet have sufficient data about heteroploidy in early human conceptions to choose an appropriate model system.

ACKNOWLEDGMENTS

This chapter was prepared, in part, while the author was a Senior International Fellow of the Fogarty Center, NIH (TW00354). Work reported herein was supported by grants from the National Institute of Child Health and Human Development (HD 09412) and the March of Dimes Birth Defects Foundation (1-410 and 1-673).

References

Alberman, E., Elliott, M., Creasy, M., and Dhadial, R., 1975, Previous history in mothers presenting with spontaneous abortions, *Br. J. Obstet. Gynaecol.* **82:**366–373.

Barros, C., Vliegenthart, A. M., and Franklin, L. E., 1972, Polyspermic fertilization of hamster eggs *in vitro*, *J. Reprod. Fertil.* **28:**117–120.

Basler, A., 1978, Timing of meiotic stages in oocytes of the Syrian hamster (*Mesocricetus auratus*) and analysis of induced chromosome aberrations, *Hum. Genet.* **42:**67–77.

Basler, A., Buselmaier, B., and Rohrborn, G., 1976, Elimination of spontaneous and chemically induced chromosome aberrations in mice during early embryo genesis, *Hum. Genet.* **33:**121–130.

Beatty, R. A., 1957, *Parthenogenesis and Polyploidy in Mammalian Development*, Cambridge University Press, London, p. 52.

Beatty, R. A., and Fischberg, M., 1951, Heteroploidy in mammals. I. Spontaneous heteroploidy in pre-implantation mouse eggs, *J. Genet.* **50:**345–359.

Beatty, R. A., Lim, M. C, and Coulter, V. J., 1975, A quantitative study of the second meiotic metaphase in male mice, *Cytogenet. Cell Genet.* **15:**256–275.

Binkert, F., and Schmid, W., 1977, Pre-implantation embryos of Chinese hamster. I. Incidence of karyotype anomalies in 226 control embryos, *Mut. Res.* **46:**63–75.

Boué, J., Boué, A., and Lazar, P., 1975, Retrospective and prospective epidemiological studies of 1500 karyotyped spontaneous human abortions, *Teratology* **12:**11–26.

Chebotar, N. A., 1978, The increase in the frequency of spontaneous chromosome aberrations in mice with increase age, *Genetika* **14:**551–553 (Russian).

Donahue, R. P., 1972, Cytogenetic analysis of the first cleavage division in mouse embryos, *Proc. Natl. Acad. Sci.* **69:**74–77.

Fabricant, J. D., and Schneider, E. L., 1978, Studies of the genetic and immunologic components of the maternal age effect, *Dev. Biol.* **66:**337–343.

Fechheimer, N. S., 1971, Cytogenetic considerations in animal breeding, *Ann. Genet. Sel. Anim.* **3:**43–58.

Fechheimer, N. S., and Beatty, R. A., 1974, Chromosomal abnormalities and sex ratio in rabbit blastocysts, *J. Reprod. Fertil.* **27:**331–341.

Fraser, L. R., and Maudlin, I., 1978, Relationship between sperm concentration and the incidence of polyspermy in mouse embryos fertilized *in vitro, J. Reprod. Fertil.* **52:**103–106.

Fraser, L. R., Zanellotti, H. M., Paton, G. R., and Drury, L. M., 1976, Increased incidence of triploidy in embryos derived from mouse eggs fertilized *in vitro, Nature* **250:**39–40.

Fujimoto, S., Pahlavan, N., and Dukelow, W. R., 1974, Chromosome abnormalities in rabbit preimplantation blastocysts induced by superovulation, *J. Reprod. Fertil.* **40:**177–181.

Golbus, M. S., Longhman, N. D., Epstein, C. J., Halbason, G., Stephens, J. D., and Hall, B. D., 1979, Prenatal genetic diagnosis in 3000 amniocourses, *N. Engl. J. Med.* **300:**157–163.

Goodlin, R. C., 1965, Non-disjunction and maternal age in the mouse, *J. Reprod. Fertil.* **9:**355–356.

Gosden, R. G., 1973, Chromosomal anomalies of preimplantation mouse embryos in relation to maternal age, *J. Reprod. Fertil.* 35:351–354.

Hansmann, I., and Probeck, H. D., 1979, Chromosome imbalance in ovulated oocytes from syrian hamsters (*Mesocricetus auratus*) and Chinese hamsters (*Cricetulus grisens*), *Cytogenet. Cell Genet.* **23:**70–76.

Hassold, T. J., 1978, Cytogenetic studies of successive spontaneous abortions occurring to the same couple, *Am. J. Hum. Genet.* **30:**82A.

Hassold, T. J., Matsuyama, A., Newlands, I. M., Matsuura, J. S., Jacobs, P. A., Manuel B., and Tsuei, J., 1978, A cytogenetic study of spontaneous abortions in Hawaii, *Ann. Hum. Genet.* **41:**443–454.

Hertig, A. T., Rock, J., Adams, E. C., and Menkin, M. D., 1959, Thirty-four fertilized ova, good, bad, and indifferent, recovered from 210 women of known fertility, *Pediatrics* **23:**202–211.

Hofsaess, F. R., and Meacham, T. N., 1971, Chromosome abnormalities of early rabbit embryos, *J. Exp. Zool.* **177:**9–11.

Hook, E. B., and Fabia, J. J., 1978, Frequency of Down Syndrome by single year maternal age interval: Results of a Massachusetts study, *Teratology,* **17:**220–223.

Hulten, M., and Linsten, J., 1970, The behavior of structural aberrations at male meiosis, in: *Human Population Cytogenetics* (P. A. Jacobs, W. H. Price, and P. Law, eds.) University of Edinburgh Pfizer Medical Monographs, pp. 24–61.

Jacobs, P. A., 1977, Epidemiology of chromosome abnormalities in man, *Am J. Epidemiol.* **105:**180–191.

Jacobs, P. A., and Morton, N. E., 1977, Origin of human trisomies and polyploids, *Hum. Hered.* **27:**59–72.

Jagiello, G. M., Miller, W. A., Ducayen, M. B., and Lin, J. S., 1974, Chiasma frequency and disjunctional behavior of ewe and cow oocytes matured *in vitro, Biol. Reprod.* **10:**354–363.

Kajii, T., 1973, Chromosome anomalies in induced abortions, in: *Chromosomal Errors in Relation to Reproductive Failure* (A. Boué and C. Thibault, eds.), INSERM, Paris, pp. 57–66.

Kajii, T., and Ferrier, A., 1978, Cytogenetics of aborters and abortuses, *Am. J. Obstet. Gynecol.* **131:**33–38.

Kajii, T., Ohama, K., and Mikamo, K., 1978, Anatomic and chromosomal anomalies in 944 induced abortuses, *Hum. Genet.* **43:**247–258.

Karp, L. E., and Smith, W. D., 1975, Experimental production of aneuploidy in mouse oocytes, *Gynecol. Invest.* **6**:337–341.

Kaufman, M. H., 1973, Analysis of the first cleavage division to determine the sex-ratio and incidence of chromosome anomalies to conception in the mouse, *J. Reprod. Fertil.* **35**:67–72.

Lauritsen, J. G., 1976, Aetiology of spontaneous abortion. A cytogenetic study of 288 abortuses and their parents, *Acta Obstet. Gynecol. Scand. (Suppl.)* **52**:1–29.

Lauritsen, J. G., and Friedrich. U., 1976, Origin of the extra chromosome in trisomy 16, *Clin. Genet.* **10**:156–160.

Long, S. E., and Williams, C. V., 1980, Frequency of chromosome abnormalities in early embryos of the domestic sheep (*Ovis aries*), J. Reprod.Fertil. **58**:197–201.

Luthardt, F. W., 1976, Cytogenetic analysis of oocytes and early preimplantation embryos from XO mice, *Dev. Biol.* **54**:73–81.

McFeely, R. A., 1967, Chromosome abnormalities in early embryos of the pig, *J. Reprod. Fertil.* **13**:579–581.

McFeely, R. A., 1975, A review of cytogenetics in equine reproduction, *J. Reprod. Fertil. (Suppl.)* **23**:371–374.

McGaughey, R. W., and Polge, C., 1971, Cytogenetic analysis of pig oocytes matured *in vitro*, *J. Exp. Zool.* **176**:383–395.

Martin, P. A., and Shaver, E. L., 1972, Sperm aging *in utero* and chromosomal anomalies in rabbit blastocysts, *Dev. Biol.* **28**:480–486.

Martin, R. H., Dill, F. J., and Miller, J. R., 1976, Nondisjunction in aging female mice, *Cytogenet. Cell Genet.* **17**:150–160.

Maudlin, I., and Fraser, L. R., 1977, The effect of PMSG dose on the incidence of chromosomal anomalies in mouse embryos fertilized *in vitro*, *J. Reprod. Fertil.* **50**;275–280.

Maudlin, I. and Fraser, L. R., 1978a, The effect of sperm and egg genotype on the incidence of chromosome anomalies in mouse embryos fertilized *in vitro*, *J. Reprod. Fertil.* **52**:107–112.

Maudlin, I., and Fraser, L. R., 1978b, Maternal age and the incidence of aneuploidy in first-cleavage mouse embryos, *J. Reprod. Fertil.* **54**:423–426.

Moon, R. G., Rashad, M. N., and Mi, M. P., 1975, An example of polyploidy in pig blastocysts, *J. Reprod. Fertil.* **45**:147–149.

Mulcahy, M., and Jenkyn, J., 1972, Results of 538 chromosome studies on patients referred for cytogenetic analysis, *Med. J. Aust.* **2**:1333–1338.

Pawloitzki, I. H., and Pearson, P. L., 1972, Chromosome aneuploidy in human spermatozoa, *Humangenetik* **16**:119–122.

Polani, P. E., and Jagiello, G. M., 1976, Chiasmata, meiotic univalents, and age in relation to aneuploid imbalance in mice, *Cytogenet. Cell Genet.* **16**:505–529.

Rohrborn, G., 1972, Frequencies of spontaneous non-disjunction in metaphase II. Oocytes of mice, *Humangenetik* **16**:123–125.

Rohrborn, G., Kuhn, O., Hansmann, I., and Thon, K., 1971, Induced chromosome aberrations in early embryogenesis of mice, *Humangenetik* **11**;316–322.

Sandler, L., and Hecht, F., 1973, Genetic effects of aneuploidy, *Am. J. Hum. Genet.* **25**:332–339.

Shaver, E. L., 1970, The chromosome complement of blastocyts from rabbits injected with various doses of HCG before ovulation, *J. Reprod. Fertil.* **23**:335–337.

Shaver, E. L., 1975, Pentobarbitol sodium and chromosome abnormalities in rabbit blastocysts, *Experientia* **31**:1212–1213.

Shaver, E. L., and Carr, D. H., 1967, Chromosome abnormalities in rabbit blastocysts following delayed fertilization, *j. Reprod. Fertil.* **14**:415–420.

Shaver, E. L., and Carr, D. H., 1969, The chromosome complement of rabbit blastocysts in relation to the time of mating and ovulation, *Can. J. Genet. Cytol.* **11**:287–293.

Skakkebaek, N. E., Bryant, J. I., and Philip, J., 1973, Studies on meiotic chromosomes in infertile men and controls with normal karotypes, *J. Reprod. Fertil.* **35**:23–36.

Speed, R. M., 1977, The effects of ageing on the meiotic chromosomes of male and female mice, *Chromosoma* **64**:241–254.

Stein, Z., Susser, M., Warburton, D., Wittes, J., and Kline, J., 1975, Spontaneous abortion as a screening device, *Am. J. Epidemiol.* **102**:275–290.

Sutherland, G. R., Carter, R. F., Bauld, R., Smith I. I., and Bain, A. D., 1978, Chromosome studies at the paediatric necropsy, *Ann. Hum. Genet.* **42**:173–181.

Takagi, N., and Sasaki, M., 1976, Digynic triploidy after superovulation in mice, *Nature* **264**:278–281.

Uchida, I. A., and Freeman, C. P. V., 1977, Radiation-induced nondisjunction in oocytes of aged mice, *Nature* **265**:186–187.

Vickers, A. D., 1969, Delayed fertilization and chromosomal anomalies in mouse embryos, *J. Reprod. Fertil.* **20**:69–76.

Warburton, D., Yu, C., Kline, J., and Stein, Z., 1978, Mosaic autosomal trisomy in cultures from spontaneous abortions, *Am. J. Hum. Genet.* **30**:609–617.

Warkaney, J., 1978, Terathanasia, *Teratology* **17**:187–192.

Widmeyer, M. A., and Shaver, E.L., 1972, Estrogen, progesterone, and chromosomal abnormalities in rabbit blastocysts, *Teratology* **6**:207–214.

Yamamoto, M., and Ingalls, T. H., 1972, Delayed fertilization and chromosome anomalies in the hamster embryo, *Science* **176**:518–521.

Yamamoto, M., and Watanabe, G., 1979, Epidemiology of gross chromosomal anomalies at the early embryonic stage of pregnancy. *Contr. Epidemiol. Biostat.* **1**:101.

Yamamoto, M., Endo, A., and Watanabe, G., 1973, Maternal age dependence of chromosome anomalies. *Nature New Biol.* **241**:141–142.

10

THE EFFECTS OF CHROMOSOMAL ANEUPLOIDY ON EARLY DEVELOPMENT
Experimental Approaches

CHARLES J. EPSTEIN

While chromosome imbalance (aneuploidy) is a frequent outcome of conception and a cause of embryonic and fetal death (Golbus, Chapter 9, this volume), very little work had been done until very recently on the effects of chromosome abnormalities during the preimplantation period of development. The major reasons for this lack of investigation have been the following: the frequencies of spontaneous aneuploidy in convenient experimental animals, particularly the mouse, are relatively low; techniques for identifying individual chromosomes were not available; nondestructive methods for identifying the aneuploid embryos did not exist. However, the recent development of staining techniques that permit specific chromosome identification and of two experimental approaches described in this chapter now make it possible to use the mouse as a subject for the systematic study of early embryonic aneuploidy.

The great advances in the study of the genetics of lower organisms ranging from viruses to *Drosophila* and plants have depended in large part on the ability of investigators to manipulate the genome so as to be able to "construct" organisms with the desired genetic properties. Among the manipulations used has been the creation of various states of genetic imbalance involving the addition or removal of whole chromosomes or of major segments of chromosomes. While it is still not possible to manipulate

CHARLES J. EPSTEIN • Departments of Pediatrics and of Biochemistry and Biophysics, University of California, San Francisco, California 94143.

the mammalian genome to the same degree as in these lower organisms, a method has now been developed that permits the production of mouse embryos monosomic or trisomic for any of the 19 different autosomes (nonsex chromosomes) in the chromosomal complement.

Products of Aneuploid Mouse Embryos

The generation of aneuploid mouse embryos relies upon the existence of numerous Robertsonian translocation (fusion) metacentric chromosomes in various strains of feral mice (Campanna *et al.*, 1976; Gropp and Winking, 1981). The prototype of these wild mice is the tobacco mouse (*M. poschiavinus*), which has 26 rather than 40 chromosomes, the reduction in number being accomplished by the formation of seven pairs of fusion chromosomes. Because this and other feral strains are interfertile with laboratory mice, it has been possible to transfer many of the naturally occurring translocation chromosomes to laboratory mice and to generate stocks homozygous for an individual metacentric chromosome. Some of these stocks are being inbred so that it will be possible to work with defined genetic backgrounds. As the present time, over 45 different metacentric chromosomes involving all autosomes in a variety of combinations have been identified.

Although animals, particularly females, carrying a single Robertsonian translocation chromosome will have chromosomally imbalanced progeny, the frequency of aneuploidy among their offspring is quite variable and usually not very great. However, the development of a method that employs animals doubly heterozygous for two different metacentric chromosomes has now made it possible to consistently generate aneuploid mouse embryos with high frequency. This method was independently introduced by Gropp and his collaborators (1975) and by White and Tjio and their collaborators (1974). It is based on the fact that the presence of two metacentric chromosomes that have one arm in common (Figure 1) results in a high frequency of unbalanced segregations in which neither or both metacentrics are passed to a gamete. When combined with a normal gamete, this results in monosomy or trisomy, respectively, for the specific chromosome present in both of the metacentrics. For experimental purposes it is generally desirable to have the male carry the translocation chromosomes, as he can be mated to a large number of normal and usually superovulated females that can then be sacrificed to recover the aneuploid embryos. However, some combinations of metacentrics result in male sterility, and then it is necessary to resort to the more costly use of double-metacentric-bearing females, each of which can be used for only a single experiment.

In addition to the high frequency of aneuploid progeny (see Table I), the double-metacentric method greatly facilitates the assessment of the chromosomal state of the embryos. By counting the number of metacentric

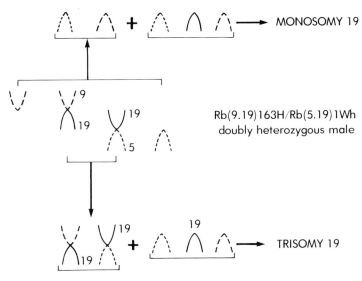

Figure 1. The production of aneuploid mouse embryos. An animal (preferably male) doubly heterozygous for two different Robertsonian fusion metacentric chromosomes that have a chromosome arm in common (in this example, chromosome 19) is mated to a chromosomally normal partner. The relevant chromosomes in the male are illustrated in the center, and two possible and complementary meiotic segregation products are shown at the top and bottom. The gamete carrying the two metacentric chromosomes (bottom) will, when combined with a normal gamete, produce a zygote trisomic for chromosome 19. The complementary gamete (top) will produce a zygote with monosomy 19. Note that the combination of metacentrics used to produce aneuploidy for chromosome 19 in this illustration differs from that shown in Table I; both are equally effective.

Table I
Frequency of Aneuploid Preimplantation Mouse Embryos

Chromosome	Male double heterozygote	Female	Days after mating plug	Monosomy (%)	Trisomy (%)
1	Rb(1.3)1Bnr/	ICR	3	16	16
	Rb(1.10)10Bnr	ICR	4	9	17
12	Rb(8.12)5Bnr/	ICR	3	14	15
	Rb(4.12)9Bnr	ICR	4	13	13
17	Rb(2.17)11Rma/	ICR	3	9	22
	Rb(8.17)1 Iem	ICR	4	8	13
19	Rb(9.19)163H/	ICR	3	18	20
	Rb(8.19)1Ct	C57BL/6J		16	20
		ICR	4	2	24
		C57BL/6J		1	19

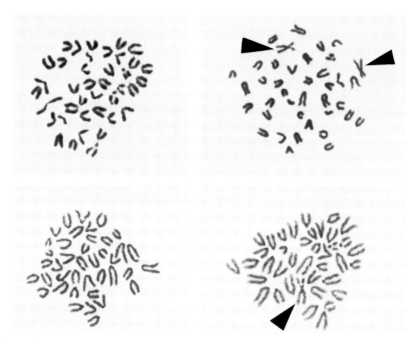

Figure 2. Metaphase spreads from monosomy-19 (upper left), trisomy-19 (upper right), and euploid (lower right) progeny of mating designed to produce aneuploidy for chromosome 19. The chromosome constitutions of the embryos are conveniently determined by counting the number of metacentric chromosomes (arrowheads) (0, 2, and 1, respectively) and the number of chromosome arms (39, 41, and 40, respectively). A normal BALB/c metaphase with 40 chromosomes and without a metacentric chromosome is shown for comparison (lower left).

chromosomes and the total number of chromosome arms, discrimination among monosomic, euploid, and trisomic chromosome constitutions is possible even in unbanded preparations. Two metacentrics and 41 total arms (39 chromosomes in all) indicate trisomy, and 39 arms with no metacentrics (again 39 chromosomes total) indicate monosomy (Figure 2). Moreoever, by virtue of the properties of the breeding scheme used for their production, the resultant aneuploidies involve only the specific chromosome contained on both of the metacentrics.

The Consequences of Monosomy

In an extensive series of investigations, Gropp and his collaborators (1974, 1975, 1976) have shown that mouse embryos trisomic for any of the autosomes survive beyond the time of implantation, with the earliest lethality occurring about 10–12 days after fertilization. The time of death and the combination of developmental abnormalities are specific for each of the trisomies. By contrast, very few, if any, monosomic embryos are detectable

after implantation. A similar situation also occurs in man. Among spontaneous abortions, the frequency of autosomal trisomies was 26%, but only
0.1% monosomies were found (Hassold et al., 1978).

With respect to the mouse, and presumably man as well, two hypotheses
to explain the discrepancy between the frequencies of monosomics and
trisomics can be advanced: either nullisomic sperm (sperm lacking an
autosome) are incapable of fertilizing eggs, or monosomic embryos die prior
to or during the time of implantation. Using the approach described here, we
have investigated these two possibilities. The data, which have already been
published in detail (Epstein and Travis, 1979), are summarized in Table I. As
the breeding scheme used predicts equal numbers of monosomic and trisomic
progeny, the actual observation of such equality in Day 3 embryos (late
morulae and early blastocysts) bred to be aneuploid for chromosome 1, 12, or
19 indicates that nullisomic sperm are capable of fertilizing normal eggs and
that monosomic embryos can survive in expected numbers until at least the
time of blastulation.

During the 24 hr following blastulation there is a precipitous decline in
the viability of monosomy-19 embryos, with virtually none surviving to the
late blastocyst stage. A lesser decline is also noted among embryos monosomic
for chromosome 1. The death of the monosomy-19 embryos cannot be
attributed to the hemizygous expression of recessive lethal genes, for the same
results were obtained when the single chromosome 19 in the monosomic
embryos was contributed by either outbred ICR or highly inbred C57BL/6J
females. Although death does not occur until after blastulation, determination
of cell numbers in monosomy-19 embryos and their normal and trisomic
littermates reveals a significant lag in growth by the morula stage, when the
latter two groups have a mean of 21–22 cells per embryo and the monosomic
embryos only 15 (Magnuson and Epstein, unpublished data). Contrary to
previous suggestions, the severity or time of lethality of the aneuploid state
does not seem to be a direct function of the size of the chromosome involved
nor of the amount of euchromatin (as assessed by banding studies) that it
appears to have (Epstein and Travis, 1979).

When death of an embryo occurs at a stage as early as the blastocyst, it is
possible that the genetic defect has resulted in general cell lethality. Such has
been suggested to be the case in embryos homozygous for the t^{12} mutation. On
the other hand, it is also possible that the problem is one of overall embryonic
organization and formation, with the individual cells themselves still being
capable of some degree of viability and function. One method for resolving
this question is by the construction of aggregation chimeras in which
monosomic and normal embryos are combined at the 8- to 16-cell stage and
reimplanted in foster mothers (Figure 3). The reimplanted embryos are then
removed at a later stage and examined for the presence of aneuploid cells. In
carrying out the latter, the existence of a chimeric state is first demonstrated

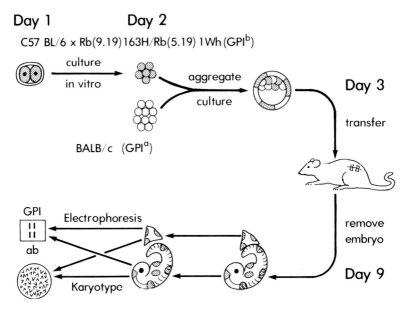

Figure 3. The construction of aggregation chimeras containing cells aneuploid for chromosome 19. Potentially aneuploid embryos (speckled), which are of glucose phosphate isomerase (GPI) electrophoretic type b, are combined with normal BALB/c embryos of type a. Because of the tendency of the former embryos to grow more rapidly, they are isolated a day earlier and cultured overnight to retard cleavage slightly. The aggregated embryos are reimplanted into a foster mother at Day 3 (counting the day of the mating plug as Day 0) and removed at Day 9. Both embryonic and extraembryonic tissues are analyzed, and the existence of the chimeric state is established by the presence of both GPI variants. The chromosomal status of the chimeras is determined by karyotype analysis, and the relative proportions of aneuploid and normal cells are estimated from both the electrophoretic and the karyotypic analyses.

by the finding of electrophoretic markers (generally variants of glucose phosphate isomerase) characteristic of each of the embryonic inputs into the chimera, and the chromosomal status of the chimeras is verified by direct cytogenetic analysis. Preliminary studies have demonstrated that monosomy-19 cells can be "rescued" in such chimeras until at least Day 8–9, the egg cylinder stage, and are present in both embryonic and extraembryonic tissues (Magnuson and Epstein, unpublished data). Accordingly, monosomy 19 cannot be considered as a cell lethal, at least during the preimplantation period.

Identical Twin Embryos

All of the studies on aneuploid preimplantation embryos carried out thus far by ourselves and others (see particularly Dyban and Baranov, 1978) have required the destruction of the embryo at the time of karyotype preparation. While satisfactory for the types of studies reported, this technique does not permit deeper investigations of the molecular and functional consequences of the aneuploid state. For such studies to be possible, it is necessary to have a method that permits cytogenetic characterization in a nondestructive manner. While direct embryonic characterization is perhaps feasible in large blastocysts of the size that occurs in rabbits, for which a biopsy can be performed by removal of a small amount of trophectoderm, the small size of the mouse embryo precludes use of this technique. However, this difficulty can be circumvented by an approach first employed for the biochemical analysis of embryos of known sex (Epstein *et al.*, 1978a) (Figure 4). The blastomeres of two-cell embryos are separated (by softening the zona pellucida with Pronase and pipetting) and cultured in parallel. The resulting identical twin embryos, which are capable of forming blastocysts (Figure 5), have half the number of cells of normal embryos. At any stage along the way, one of the twin embryos can be removed from culture and used for whatever studies are required; the other embryo is karyotyped at the morula or blastocyst stage. The efficiency of this procedure is relatively high: 71% of blastomere pairs

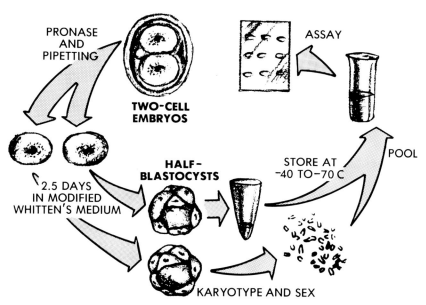

Figure 4. The preparation of identical twin "half-embryos." The blastomeres of two-cell embryos are separated and cultured under oil in the wells of microtiter plates. One of the twin embryos can be used for genotypic assignment (usually by karyotyping) and the other for biochemical assay. The details of the procedure are given in Epstein *et al.* (1978a). (Reprinted with permission from Epstein *et al.*, 1978b.)

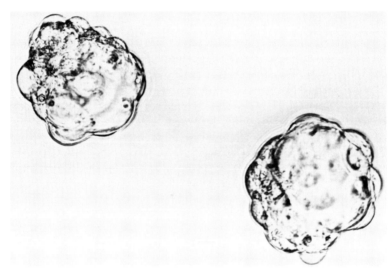

Figure 5. Identical twin "half-embryos" at the blastocyst stage.

develop to blastocysts and 47% of the pairs are characterizable cytogenetically, yielding an overall efficiency of 33%.

In its initial use, this method permitted the demonstration, based on measurements of hypoxanthine guanine phosphoribosyltransferase activity, that both X chromosomes function in female mouse embryos prior to the time of blastulation (Epstein *et al.*, 1978a). The application of this approach to the study of aneuploid embryos is quite straightforward, as it involves only the direct analysis of the embryonic karyotype. However, by incorporating appropriate cytogenetic or biochemical markers, this method can also be made applicable to the investigation of other genetic abnormalities affecting early embryonic development, particularly those produced by homozygosity for recessive genes. In these instances it will be possible to identify specifically the affected embryos and to separate them for analytical purposes from heterozygous and normal littermates.

Conclusions

It has recently become possible to manipulate the chromosomes of the mouse to produce aneuploid embryos of desired types in high frequency. This has permitted the elucidation of some of the properties of aneuploid embryos during the preimplantation period. In combination with techniques for preparing identical twin embryos and for the biochemical, immunological, and physiological analysis of these embryos, the systematic investigation of the early molecular and functional consequences of aneuploidy is now feasible.

ACKNOWLEDGMENTS

This work was supported by Grants HD-03132 and GM-24309 from the National Institutes of Health. The author is an investigator of the Howard Hughes Medical Institute.

The author expresses his appreciation to Mr. Bruce Travis for preparing Figures 4 and 5.

References

Campanna, E., Gropp, A., Winking, H., Noack, G., and Civitelli, M. V., 1976, Robertsonian metacentrics in the mouse, *Chromosoma* **58**:341–353.

Dyban, A. P., and Baranov, V. S., 1978, *The Cytogenetics of Mammalian Embryogenesis*, Nauka, Moscow (in Russian).

Epstein, C. J., and Travis, B., 1979, Preimplantation lethality of monosomy for mouse chromosome 19, *Nature (London)* **280**:144–145.

Epstein, C. J., Smith, S., Travis, B., and Tucker, G., 1978a, Both X-chromosomes function before visible X-chromosome inactivation in female mouse embryos, *Nature (London)* **274**: 500–503.

Epstein, C. J., Travis, B., Tucker, G., and Smith, S., 1978b, The direct demonstration of an X-chromosome dosage effect prior to inactivation, in: *Genetic Mosaics and Chimeras in Mammals* (L. B. Russell, ed.), Plenum Press, New York, pp. 261–267.

Gropp, A., and Winking, H., 1981, Robertsonian translocations: Cytology, meiosis, segregation patterns and biological consequences of heterozygosity, in: *Proceedings of the Symposium on the House Mouse*, The Zoological Society, London, in press.

Gropp, A., Giers, D., and Kolbus, V., 1974, Trisomy in the fetal back cross progeny of male and female metacentric heterozygotes of the mouse, I, *Cytogenet. Cell Genet.* **13**:511–535.

Gropp, A., Kolbus, V., and Giers, D., 1975, Systematic approach to the study of trisomy in the mouse, II, *Cytogenet. Cell Genet.* **14**:42–62.

Gropp, A., Putz, B., and Zimmerman, U., 1976, Autosomal monosomy and trisomy causing developmental failure, *Curr. Top. Pathol.* **62**:177–192.

Hassold, T. J., Matsuyama, A., Newlands, I. M., Matsuura, J. S., Jacobs, P. A., Manuel B., and Tsuei, J., 1978, A cytogenetic study of spontaneous abortions in Hawaii, *Ann. Hum. Genet.* **41**:443–454.

White, B. J., Tjio, J. H., Van de Water, L. C., and Crandall, C., 1974, Trisomy 19 in the laboratory mouse. I. Frequency in different crosses at specific developmental stages and relationship of trisomy to cleft palate, *Cytogenet. Cell Genet.* **13**:217–231.

11

BLASTOCYST FLUID FORMATION

DALE JOHN BENOS and JOHN D. BIGGERS

All mammalian blastocysts undergo some expansion prior to implantation, but the amount varies between species. Blastocysts of the human, mouse, and rat display minimal volume changes, while those of the rabbit and pig undergo enormous increases. Figure 1 presents growth curves for preimplantation rabbit blastocysts. The blastocoelic cavity increases from about 70 nl on Day 4 postcoitus (p.c.) to almost 80 μl on Day 7 p.c., the day of implantation. This increase in size stems largely from fluid accumulation, although cell multiplication also occurs (Daniel, 1964). Because the blastocyst consists almost entirely of a single-cell-thick epithelium, the trophectoderm, it is ideally suited for the study of developmental aspects of epithelial solute and water movements.

This chapter initially summarizes several important references on the transport of substances across the wall of the blastocyst. We will then focus on recent experiments designed to elucidate the molecular basis of solute transport in preimplantation rabbit blastocysts. The experiments will be discussed under three main headings: (1) the number of active transport "pump" sites (Benos, 1981b), (2) the relationship between oxidative metabolism and active transport (Benos and Balaban, 1980), and (3) developmental aspects of solute transport mechanisms, in particular, amiloride-sensitive Na entry, Na-dependent glucose and amino acid uptake, and nonelectrolyte permeability (Benos, 1981a).

Previous work by several different laboratories has established that the rabbit trophectoderm can actively transport solutes, and that the massive

DALE JOHN BENOS and JOHN D. BIGGERS • Department of Physiology and Biophysics, Laboratory of Human Reproduction and Reproductive Biology, Harvard Medical School, Boston, Massachusetts 02115.

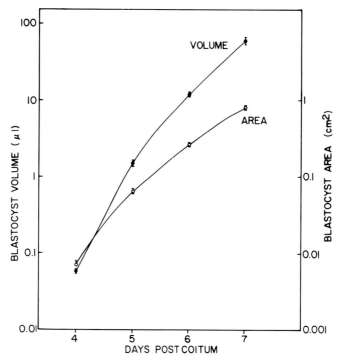

Figure 1. Growth curves for preimplantation rabbit blastocysts. Each point represents the mean of at least 40 separate blastocysts. Area and volume measurements were made as described in Benos and Balaban (1980).

fluid accumulation seen during the preimplantation period of development is a direct result of these processes (see Biggers and Powers, 1979, for a recent review). Smith (1970) showed that fluid accumulation was inhibited if the embryos were cooled to $0°C$ or if they were incubated for at least 2 hr in a solution containing a very high concentration of the Na^+/K^+-activated adenosine triphosphate (Na^+/K^+ ATPase) inhibitor, ouabain. Both Gamow and Daniel (1970) and Cross and Brinster (1970) demonstrated that a transepithelial potential difference existed across the rabbit trophectoderm, and that this potential difference could be reduced to zero if the blastocysts were exposed to dinitrophenol, cyanide, iodoacetate, or anoxic conditions. Cross (1971, 1973, 1974) measured unidirectional tracer Na^+ and Cl^- fluxes in conjunction with short-circuit current measurements in Day 6 p.c. blastocysts, and concluded that Na^+, Cl^-, and HCO_3^- are actively transported from the medium into the blastocoelic cavity. Borland et al. (1976) used electron-probe microanalysis to measure the concentration of several elements in micro-droplet samples of blastocoele fluid. This work showed that the rate of fluid accumulation was directly related to the rate of net Na^+ and Cl^- accumulation.

Further, and very importantly, the rate of both solute and H_2O accumulation, expressed either per unit surface area or per cell, increased with developmental age. Later, Biggers, *et al.* (1978) presented experiments that showed that the microinjection of ouabain into the blastocoelic cavity of Day 6 p.c. rabbit blastocysts would inhibit fluid accumulation.

The evidence that exists at present indicates that the formation of the blastocoelic fluid involves the active transport of ions and possibly, other solutes across the trophoblast wall. Water presumably follows the gradients established by the active solute transport mechanism. Fluid transport is isotonic (Borland *et al.*, 1977), and the active transport of NaCl is of sufficient magnitude to account for the water movements (Borland *et al.*, 1976).

If the trophectoderm were impermeable to water, then clearly osmosis resulting from active solute transport could not account for net fluid accumulation. Recently, Borland and Biggers (1981) have determined the hydraulic conductivity (L_p) of rabbit blastocysts at Days 5 and 6 p.c. When the embryos were incubated in a medium made hypertonic with 100 mM sucrose at 37° C, the L_p averaged 80×10^{-7} cm sec^{-1} atm^{-1}. From this value an average osmotic permeability coefficient (P_f) for rabbit trophectoderm can be calculated using the formula

$$P_f = L_p RT / V_{H_2O}$$

where R is the gas constant, T is the absolute temperature, and V_{H_2O} is the partial molar volume for water. The result is 1.13×10^{-2} cm sec^{-1}. This value for P_f is comparable to that obtained for rat jejunum, and is much higher than that of rabbit gall bladder, frog skin, toad urinary bladder (see House, 1974), or fertilized mouse ova (Leibo, 1980).

Na^+/K^+ ATPase and Blastocyst Fluid Accumulation

As fluid accumulation by the blastocyst can be inhibited by ouabain, and as ouabain inhibits net transepithelial Na^+ flux in most epithelia, there should be a component of unidirectional Na^+ influx across the trophectoderm that is inhibited in a dose-dependent fashion by ouabain. Figure 2 demonstrates that this is indeed the case in Day 6 p.c. rabbit blastocysts. This figure relates the percent inhibition of the unidirectional, transtrophectodermal influx of $^{22}Na^+$ versus different concentrations of ouabain injected into the blastocoelic cavity. The $^{22}Na^+$ influxes were measured between 30 and 45 min after ouabain injection. One hundred percent inhibition was operationally defined as that produced by a concentration of 0.1 mM ouabain in the blastocoele fluid. The magnitude of this fluid represents approximately 50% of the total $^{22}Na^+$ influx. The results demonstrate that the $K_{1/2}$ for ouabain, defined as the concentration of ouabain producing 50% inhibition, is around 0.1 μM.

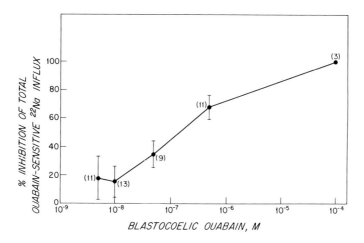

Figure 2. Percent inhibition of ouabain-sensitive $^{22}Na^+$ influx versus blastocoelic ouabain concentration in Day 6 p.c. rabbit embryos. The total ouabain-sensitive Na^+ influx was operationally defined as that produced by 10^{-4} M ouabain. Fluxes were measured 30–45 min after microinjection of ouabain.

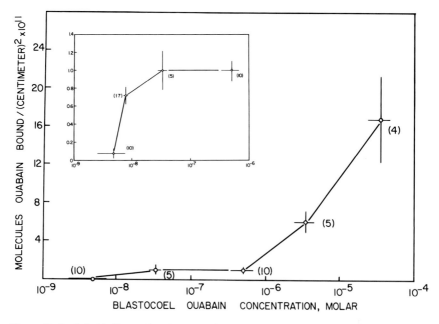

Figure 3. Ouabain binding to Day 6 p.c. rabbit embryos as a function of blastocoelic ouabain concentration. (Reproduced by permission of Academic Press from Benos, 1981b.)

As ouabain can inhibit Na^+ influxes in blastocysts, it is reasonable to presume that the number of pump sites can be determined by measuring the extent of $[^3H]$ouabain binding to the tissue, assuming a stoichiometry of one ouabain molecule per Na^+/K^+ ATPase molecule. However, in any binding study, a range of substrate concentrations leading to minimal nonspecific (i.e., nonpump-associated) binding must be chosen. Figure 3 plots the number of ouabain molecules bound per square centimeter of blastocyst area (corrected for extracellular space trapping) as a function of the blastocoelic ouabain concentration. In these experiments, each blastocyst was exposed to ouabain for at least 2 hr. After this time, each blastocyst was thoroughly washed with ice-cold tracer-free Krebs–Ringer bicarbonate buffer. The insert of Figure 3 is an expanded plot of the binding at low ouabain concentrations. At concentrations up to $0.05\,\mu M$ ouabain, the binding increases. Between 0.05 and $0.5\,\mu M$, the amount of ouabain bound is independent of concentration. Above 0.5 μM, the amount of ouabain bound is again dose dependent. It has been shown that extracellular K^+ competes with ouabain for specific binding to the Na^+/K^+ ATPase pool, and has no effect upon the nonspecific component of binding (Baker and Willis, 1970). In other experiments, it was found that raising the blastocoelic K^+ concentration antagonized the rate of ouabain binding when the concentration of ouabain was less than $0.5\,\mu M$, but had no effect on the rate of binding at higher concentrations. Furthermore, K^+ does not affect the equilibrium levels of binding. The results indicate that the binding observed at ouabain concentrations above 0.5 μM is largely nonspecific. To measure the number of pump sites in the rabbit blastocyst, the concentration of blastocoelic ouabain chosen was 0.5 μM with an exposure time of 2 hr. If these conditions cause complete and specific saturation of all basolateral Na^+/K^+ ATPase molecules, the magnitude of the ouabain-sensitive Na^+ influx should be identical to that measured when higher ouabain concentrations are used. In fact, this proves to be the case: the ouabain sensitive Na^+ influx measured subsequent to injection 0.5 μM ouabain and 2-hr incubation is the same as that measured after 0.1 mM ouabain. The magnitude of this flux is around $0.3\,\mu$mole cm^{-2} hr^{-1} for Day 6 p.c. blastocysts.

The number of molecules of $[^3H]$ouabain bound per blastocyst on Days 4–7 p.c. is shown in Figure 4A. Statistical analysis shows that the increase in the number of molecules is biphasic ($p < 0.001$). The number of molecules bound increases about 50-fold between Days 4 and 5 p.c., changes little between Days 5 and 6, and then increases about 5-fold by Day 7. The surface area of the blastocyst does not increase in a similar biphasic way (Figure 4A), so that when the results are expressed as the number of ouabain molecules bound per unit area there is a significant drop between Days 5 and 6 (Figure 4B). These results suggest that there are two phases of appearance of Na^+/K^+ ATPase, one between Days 4 and 5 and another after Day 6. Because the

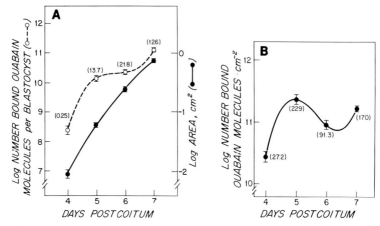

Figure 4. (A) Log number of ouabain molecules bound per blastocyst as a function of age. The surface area per blastocyst at different ages is also shown. (B) Log number of ouabain molecules bound per unit surface area of blastocyst as a function of age. The numbers in parentheses refer to the average number of ouabain molecules in billions. The data were fitted by orthogonal polynomial regression analysis. The minimum order of polynomial to which the ouabain binding data correspond is 3, while that for the surface area data is 2. The number of blastocysts used for measuring ouabain binding were 5, 11, 10, and 7 for Day 3, 5, 6, and 7 p.c. embryos, respectively. These data were taken from Benos (1981b) and are reproduced here by permission of Academic Press. Surface area data are from Figure 1.

trophoblast cells continue to divide between Days 5 and 6, the density of Na^+/K^+ ATPase molecules per unit area diminishes during this time.

Unidirectional $^{22}Na^+$ influxes were measured in the absence and presence of ouabain in different-aged blastocysts to assess the magnitude of the ouabain-sensitive component of transepithelial Na^+ transport. These tracer fluxes were compared to the net Na^+ flux estimates of Borland et al. (1976) (Table I). It can be seen that both the ouabain-sensitive component of this

Table I

Fluid Accumulation, Net and Ouabain-Sensitive Na^+ Influxes in Preimplantation Rabbit Blastocysts

Days postcoitus	Fluid accumulation rate[a] (μl cm^{-2} hr^{-1})	Net Na^+ accumulation rate[a] (μmole cm^{-2} hr^{-1})	Ouabain-sensitive $^{22}Na^+$ influx[b] (μmole cm^{-2} hr^{-1})
4	7.57	0.098	—
5	26.05	0.342	0.20
6	32.26	0.452	0.33
7	70.98	0.820	1.3

[a] From Borland et al. (1976).
[b] From Benos (1981b).

unidirectional Na^+ influx and the estimated net flux of Na^+ increased with developmental age. It can be concluded that the increased active transport of Na^+, and hence fluid accumulation, observed with age results from both an increased number of pump sites and an increased capacity of each site to transport Na^+.

Oxygen Consumption and Active Transport

Measurements of blastocyst oxygen consumption in the absence and presence of ouabain have also been performed in order to ascertain the degree of coupling between the aerobic conversion of energy and active ion transport (Benos and Balaban, 1980). A linear relationship between the rate of oxygen consumption and active sodium transport has been observed in many transporting epithelia. As transepithelial fluid transport across the rabbit trophectoderm is, at least in part, mediated by the Na^+/K^+ ATPase (Biggers *et al.*, 1978), and as there is a large, ouabain-sensitive component to Na^+ influxes (Benos, 1981b), the relative metabolic cost of active Na^+ transport in the developing blastocyst can be determined by measuring the oxygen consumption Q_{O_2} of blastocysts incubated in Krebs Ringer, before and after injection with ouabain. If ATP is the energy source for active sodium transport, as is the case for all epithelia heretofore studied, a decrease in active transport produced by ouabain would result in a decrease in the rate of ATP hydrolysis, which in turn would result in an increase in the intracellular ATP $(ADP + P_i)$ ratio. This in turn would be manifest as a decrease in the rate of blastocyst oxygen consumption. Table II compares the inhibition of $^{22}Na^+$ influx in Day 6 p.c. blastocysts produced by either ouabain or KCN. Maximal inhibition of Na^+ influx by ouabain averaged 0.33μmole cm^{-2} hr^{-1}, a value not significantly different from the 0.36μ mole cm^{-2} hr^{-1} inhibition produced by 0.1 mM KCN. Oxygen consumption by rabbit blastocysts is completely abolished by this concentration of cyanide (Benos and Balaban, 1980). The combination of cyanide and ouabain does not induce any significant change in the $^{22}Na^+$ influx inhibition as compared to that produced by either agent alone. Therefore, when oxidative metabolism is reduced to zero, active sodium

Table II

The Effect of Ouabain and KCN on $^{22}Na^+$ Influxes in
Day 6 p.c. Rabbit Blastocysts

	n	J_{Na}^i (μmole cm^{-2} hr^{-1})
Control	9	0.71 ± 0.13
5×10^{-3} M ouabain	9	0.38 ± 0.03
1×10^{-4} M KCN	10	0.35 ± 0.06
KCN + ouabain	3	0.31 ± 0.08

transport is completely inhibited. Furthermore, when active Na^+ transport is inhibited, the reduction in Q_{O_2} is correlated with the degree of inhibition.

Ouabain depressed the Q_{O_2} of blastocysts of all ages, but the percent inhibition was different for different-aged embryos. The results of these experiments are summarized in Figure 5. The ouabain-sensitive Q_{O_2} (expressed as a percentage of total Q_{O_2}) is plotted as a function of blastocyst age. Ouabain inhibited the Q_{O_2} or Day 4 p.c. embryos by 43%, of Day 5 embryos by 62%, of Day 6 embryos by 70%, and of Day 7 embryos by only 16%. The absolute values of Q_{O_2} averaged $4 \mu l \, O_2 \, cm^{-2} \, hr^{-1}$ for Day 4 and 5 rabbit blastocysts, and $2.7 \mu l \, O_2 \, cm^{-2} \, hr^{-1}$ for Day 6 and 7 embryos. Between Days 4 and 6, the respiration that supports Na^+/K^+ ATPase activity is as high as in the mammalian kidney, which is highly specialized for active transport (Balaban et al., 1980). The most obvious physiological function occurring during this Day 4–6 period is blastocyst expansion via fluid accumulation, and from these measurements it appears that the energy requirements used for active transport predominate. The change in the coupling of respiration to transport

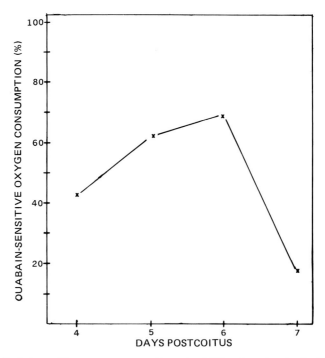

Figure 5. Ouabain-sensitive oxygen consumption rate of different-aged preimplantation rabbit blastocysts. The data are expressed as percent of total Q_{O_2} (Reproduced by permission of the Society for the Study of Reproduction from Benos and Balaban, 1980.)

at Day 7 may reflect a shift in the utilization of the energy derived from oxidative metabolism from one of fluid transport to the support of other functions of the trophectoderm and inner cell mass that begin at this time.

Developmental Aspects of Solute Transport in Blastocysts

There are several characteristics of the rabbit trophectoderm indicating that important developmental changes in transport properties are occurring during the preimplantation period, particularly between Day 6 and Day 7 p.c. It is now well established that (1) the rate of fluid and solute transport increases with age as well as significant fluctuations occurring in the number of pump sites per cell (Borland et al., 1976; Benos, 1981b); (2) the ouabain-sensitive oxygen consumption sharply decreases between Day 6 and Day 7 (Benos and Balaban, 1980); and (3) the transepithelial potential difference increases in magnitude and reverses polarity between Day 6 and Day 7 (Powers et al., 1977). Other changes have also been detected in preliminary studies and will be briefly summarized.

Amiloride Sensitivity

Table III presents $^{22}Na^+$ influx measurements in Day 6 and 7 embryos in the absence and presence of the pyrazine diuretic, amiloride (Benos, 1981b). Amiloride is a specific inhibitor of transepithelial Na^+ transport in many epithelia (see Benos et al., 1979), and works by blocking the entry of Na^+ into the cellular compartment. The results show that amiloride had no effect on Na^+ influx in the Day 6 embryo, but inhibited this flux by 72% in the Day 7 blastocysts. These observations support the notion that there is an amiloride-sensitive Na^+ entry protein that is either activated or synthesized de novo and inserted in the apical membrane 6 or 7 days after fertilization in the rabbit. Interestingly, a similar appearance of an amiloride-sensitive component of

Table III
The Effect of Amiloride on Unidirectional $^{22}Na^+$ Influxes in Day 6 and 7 p.c. Rabbit Blastocysts[a]

	J^i_{Na} (μmole cm^{-2} hr^{-1})		
	Control	10^{-4} M amiloride	p
Day 6	0.50 ± 0.05 (N = 8)	0.51 ± 0.03 (N = 8)	>0.5
Day 7	3.9 ± 1.1 (N = 9)	1.1 ±0.2 (N = 11)	<0.025

[a]Data taken from Benos (1981b).

Table IV

Sodium Dependence of Glucose Uptake into Different-Aged Preimplantation
Rabbit Blastocyst Trophectoderm[a,b]

	Glucose uptake (pmole cm^{-2} hr^{-1})		
	Day 5 p.c.	Day 6 p.c.	Day 7 p.c.
Na^+-containing medium	0.22 ± 0.03	0.20 ± 0.05	0.49 ± 0.24
	($N = 4$)	($N = 8$)	($N = 11$)
Na^+-free medium	0.22 ± 0.03	0.17 ± 0.05	0.53 ± 0.12
	($N = 10$)	($N = 5$)	($N = 19$)
Probability, mean values are equal	>0.5	>0.5	>0.5

[a] Data taken from Benos (1981a).
[b] Glucose concentration 0.7 μM.

sodium transport across postnatal lamb and pig distal colon has been
reported (Hills *et al.*, 1980). In these tissues, Na^+ transport began to display
amiloride sensitivity between the first and the second weeks after birth. These
authors suggest that increased plasma levels of cortisol and/or aldosterone
may be responsible for this activity.

Glucose and Methionine Uptake

The Na^+ dependence of total tissue uptake of glucose and methionine was
also studied at different preimplantation stages (Benos, 1981a). Table IV
summarizes the glucose experiments. Although there are significant differences in the absolute rates of [^{3}H] glucose uptake between Day 5, 6, and 7
embryos, there is no dependence of this process on external sodium (choline
was used as a replacement ion). This should be contrasted with the results
obtained with methionine (Figure 6). Methionine uptake was about 10^4-fold

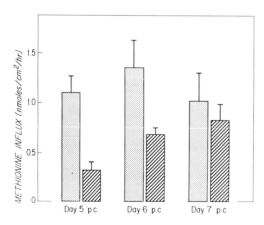

Figure 6. [^{3}H]methionine uptake into
different-aged preimplantation rabbit
blastocysts in the presence (stippled
bars) and absence (hatched bars) of
external sodium. An equimolar quantity of choline chloride was used to
substitute for the NaCl. Probabilities
that the difference between mean methionine uptake rates plus and minus
sodium was significant are $p < 0.005$,
$p < 0.025$ and $p < 0.5$ for Day 5, 6,
and 7 p.c. embryos, respectively.
(From Benos, 1981a.)

greater than that of glucose at all developmental ages. At Day 5, the total [³H]methionine uptake was diminished over 70% when the external Na⁺ concentration was reduced to zero. The Na⁺-dependent uptake was reduced to 50% by Day 6. By Day 7, [³H]methionine uptake was independent of the external Na⁺ concentration.

Urea Permeability

The transepithelial influx of the small, hydrophilic molecule urea was also measured (Benos, 1981a). In some epithelia (e.g., frog skin; Mandel and Curran, 1972), transepithelial urea fluxes occur only through the pathway between adjacent cells (the paracellular pathway), while in others (e.g., toad urinary bladder; Levine *et al.*, 1973) there exists a saturable, phloretin-sensitive urea cellular entry mechanism. Figure 7A presents measurements of

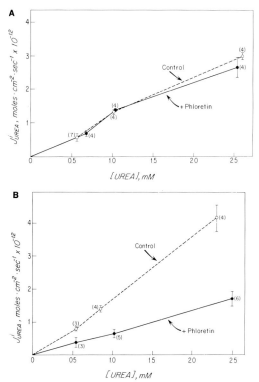

Figure 7. (A) [¹⁴C]urea influx versus external urea concentration in the absence and presence of 5×10^{-4} M phloretin in Day 6 p.c. rabbit embryos. (B) [¹⁴C]urea influx versus external urea concentration in the absence and presence of 5×10^{-4} M phloretin in Day 7 p.c. rabbit embryos. (Reproduced by permission of the Physiological Society from Benos, 1981a.)

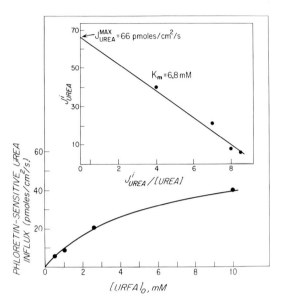

Figure 8. Phloretin-sensitive transepithelial urea influx versus external urea concentration. The inset is a single reciprocal plot (Eadie) of the same flux data. (From Benos, 1981a.)

unidirectional transepithelial $[^{14}C]$urea influxes versus external urea concentration in Day 6 blastocysts in the absence and presence of 0.5 mM phloretin. Phloretin had no effect on urea influx at any concentration of external urea. Figure 7B shows an identical plot for Day 7 blastocysts. Phloretin significantly inhibited the urea flux at all urea concentrations. If the difference between the urea flux determined in the presence and absence of phloretin is plotted against the urea concentration (Figure 8), the resultant curve is a rectangular hyperbola. By appropriate transformations, the kinetic constants V_{max} and K_m can be determined. For Day 7 blastocysts, these values are 66 pmoles cm^{-2}sec^{-1} and 6.8 mM, respectively (see inset of Figure 8). Thus, it appears that the rabbit blastocyst acquires a phloretin-sensitive, urea entry pathway between Day 6 and Day 7 p.c.

Transepithelial Electrical Resistance Measurements

Table V presents a compilation of relevant physiological characteristics of the two classes of transporting epithelia, the so-called electrically "tight" and "leaky" tissues (Diamond, 1977). Although not all of these properties have been examined in preimplantation rabbit blastocysts, some tentative observations and conclusions can be drawn. First of all, measurements of transepithelial electrical resistances of Day 4 and 6 rabbit embryos have been made (Benos, 1981a). These were done by first impaling a blastocyst with two

Table V
Characteristics of "Tight" and "Leaky" Transporting Epithelia

Property	"Tight"	"Leaky"
Potential difference	High (>20 mV)	Low (<20 mV)
Transepithelial electrical resistance	High ($>300 \, \Omega \cdot cm^2$)	Low ($<300 \, \Omega \cdot cm^2$)
Can support large gradients of concentration and osmolality?	Yes	No
Water permeability	Low	High
ADH sensitivity	Yes	No
Aldosterone sensitivity	Yes	No
Coupled Na^+-nonelectrolyte apical entry mechanism?	No	Yes
Coupled $Na+Cl$ apical entry mechanism?	No	Usually
Amiloride-sensitive Na^+ flux?	Yes	No

microelectrodes, one for injecting current, the other for recording voltage. A 5-min train of bipolar current pulses of amplitude 0.3–500 μA and 5-sec duration was delivered. From the measured blastocyst area, the transepithelial electrical resistance of six Day 4 blastocysts averaged $8.4 \pm 5.5 \, \Omega \cdot cm^2$ (range 1–35 $\Omega \cdot cm^2$), while that measured in three Day 6 blastocysts was 1758 ± 833 $\Omega \cdot cm^2$. It is apparent that the electrical resistance of the rabbit trophectoderm dramatically increases between Day 4 and Day 6 p.c. In light of these findings, the rabbit trophectoderm epithelium appears to differentiate from an electrically "leaky" to an electrically "tight" epithelium between the early and the late blastocyst stages. The early (Day 4) embryo has a very low transepithelial resistance, a low transepithelial potential, does not possess an amiloride-sensitive Na^+ entry pathway, and has a Na^+-dependent glucose or amino acid uptake system. Late blastocysts (Day 6–7), on the other hand, have high transepithelial resistances and potentials, possess an amiloride-sensitive Na^+ entry pathway, and have no Na^+-dependent glucose or amino acid uptake systems.

Conclusions

The evidence that has been reviewed indicates that the isotonic fluid accumulation of the rabbit blastocyst occurs as a result of active solute transport processes. The membrane-bound enzyme, Na^+/K^+ ATPase, plays a crucial role in transepithelial fluid movements during the preimplantation period. Much of the metabolic energy derived from oxidative processes directly supports the activity of the Na^+/K^+ ATPase. The trophectoderm epithelium, in addition to its fluid-transporting function, displays marked changes in its solute transport characteristics during development. These changes include the acquistion of an amiloride-sensitive component to Na^+ influx, the acquistion of a phloretin-sensitive component to urea influx, and the loss of a Na^+-dependent methionine uptake system. The rabbit blastocyst differentiations from a "leaky" to a "tight" transporting epithelium during preimplantation development. It is apparent that the transport activity of the preimplantation rabbit blastocyst (and presumably of all mammalian blastocysts) is high, and also that this tissue may well be a useful model not only for understanding epithelial transport function in general, but also for understanding the physiological events associated with normal embryonic development.

ACKNOWLEDGMENTS

The invaluable technical assistance of Ms. Marie Angela Blazonis is gratefully acknowledged. We also thank Ms. Diane Staples for typing the manuscript. This work was supported by NIH Grant HD 12353 and by funds from the Andrew W. Mellon Foundation.

References

Baker, P. F., and Willis, J. S., 1970, Potassium ions and the binding of cardiac glycosides to mammalian cells, *Nature (London)* **266**:521–523.

Balaban, R. S., Mandel, L. J., Soltoff, S. P., and Storey, J. M., 1980, Coupling of active ion transport and aerobic respiratory rate in isolated renal tubules, *Proc. Natl. Acad. Sci. USA* **22**:447–451.

Benos, D. J., 1981a, Developmental changes in epithelial transport characteristics of preimplantation rabbit blastocysts, *J. Physiol. (London)*, in press.

Benos, D. J., 1981b, Ouabain binding to preimplantation rabbit blastocysts, *Dev. Biol.* **83**:69–78.

Benos, D. J., and Balaban, R. S., 1980. The energy requirements for active ion transport of the developing mammalian blastocyst, *Biol. Reprod.* **23**:941–947.

Benos, D. J., Mandel, L. J., and Balaban, R. S., 1979, On the mechanism of the amiloride-sensitive entry site interaction of anuran epithelia, *J. Gen. Physiol.* **73**:307–326.

Biggers, J. D., and Powers, R. D., 1979, Na transport and swelling of the mammalian blastocyst: Effect of amiloride, in: *Amiloride and Epithelial Sodium Transport* (A. W. Cuthbert, G. M. Fanelli, Jr., and A. Scriabine, eds.), Urban & Schwarzenberg, Munich, pp. 167–179.

Biggers, J. D., Borland, R. M., and Lechene, C. P., 1978, Ouabain-sensitive fluid accumulation and ion transport by rabbit blastocysts, *J. Physiol. (London)* **280**:319–330.

Borland, R. M., and Biggers, J. D., 1981, Water permeability of the rabbit blastocyst *in vitro*, manuscript in preparation.

Borland, R. M., Biggers, J. D., and Lechene, C. P., 1976, Kinetic aspects of rabbit blastocoele fluid accumulation: An application of electron probe analysis, *Dev. Biol.* **50**:201–211.

Borland, R. M., Biggers, J. D., and Lechene, C. P., 1977, Fluid transport by rabbit preimplantation blastocysts, *J. Reprod. Fertil.* **51**:131–135.

Cross, M. H., 1971, Rabbit blastocoele perfusion technique, *Nature (London)* **232**:635–637.

Cross, M. H., 1973, Active sodium and chloride transport across the rabbit blastocoele wall, *Biol. Reprod.* **8:**566–575.

Cross, M. H., 1974, Rabbit blastocoele bicarbonate: accumulation rate, *Biol. Reprod.* **11:**654–662.

Cross, M. H., and Brinster, R. L., 1970, Influence of ions, inhibitors and anoxia on transtrophoblast potential of rabbit blastocysts, *Exp. Cell Res.* **62:**303–309.

Daniel, J. C., 1964, Early growth of the rabbit trophoblast, *Am. Nat.* **98:**85–98.

Diamond, J. M., 1977, The epithelial junction: Bridge, gate, and fence, *Physiologist* **20:**10–18.

Gamow, G., and Daniel, J. C., 1970, Fluid transport in the rabbit blastocyst, *Wilhelm Roux Arch. Entwicklungsmech. Org.* **164:**261–278.

Hills, F., James, P. S., Paterson, J. Y. F., and Smith, M. W., 1980, Delayed development of amiloride-sensitive sodium transport in lamb distal colon, *J. Physiol. (London)* **303:**371–384.

House, C. R., 1974, *Water Transport in Cells and Tissues*, Arnold, London.

Leibo, S. P., 1980, Water permeability and its activation energy of fertilized and unfertilized mouse ova, *J. Membr. Biol.* **53:**179–188.

Levine, S., Franki, N., and Hays, R. M., 1973, Effect of phloretin on water and solute movement in the toad bladder, *J. Clin. Invest.* **52:**1435–1442.

Mandel, L. J., and Curran, P. F., 1972, Response of the frog skin to steady-state voltage clamping. I. The shunt pathway, *J. Gen. Physiol.* **59:**503–518.

Powers, R. D., Borland, R. M., and Biggers, J. D., 1977, Acquisition of amiloride-sensitive rheogenic Na^+-transport in the rabbit blastocyst, *Nature (London)* **270:**603–604.

Smith, M. W., 1970, Active transport in the rabbit blastocyst, *Experientia* **26:**736–738.

12

WATER AND ELECTROLYTE TRANSPORT BY PIG CHORIOALLANTOIS

FULLER W. BAZER, M. H. GOLDSTEIN, and D. H. BARRON

Developing pig embryos enter the uterus on Day 3 of pregnancy (day of onset of estrus and mating = Day 0) and undergo hatching from the zona pellucida on about Day 7. By about Day 10.5 to 11.5 the blastocysts achieve a diameter of 5–12 mm and appear as fluid-filled spheres. It is assumed that these expanded spherical pig blastocysts actively accumulate water as described for those of rabbits (Biggers and Borland, 1976; see Benos and Biggers, this volume) and mice (DiZio and Tasca, 1974); however, direct evidence for the mechanism(s) of fluid accumulation in pig blastocysts is not available.

Between Days 11.5 and 16 of pregnancy, pig blastocysts undergo rapid elongation to form a threadlike cylinder of about 800 mm in length and less than 1 mm in diameter (Anderson, 1978). Through this process of trophoblast elongation, the blastocyst achieves contact over a large surface area of the uterine endometrium and the process of placentation begins. Placentation or central implantation refers to the process of adhesion through a microvillous junction between the trophectoderm of the blastocyst and the endometrial surface epithelium. Placentation in the pig is, therefore, a noninvasive process.

The elongated blastocysts then expand through the accumulation of water within membranes derived from evaginations of the embryonic gut. First, the yolk sac accumulates fluid and is transiently involved in bringing the

FULLER W. BAZER • Department of Animal Science, University of Florida, Gainesville, Florida 32611. M. H. GOLDSTEIN • Department of Physiology, University of Florida, Gainesville, Florida 32611. D. H. BARRON • Department of Obstetrics and Gynecology, University of Florida, Gainesville, Florida 32611.

trophoblast into apposition with the uterine wall between Days 17 and 22 of gestation. After Day 22, the yolk sac becomes a vestigial structure.

The allantoic sac forms form an evagination of the hindgut and expands rapidly between Days 18 and 30 of gestation to almost completely fill the extraembryonic coelom. The driving force for expansion of the allantois, and in turn the chorioallantois, appears to be water accumulation from about 1 ml on Day 18 to an average of 200–250 ml on Day 30 of gestation (Knight et al., 1977; Goldstein et al., 1980).

The anatomical studies of Bremer (1916) and Davies (1952) suggested that the allantoic sac serves as a reservoir for fetal excretion, i.e., urine, and they proposed that the mesonephric glomeruli were the source of allantoic fluid. However, they failed to recognize that the urinary system does not produce water, but only redistributes that water that is available to it. McCance and Dickerson (1957) concluded that allantoic fluid is of maternal origin and is derived from secretion of water into the allantoic sac by the allantoic membrane. Demonstrations of active transport of water and other nutrients into the blastocoelic cavity of rabbit (Tuft and Boving, 1970; Biggers and Borland, 1976) and mouse (DiZio and Tasca, 1974) preimplantation blastocysts further support the concept that active-transport processes exist in the chorioallantoic membranes of species having epitheliochorial-type placenta.

The significance of changes in allantoic fluid volume appears to be severalfold. In the case of epitheliochorial placentation, increasing allantoic fluid volume appears to be essential for expanding the chorioallantoic membranes and supporting their apposition with the maternal endometrium. Maximal placental surface area is essential for adequate nutrient and waste exchange in species having this type of placenta. The allantoic fluid is rich in electrolytes, sugars, and proteins and appears to serve as a nutrient reservoir rather than a reservoir for fetal waste. In this respect one must recall that the allantoic epithelium is derived from the hindgut and is, therefore, an absorptive epithelium.

Although amniotic fluid will not be discussed and its source is not clear, it does serve at least a protective role for the fetus. That is, it allows the embryo/fetus to develop in a liquid environment and therefore in a symmetrical fashion, as the forces of gravity and surrounding tissues are negated by the supporting amniotic fluid. As shown by Goldstein et al. (1980), changes in volume and electrolyte composition of allantoic and amniotic fluids are clearly different throughout gestation.

Porcine Allantoic Fluid Volume and Composition

Studies by Wislocki (1935), Knight et al. (1977), and Goldstein et al. (1980) indicate that allantoic fluid volume increases from Day 20 (3.7 ± 3 ml) to Day 30 (189.0 ± 7.4 ml), decreases to Day 45 (74.7 ± 7.4 ml), and then increases again to Day 58 (451.3 ± 53.5 ml). Thereafter, it decreases to Day 112 (23.8 ± 5.5 ml). A comparison of electrolyte concentrations of maternal plasma and allantoic fluid suggests that allantoic fluid is not a dialysate of serum. In fact, osmotic gradients (McCarthy, 1946; McCance and Widdowson, 1953; Meschia et al., 1957; Meschia, 1955; Battaglia et al., 1959) and hydrostatic differences in monkey (Ramsey et al., 1959), human (Hellman et al., 1957; Prystowsky, 1958), and ewe (Barcroft and Barron, 1946; Reynolds, 1960; Davies, 1952) favor exchange of fluids in a fetal-to-maternal direction.

As stated above, McCance and Dickerson (1957) concluded that allantoic fluid was of maternal origin. Crawford and McCance (1960) later reported a net flux of sodium from the allantois toward the maternal tissue and suggested that sodium was essential for maintenance of the short-circuit current and potential difference across the porcine chorioallantois. Furthermore, Goldstein (1977) found that ouabain, Na^+/K^+ ATPase inhibitor, blocked maintenance of a potential difference and short-circuit current by pig chorioallantois maintained in a Ussing double chamber.

As shown in Table I, allantoic fluid volume and total allantoic fluid glucose and fructose all follow a similar pattern of accumulation between Days 21 and Days 30 and 40 of pregnancy. This suggests that water and

Table I

Allantoic Fluid Volume, Total Glucose, and Total Fructose (x ± S.E.M.) on Days 21, 30, and 40 of Gestation in Swine

	Allantoic fluid volume (ml)	Total glucose (mg)	Total fructose (mg)
Control			
Day 21	1.4 ± 0.1 (34)[a]	ND[b]	ND
Day 30	171.8 ± 7.3 (54)	63.6 ± 3.8 (44)	318.3 ± 25.5 (43)
Day 40	47.5 ± 5.1 (34)	4.1 ± 0.5 (29)	98.4 ± 15.8 (31)
UOVX[c]			
Day 21	2.4 ± 0.3 (27)	ND	ND
Day 30	220.6 ± 7.5 (34)	78.0 ± 2.8 (24)	446.7 ± 12.2 (24)
Day 40	48.1 ± 7.4 (25)	4.3 ± 0.8 (23)	80.3 ± 15.2 (24)
BOVX[d]			
Day 21	1.5 ± 0.1 (31)	ND	ND
Day 30	204.2 ± 15.2 (23)	68.1 ± 5.8 (33)	432.0 ± 42.9 (33)
Day 40	109.6 ± 14.4[e] (28)	21.7 ± 4.1[f] (27)	391.6 ± 60.4[f] (28)

[a] Number of gilts in parentheses.
[b] Samples obtained on Day 21 were not analyzed for glucose and fructose.
[c] Gilts unilaterally ovariectomized on Day 4 of pregnancy.
[d] Bilaterally ovariectomized gilts treated with 3.3 mg progesterone and 1.7 μg estrone/kg per day from Day 4 of pregnancy.
[e] Significantly different ($p < 0.05$) from values for control and UOVX gilts.
[f] Significantly different ($p < 0.01$) from values for control and UOVX gilts.

glucose transport may be affected by similar mechanisms. Fructose is produced from glucose by the chorioallantois and is, therefore, quantitatively positively correlated with glucose content (Alexander *et al.*, 1955).

Some speculation is necessary with regard to the possible mechanisms of the observed rapid changes in allantoic fluid volume and composition. We propose that early in gestation, i.e., Days 16 and 18, progesterone may promote the synthesis and/or activation of transport enzymes, e.g., Na^+/K^+ ATPase, in the chorioallantoic membrane. By Day 18, enzymatic activity begins and sodium is pumped out of the allantoic fluid with negative ions (chloride and bicarbonate) following passively to maintain electroneutrality. Thus, the sodium concentration ($[Na^+]$) in allantoic fluid, which is essentially identical to maternal plasma at Day 20 (135 vs 152 meq/liter, respectively), decreases dramatically to Day 30, when allantoic fluid $[Na^+]$ is about 9 meq/liter compared to 153 meq/liter for maternal plasma (Goldstein *et al.*, 1980). Therefore, a concentration gradient is established across the chorioallantois due to Na^+/K^+ ATPase (pump) activity. It is assumed that the rate of active transport of sodium across the chorioallantois in the maternal direction is greater than the rate of passive sodium diffusion in the maternal-to-placental direction. In addition, a high progesterone/estrogen ratio may result in chorioallantoic membrane of low resistance to sodium flux in a maternal-to-placental direction. As sodium flows down its concentration gradient, a negative ion and water or glucose would follow. The water and glucose would accumulate in the allantoic sac while the sodium would be pumped in a maternal direction to maintain the $[Na^+]$ gradient.

The accumulation of allantoic fluid and fructose between Days 20 and 30, for example, would not occur without estrogens, which may decrease the permeability of the chorioallantois by decreasing the passive flow of ions across the membrane. With decreased permeability, i.e., decreased "leakiness' or increased resistance, of the chorioallantois, the active pumping of ions can establish greater ionic gradients.

It is assumed, therefore, that excessive progesterone and excessive estrogen can both impede accumulation of water and glucose in the chorioallantoic sac. A progesterone excess would lead to a chorioallantois of low resistance, which would preclude establishment of concentration gradients necessary for efficient transport. An estrogen excess, on the other hand, would result in a high membrane resistance to the flow of sodium-coupled water and glucose into the chorioallantoic sac and the cessation of their accumulation within the allantoic sac.

Because of observed temporal relationships between changes in progesterone/estrogen ratio and allantoic fluid volume of pigs and known effects of lactogenic hormones, i.e., prolactin and placental lactogen, on osmoregulation, the effects of these steroid and protein hormones on transport properties of the pig chorioallantois have been evaluated.

Effect of Estrogen and Progesterone on
Allantoic Fluid Volume and Composition

In pigs, there are two periods in gestation when the progesterone/estrogen ratio is decreasing, i.e., between Days 15 and 30 and between Days 50 and term (Robertson and King, 1974; Knight *et al.*, 1977). Allantoic fluid volume increases during each of these periods and then ceases to accumulate or actually decreases as the progesterone/estrogen ratio narrows. For example, the first period of allantoic fluid accumulation begins on about Day 20 and reaches an initial peak on Day 30, when the first estrogen peak occurs. The second peak in allantoic fluid occurs between Days 55 and 60, when initiation of the second rise in estrogen becomes evident. After Day 60, placental estrogen production increases to term and allantoic fluid volume steadily declines (Knight *et al.*, 1977).

Knight *et al.* (1974) injected pregnant gilts that were either sham operated or bilaterally ovariectomized on Day 4 with either high (3.3 mg/kg per day) or low (1.1 mg/kg per day) progesterone from Day 4 to Day 40 of gestation. Allantoic fluid volume was significantly greater in sham-operated and ovariectomized gilts receiving the greater dosage of progesterone. These data suggest that the high level of progesterone allowed for a greater progesterone/estrogen ratio that in turn would continue to favor allantoic fluid accumulation after Day 30, when it normally ceases to accumulate. Allantoic fluid volume in ovariectomized gilts was 94.4 ± 13.9 and 177.4 ± 20.4 ml for the low- and high-progesterone groups, respectively.

In a subsequent experiment, 27 gilts were assigned to three treatment groups, three gilts of each group being hysterectomized on Days 21, 30, and 40 of gestation. Control gilts (group I) received corn oil daily from Day 4 until hysterectomy. In Group II, gilts were unilaterally ovariectomized on Day 4. Group III gilts were bilaterally ovariectomized on Day 4 of gestation and injected subcutaneously daily with 3.3 mg progesterone and $1.7\,\mu g$ estrone in corn oil per kilogram body weight until hysterectomy.

The hypothesis tested was that a narrow progesterone/estrogen ratio would be achieved early in gestation in the unilaterally ovariectomized gilts and, therefore, allantoic fluid volume would be increased over that of control and progesterone plus estrogen-treated gilts on Days 21 and 30. The ovariectomized, progesterone plus estrogen-treated gilts were expected to have conceptuses with greater allantoic fluid volume on Day 40 compared to the other two treatment groups, because of maintenance of a ratio between the two steroids that would favor continued accumulation of allantoic fluid. Glucose and fructose concentrations were also measured in allantoic fluid samples, and total glucose and total fructose for each conceptus were calculated by multiplying allantoic fluid volume by concentration of the respective sugars.

Data from this study are summarized in Table I. Allantoic fluid volume was not significantly ($p < 0.10$) affected by treatment on either Day 21 or 30. Furthermore, total glucose and total fructose in allantoic fluid were also similar for the three treatment groups on Day 30. On Day 40, however, allantoic fluid volume ($p < 0.05$), total allantoic fluid glucose ($p < 0.05$), and total allantoic fluid fructose ($p < 0.01$) were greater in progesterone plus estrogen-treated gilts than from gilts in the other two treatment groups.

These data support the concept that altering the progesterone/estrogen ratio can affect allantoic fluid volume. In addition, one may speculate that water and glucose transport across the chorioallantoic membrane may be affected by similar mechanisms. Fructose is presumed to increase due to increased glucose availability to the fetal–placental unit of the pig as has been reported for sheep (Alexander et al., 1955). Consequently, total fructose in allantoic fluid changes in a pattern directly related to that for glucose. One must also consider that fructose is a sequesterable sugar and hence does not move from the fetal–placental unit to the maternal circulation as does glucose (Alexander et al., 1955). Consequently, total glucose in allantoic fluid decreased from 68.1 ± 5.8 mg to 21.7 ± 4.1 mg between Days 30 and 40 in the progesterone plus estrogen-treated gilts, while fructose decreased very little between Day 30 (432.0 ± 42.9 mg) and Day 40 (391.6 ± 60.4 mg) of gestation.

The effect of exogenous steroids on allantoic fluid volume of bilaterally ovariectomized sheep and goats has also been reported. In two studies, Alexander and Williams (1966, 1968) showed that in pregnant ewes ovariectomized 2 weeks after mating, accumulation of allantoic fluid to Day 60 was inversely related to the dose of progesterone given. Ewes receiving the low dosages of progesterone (0.1 and 0.15 mg/kg per day) had conceptuses with allantoic fluid volumes 10-fold higher than those from ewes receiving 0.45 to 1.35 mg progesterone/kg per day and sham-operated control ewes. In a second experiment, either unilaterally or bilaterally ovariectomized ewes received progesterone as in the first experiment, and some ewes received $10 \mu g$ of estradiol per day. Similar to results in the first experiment, low doses of progesterone resulted in greater allantoic fluid volumes; however, those receiving $10 \mu g$ estradiol along with low dosages of progesterone did not have elevated allantoic fluid volumes. Sodium and potassium concentrations tended to be positively associated with allantoic fluid volume.

McGovern (1976) reported the effect of administering either 0.35 or 0.76 mg progesterone/kg per day to goats bilaterally ovariectomized on Day 25 and treated to either Day 56 or 57 of pregnancy. Untreated pregnant goats served as controls. Allantoic fluid volumes were 77.0 ± 13.5, 81.4 ± 18.2, and 251.5 ± 66.5 ml for the control, high-progesterone, and low-progesterone groups, respectively. As in sheep, sodium and potassium concentrations were positively associated with elevated allantoic fluid volumes in the low-progesterone group.

Amniotic fluid volume has not been altered by the progesterone plus estrogen treatment regimes that affect allantoic fluid volume in ovariectomized pigs, sheep, and goats. One must suspect, therefore, that control of volume in these two fluid pools is under control of different endocrine mechanisms.

Effect of Lactogenic Hormones on Transport Properties of the Porcine Chorioallantoic Membrane

Riddle (1963) provided a thorough review of known osmoregulatory roles of prolactin. Prolactin in mammals affects water and ion movement across renal tubules (Stanley and Fleming, 1967) and intestine (Utida *et al.*, 1972; Ramsey and Bern, 1972; Mainoya *et al.*, 1974; Mainoya, 1975). Prolactin is present in large amounts in human amniotic fluid (Friesen *et al.*, 1969; Josimovich *et al.*, 1974), but only in the guinea pig has prolactin been shown to affect water movement across the chorioamnion (Holt and Perks, 1975; Manku *et al.*, 1975).

Human placental lactogen is produced by the syncytiotrophoblast (Beck and Currie, 1967) and has been implicated in the transfer of amino acids from the maternal circulation to that of the fetal–placental unit.

The following sections describe effects of human placental lactogen, prolactin, estrogen, progesterone, and ouabain on the potential difference and short-circuit current across the procine chorioallantois.

Methods

The reproductive tracts of pregnant gilts were exposed by midventral laparotomy. With the uterine vasculature intact, an incision was made along the antimesometrial border of the uterus. The chorioallantois was then separated from the endometrium, removed, and placed in warm (37°C) Krebs Ringer solution until mounted in a Ussing chamber (Ussing and Zerahn, 1951). The potential difference across the chorioallantois was measured in millivolts with a potentiometer, and the short-circuit current was measured on a microammeter. Readings were taken at least every 5–10 min and membranes were allowed to stabilize for 1–2 hr before experiments were initiated. Details of the experimental protocol have been described by Goldstein (1977).

Electrical Properties of the Pig Chorioallantois

The observation that the potential difference (PD) across the chorioallantois changes throughout gestation has been made in goats (Meschia *et al.*, 1958), sheep (Mellor, 1970), and pigs (Crawford and McCance, 1960). Results of measurements of PD and short-circuit current (SCC) on 112 membranes at selected times during gestation were used to calculate membrane resistance

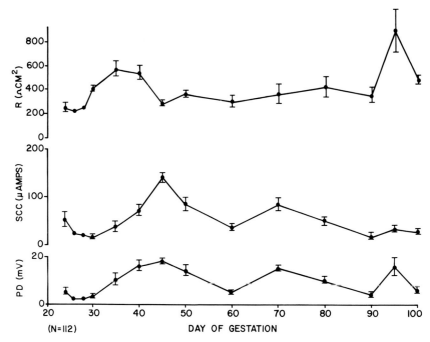

Figure 1. Changes in the electrical properties of the chorioallantois throughout gestation. Changes in the potential difference (PD; in mV); the short-circuit current (SCC; in μA), and the resistance (R; in $\Omega \cdot cm^2$) are shown from Day 24 through Day 100. Each point represents the $x \pm$ S.E., and the total number of observations (N) is shown.

(R) (Watlington *et al.*, 1970). As shown in Figure 1, R changes throughout gestation, but during periods of water movement into the allantoic sac (Days 20–30 and 50–60), R was relatively lower than during periods in gestation when water was not accumulating in the allantoic sac, e.g., Days 31–45.

A comparison of equilibrium potentials and PD across the chorioallantois on the same days indicated that: (1) sodium must be actively transported out of the allantoic fluid daily, as there is less sodium in allantoic fluid than predicted by the equilibrium potential; (2) the potassium equilibrium potential was less than the membrane potential, i.e., more negative at least on Days 28, 40, 60, and 85 of gestation, and therefore potassium must be actively transported into the allantoic fluid, as there is a greater concentration of potassium than predicted by the equilibrium potential; and (3) similar calculations suggested transport of chloride out of the allantoic fluid. It is clear from a definition of the electrochemical gradient that active transport of several ions occurs across the chorioallantois and that the degree of such activity depends upon the stage of gestation.

Ouabain

Ouabain, a cardiac glycoside, is a known inhibitor of active sodium transport in epithelia. This effect is thought to be related to inhibition of a specific enzyme system, Na^+/K^+-activated Mg^{2+}-dependent ATPase located in the cellular membrane and intimately involved in energy-dependent movement of sodium across the membrane (Skou, 1965).

The effect of adding ouabain to the chorionic surface on the PD and SCC is shown in Figure 2A,Б. Ouabain, when added to the chorionic solution in a

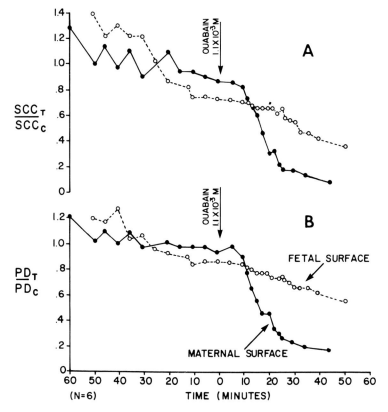

Figure 2. (A) A typical experiment on paired placentae showing the effect on the short-circuit current of adding ouabain (1.1 mM final concentration) to either the material (●) or the fetal (■) surface. Effect is plotted as the ratio SCC_T/SCC_C (SCC_T referring to the SCC at some time T during the treatment, and SCC_C being the mean SCC during the equilibrium period) versus time (minutes). (B) Effect on the potential difference of adding ouabain (1.1 mM final concentration) to either the maternal (●) or the fetal (■) surface. Effect is plotted as the ratio $PD_T PD_C$ (PD_T referring to the PD at some time t during the treatment and PD_C being the mean PD during the equilibrium period) versus time (minutes).

final concentration of 1.1 mM, reduced the PD and SCC after a delay of approximately 5–10 min. Values for both measurements declined steadily and eventually approached zero.

The effect of adding ouabain at the same concentration to the allantoic surface is also shown in Figures 2A,B. The PD and SCC were essentially unaffected. The decline in both parameters appeared to be associated with the decline in tissue viability over time.

Prolactin

The effects of adding prolactin (0.15 μM) on the PD and SCC of the chorioallantois were examined at Days 30 and 70 of gestation (Figure 3). At both times, addition of prolactin to the chorionic surface elicited a rapid stimulatory effect resulting in an increase in PD and SCC to a maximum within 2–3 min and then an ensuing decline. The overall response lasted 20–30 min, after which time the PD and SCC returned to basal levels. Addition of prolactin to the allantoic surface had no effect at Day 30.

The maximum response in SCC as a function of prolactin concentration was achieved at 0.15 μM.

Human Placental Lactogen

The effect of the addition of human placental lactogen (hPL; 3.3 μM) at Day 24 of gestation is shown in Figure 4A. Addition of hPL to the chorionic side of the chorioallantois resulted in six- and sevenfold stimulations of the PD and SCC, respectively. Maximum stimulation was attained within 2 min

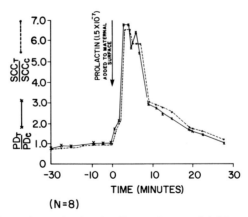

Figure 3. A typical experiment showing the effect on the potential difference and short-circuit current of adding prolactin (0.15 μM final concentration) to the maternal surface. In a similar experiment, the addition of prolactin to the fetal surface had little effect.

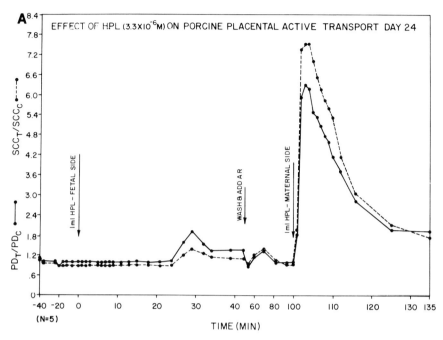

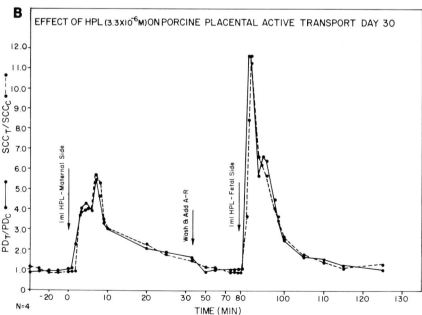

Figure 4. Typical experiments at Days 24 (A) and 30 (B) of gestation showing the effect on the potential difference and short-circuit current of adding human placental lactogen (HPL) (final concentration 3.3 μ M) to either the fetal or the maternal surface.

after addition, followed by a steady decline; measurements returned to basal levels in approximately 30 min. No effect of hPL was observed when added to the allantoic side of the membrane.

An identical experiment with hPL administered at Day 30 (Figure 4B) resulted in 6-fold increases in PD and SCC when hPL was added to the chorionic surface; almost 12-fold increases in both parameters were observed when hPL was added to the allantoic surface (Figure 4B). Both responses were characterized by a rapid increase in PD and SCC.

At Day 60 of gestation, addition of hPL to the allantoic surface resulted in fourfold increases in PD and SCC (Figure 5). Addition of hPL to the chorionic surface resulted in 13-fold increases in PD and SCC. The peak occurred within 3 min after addition of hPL, followed by the characteristic decline and return to basal level within approximately 30 min.

Addition of hPL, in the same manner, to the allantoic surface of Day 90 chorioallantois had no effect on PD and SCC (Figure 5B). When added to the chorionic surface, however, hPL caused fivefold increases in PD and SCC.

The effects of hPL on a term human amniochorion membrane obtained following cesarian section are shown in Figure 6. The same experimental protocol as used for the porcine chorioallantois was followed. Addition of hPL to the amniotic surface had no effect on PD or SCC. After washing the membrane and allowing it to stabilize for nearly 1 hr, addition of hPL to the chorionic side resulted in stimulation of both PD and SCC characterized by an irregular increase with maximum values at 30 min followed by an irregular decline. The PD and SCC did not return to basal levels for nearly 2 hr. Thus, the time course of stimulation of PD and SCC by hPL on human placental tissue is much different than that observed for porcine chorioallantois. This may be due to a tissue-specific response by a human target tissue.

The effects of hPL on PD and SCC across porcine chorioallantois and human amniochorion are summarized in Table II. In 43 experiments hPL had a marked effect on transport properties of the placental membranes. In the porcine chorioallantois, hPL stimulated the PD and SCC early in gestation when added to both fetal and maternal surfaces. By Day 60 the effect of hPL on the allantoic surface was reduced, but a response occurred when added to the chorionic surface. In late gestation the effect of hPL was only seen when added to the chorionic surface. Thus, as gestation progresses, the effect resides predominately on the chorionic surface. A similar situation was observed for human amniochorion, i.e., the effect of hPL was only observed when added to the chorionic surface. It should be pointed out that difficulty was encountered in eliciting a porcine chorioallantois response to hPL after an initial 43 experiments. Two possibilities deserve mention. First, it is possible that undetectable impurities in solutions may have developed in spite of precautions taken. The second possibility is a seasonal effect. Experiments that yielded little or no response were carried out in the spring and early summer.

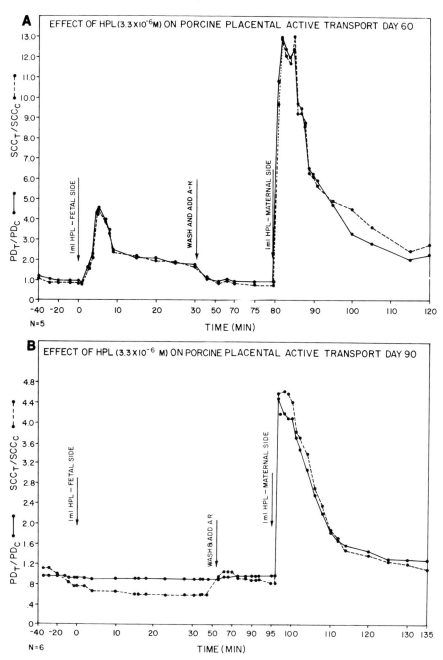

Figure 5. Typical experiments at Days 60 (A) and 90 (B) of gestation showing the effect on the potential difference and short-circuit current of adding human placental lactogen (HPL) (final concentration 3.3 μ M) either to the fetal or the maternal surface.

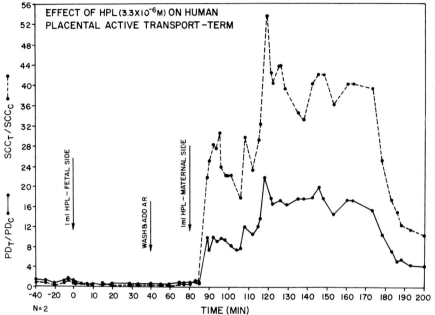

Figure 6. Graph showing the effect on the potential difference and short-circuit current of adding human placental lactogen (final concentration 3.3 μM) to the fetal and maternal surfaces of a term human amniochorion.

Although the pig is not considered a seasonal animal, this observation is of interest.

Estrone and Progesterone

Estrogen and progesterone are intimately involved in modulating many facets of reproductive function, e.g., blood flow during pregnancy, myo-

Table II

Summary of the Effects of Human Placental Lactogen on Placental Membrane

	Allantoic side	Chorionic side
Porcine chorioallantois		
Early (Day 20–30)	+ to ++	− to ++
(N = 13)		
Middle (Day 40–70)	− to +	+ to ++
(N = 20)		
Late (Day 70–100)	−	− to ++
Human amniochorion[a]		
Term (N = 2)	−	++

[a]Amniotic side rather than allantoic side in human placentae.

metrial activity, water retention, and cardiovascular and pulmonary effects (Heap *et al.*, 1973). Estrogen and progesterone have also been found to affect the permeability of phospholipid membranes (Heap *et al.*, 1971).

The effect of adding progesterone to Ringer solution in a final concentration of $0.1 \mu M$ on PD and SCC is shown in Figure 7. Progesterone, on the fetal surface, had little effect on either measurement. However, addition of progesterone to the chorionic surface of the chorioallantois resulted in a decline in both PD and SCC, the onset occurring soon after addition and the steady decline being maintained for 2 hr.

In Figure 8 the effects of the addition of estrone (1.2 nM) to the chorionic and allantoic surfaces of paired placentae are shown. Estrone had a stabilizing effect or slightly enhanced the PD and SCC when added to the allantoic surface. When added to the chorionic surface, some stabilization was seen, but this effect was not as pronounced as that on the allantoic surface. It is

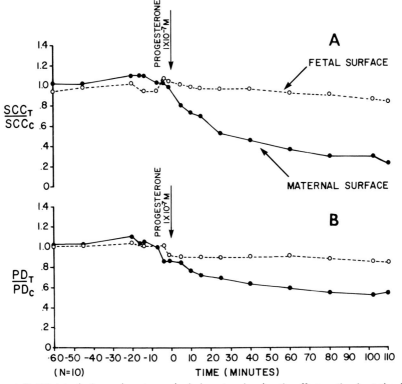

Figure 7. (A) A typical experiment on paired placentae showing the effect on the short-circuit current of adding progesterone (final concentration 0.1 μM) to the fetal and maternal surfaces. The effect is plotted as the ratio SCC_T/SCC_C versus time (see Figure 2A). (B) The same experiment as (A) but showing the effect of progesterone addition to the potential difference.

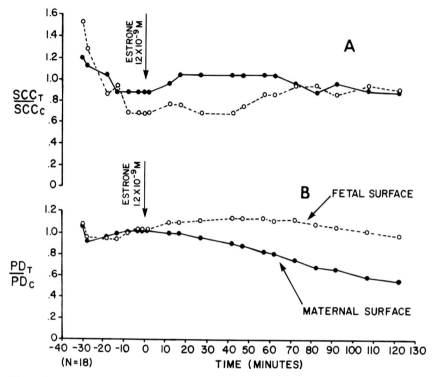

Figure 8. (A) A typical experiment on paired placentae showing the effect on the short-circuit current of adding estrone (final concentration 1.2 μM) to the fetal and maternal surfaces. The effect is plotted as SCC_T / SCC_C versus time (see Figure 2A). (B) The same experiment as (A) but showing the effect of estrone addition on the potential difference.

important to note that the addition of estrone to the allantoic surface maintained the permeability for the entire 2-hr period, while addition to the chorionic surface did not result in such a prolonged effect.

In the above experiments, the effects of progesterone were examined at Days 26, 28, 35, and 80, while the effects of estrogen were examined at Days 28, 35, 40, and 95 of gestation.

Effect of Bromocryptine on Allantoic Fluid Volume and Electrolyte Composition at Day 30 of Gestation

Prolactin has been shown to increase fluid (Ramsey and Bern, 1972) and ion transport (Mainoya, 1972) across the rat jejunum and results in decreased renal excretion of water, sodium, and potassium in rats (Lockett and Nail, 1965). Horrobin *et al.* (1971) found that prolactin injections in man were antidiuretic, resulting in sodium and potassium retention. Falconer and Rowe

(1975) demonstrated that prolactin stimulated sodium transport out of rabbit lactating mammary tissue while promoting potassium uptake, an effect presumed to result from the stimulation of the Na^+/K^+-transport ATPase by prolactin. Manku *et al.* (1975) and Holt and Perks (1975) observed that prolactin affected water movement across the guinea pig amniotic membrane.

The ergot alkaloids are known inhibitors of prolactin release from the pituitary (Meites *et al.*, 1972). They inhibit prolactin release in the cow (Karg and Schams, 1974), sheep (Kann and Denamur, 1974), sow (Kraeling *et al.*, 1979), and rat (Meites *et al.*, 1972) by two possible mechanisms of action. The first, suggested by Wuttke *et al.* (1971), is that the drug acts on the hypothalamus to increase prolactin-inhibiting factor that in turn reduces prolactin secretion. The second mechanism is a possible direct effect of the ergot alkaloids on the pituitary via an α-adrenergic or dopaminergic action (Nicoll *et al.*, 1970; Lehmeyer and MacLeod, 1972).

As previously discussed, prolactin and a structurally similar compound, hPL, were shown to stimulate the PD and SCC across the porcine chorioallantois. With knowledge that prolactin serves an osmoregulatory role in other animals and in other mammalian tissues, an experiment was designed to determine whether bromocryptine, a potent inhibitor of prolactin release from the pituitary, would affect procine allantoic fluid volume and electrolyte composition at Day 30 of gestation.

Eight sexually mature crossbred gilts were bred at 12 and 24 hr after onset of their third estrus. The first day of estrus was designated Day 0 and gilts were randomly assigned to either the control or the treatment group. Beginning on Day 15 of pregnancy, treated gilts were injected subcutaneously with bromocryptine (0.5 mg/kg per day). Control animals received a similar volume of saline. All animals were injected daily, until hysterectomized on Day 30 of pregnancy. Allantoic fluid volume was measured and samples were obtained for electrolyte analysis.

Results of this experiment are summarized in Table III. There was a significant reduction ($p < 0.025$) in allantoic fluid volume in treated animals compared to controls (152.6 vs. 208.8 ml); however, sodium, calcium, chloride, and bicarbonate concentrations were not significantly affected by treatment. Potassium ion concentration was significantly ($p < 0.05$) lower in control (13.40 ± 0.57 meq/liter) than treated (18.72 ± 0.62 meq/liter) gilts, and allantoic fluid osmolarity was significantly ($p \pm 0.05$) increased in treated animals.

Additional evidence of the effect of prolactin on ion and water movement across the chorioallantois can be gleaned by considering the total amount of electrolyte (allantoic fluid volume $\times$ concentration of ion) in allantoic fluid. Total sodium and bicarbonate were reduced, while total potassium, calcium, and chloride remained nearly the same for control and treated animals.

Table III

Effect of Bromocriptine on Allantoic Fluid Volume, Electrolyte Composition, and Osmolarity[a]

	Ion concentration		Total ion[b]	
	Control	Treatment	Control	Treatment
Allantoic fluid volume (ml)	208.82 ± 5.6	152.57 ± 6.10[c]	—	—
Na⁺ (meq/liter)	9.99 ± 0.59	10.60 ± 0.64	2.09	1.62
K⁺ (meq/liter)	13.40 ± 0.57	18.72 ± 0.62[c]	2.80	2.86
Ca²⁺ (meq/liter)	3.70 ± 0.12	6.27 ± 0.13	0.77	0.96
Cl⁻ (meq/liter)	8.89 ± 0.92	16.58 ± 0.99	1.86	2.53
HCO₃⁻ (meq/liter)	5.89 ± 0.67	6.94 ± 0.73	1.23	1.06
Osmolarity (mOsM/liter)	85.55 ± 10.54	137.09 ± 11.42[c]	—	—

[a]All concentration values represent least-squares means ± S.E.
[b]Total ion (meq) was computed from: allantoic fluid volume × ion concentration.
[c]Significantly ($p < 0.05$) different from values for control gilts.

As Manku *et al.* (1975) and Holt and Perks (1975) have shown with guinea pig amnion, these results implicate prolactin in the control of water movement across the pig placenta. The data indicate that in the absence of prolactin, less water accumulated in the allantoic cavity. This finding supported the observations of Holt and Perks (1975) that prolactin, applied to the fetal side of the guinea pig amnion in an *in vitro* experiment, promoted water retention around the fetus. Prolactin was previously shown to stimulate the PD and SCC and, in the absence of this stimulation, active transport of sodium was reduced. A decrease in the gradient for sodium in a maternal-to-fetal direction would result and less water would follow passively. The net effect would be a decrease in allantoic fluid volume, total sodium, and total bicarbonate in control as compared to treated animals, shown in Table III. This *in vivo* experiment supports the *in vitro* results, i.e., that prolactin enhances transport across the porcine chorioallantois.

Discussion and Conclusions

Inhibition of the PD and SCC across the chorioallantois by ouabain lends strong support for the presence of active-transport processes within the porcine placenta, especially for sodium and potassium. It also suggests that the PD across the chorioallantois is dependent upon the active transport of sodium, resulting in a net flux from the allantoic to the chorionic surface. These results support previous data from pig (Crawford and McCance, 1960, chick (Stewart and Terepka, 1969; Moriarity and Hobgen, 1970), and sheep (Mellor, 1970) chorioallantois.

Effects of estrone and progesterone indicate that estrogen may stabilize the membrane and maintain the PD of the placenta. Progesterone, on the other hand, decreased the PD and SCC and increased the "leakiness" of the membrane. These results are similar to those obtained by Heap *et al.* (1971) using lysosomes as a model membrane system. They found that estradiol decreased or maintained the permeability of the lysosome to potassium, whereas progesterone increased the permeability of the lysosome to potassium. The changing membrane resistance demonstrated in Figure 1 may be due, in part, to effects of these two steroids.

The effect of prolactin in stimulating the PD and SCC of the pig chorioallantois parallels its effect in other tissues. It seems reasonable that prolactin, which is so important in osmoregulation in animals lower on the phylogenetic scale, would assume a similar role for the mammalian fetus as it develops in its marine environment. This role for prolactin in controlling water movement during development has been investigated recently by Holt and Perks (1975) and Manku *et al.* (1975) working with guinea pig amniochorion.

It has also been shown that estrogen stimulates prolactin release (Lloyd *et al.*, 1975) as well as priming the uterus to respond to protein hormones (Soloff, 1975). Perhaps the effect of estrogen on the placenta may not be solely due to its own effect on permeability, but due, in addition, to promoting prolactin release from the pituitary and preparing the placenta by increasing the affinity and/or number of prolactin receptors.

hPL is structurally similar to prolactin (Niall *et al.*, 1971) and is believed to enhance amino acid availability to the fetus. Amino acid transport across the intestine is dependent upon sodium transport (Schultz and Curran, 1970; Reiser and Christiansen, 1972). Bihler and Crane (1962) and Wheeler *et al.* (1965) have shown a correlation between glucose and sodium absorption (Schultz and Zalusky, 1964; Schultz and Curran, 1970). Miller and Berndt (1974) found that amino acid transport across human term placentae was dependent upon sodium and potassium ions and was inhibited by ouabain. Recent work by Mainoya (1975) showed the hPL increased fluid and ion transport across rat intestine as did prolactin and growth hormone. Data from this study suggest that hPL may achieve its hypothesized role of increasing amino acid availability to the fetus by an effect on placental active-transport processes.

The observed response to hPL varied according to the stage of gestation. At Day 24 the response was seen only after application to the chorionic surface, whereas at Day 30 the response was seen on both surfaces—the major response occurring after application to the allantoic surface. At Day 60 the response had shifted back to the chorionic surface, and by Day 90 the response was entirely restricted to the chorionic surface.

Two studies on the action of prolactin on guinea pig amniochorion water movement demonstrated the effect occurred when the protein hormone was placed on the fetal amniotic surface (Holt and Perks, 1975; Manku *et al.*, 1975).

The dynamic changes in allantoic fluid volume and electrolyte composition found in pigs (Knight *et al.*, 1977; Goldstein *et al.*, 1980) led to the findings that the permeability of the chorioallantois changes during gestation. In addition, it has been shown that placental permeability and transport are affected by hormones, i.e., estrogen, progesterone, prolactin, and human placental lactogen. It may be that these hormones modulate or control the transport process of the chorioallantois, which ultimately affects the observed dynamic changes in allantoic fluid volume and electrolyte composition.

References

Alexander, D. P., Andrews, D. A., Huggett, A. St. G., Nixon, D. A., and Widdas, W. F., 1955, The placental transfer of sugars in the sheep: Studies with radioactive sugar, *J. Physiol.* **129:**352.

Alexander, G., and Williams, D., 1966, Progesterone and placental development in sheep, *J. Endocrinol.* **34:**241.

Alexander, G., and Williams, D., 1968, Hormonal control of amniotic and allantoic fluid volume in ovariectomized sheep, *J. Endocrinol.* **41:**477.

Anderson, L. L., 1978, Growth, protein content and distribution of early pig embryos, *Anat. Rec.* **190:**143.

Barcroft, J., and Barron, D. H., 1946, Blood pressure and pulse rate in the foetal sheep, *J. Exp. Biol.* **22:**63.

Battaglia, F. C., Prystowsky, H., Smisson, C., Hellegers, A. E., and Bruns, P., 1959, Fetal blood studies. XVI. On the changes in total osmotic pressure and sodium and potassium concentrations in amniotic fluid during the course of human gestation, *Surg. Gynecol. Obstet.* **109:**509.

Beck, J. S., and Currie, A. R., 1967, Immunofluorescence localization of growth hormone in the human pituitary gland and of a related antigen in the syncytiotrophoblast, *Vitam. Horm. (N. Y.)* **25:**89.

Biggers, J. D., and Borland, R. M., 1976, Physiological aspects of growth and development of the preimplantation mammalian embryo, *Annu. Rev. Physiol.* **48:**95.

Bihler, I., and Crane, R. K., 1962, On the mechanism of intestinal absorption of sugars, *Biochim. Biophys. Acta* **59:**78.

Bremer, J. L., 1916, The interrelations of the mesonephros, kidney and placenta in different classes animals, *Am. J. Anat.* **19:**179.

Crawford, J. D., and McCance, R. A., 1960, Sodium transport by the chorioallantoic membrane of the pig, *J. Physiol.* **151:**458.

Davies, J., 1952, Correlated anatomical and histochemical studies on the mesonephros and placenta of the sheep, *Am. J. Anat.* **91:**263.

DiZio, S. M., and Tasca, R. J., 1974, Ion dependent, ouabain sensitive reexpansion of mouse blastocysts collapsed with cytochalasin B, *Proc. Am. Soc. Cell Biol.* **63:**85 (abstract 85a).

Falconer, I. R., and Rowe, J. M., 1975, Possible mechanism for action of prolactin on mammary cell sodium transport, *Nature (London)* **256:**327.

Friesen, H., Suwa, S., and Pare, P., 1969, Synthesis and secretion of human placental lactogen and other proteins by placents, *Recent Prog. Horm. Res.* **25:**161.

Goldstein, M. H., 1977, Placental ion and water movement with emphasis on the porcine chorioallantois, M.S. thesis, University of Florida, Gainesville.

Goldstein, M. H., Bazer, F. W., and Barron, D. H., 1980, Characterization of changes in volume, osmolarity and electrolyte composition of porcine fetal fluids during gestation, *Biol. Reprod.* **22**:1168.

Heap, R. B., Symons, A. F., and Watkins, J. C., 1971, On interaction between estradiol and progesterone in aqueous solutions and in a model membrane system, *Biochim. Biophys. Acta* **233**:307.

Heap, R. B., Perry, J. S., and Challis, J. R. G., 1973, Hormonal maintenance in pregnancy, in: *Handbook of Physiology*, Section VII (R. O. Greep and E. B. Astwood, eds.), American Physiological Society, Washington, D.C., pp. 217–260.

Hellman, L. M., Tricomi, V., and Gupta, O., 1957, Pressures in the human amniotic fluid and intervillous space, *Am. J. Obstet. Gynecol.* **74**:1018.

Holt, W. F., and Perks, A. M., 1975, The effect of prolactin on water movement through the isolated amniotic membrane of the guinea pig, *Gen. Comp. Endocrinol.* **26**:153.

Horrobin, D. F., Burstyn, P. G., Lloyd, I. J., Durkin, N., Lipton, A., and Muiruri, K. L., 1971, Actions of prolactin on human renal functions, *Lancet* **2**:352.

Josimovich, J. B., Weiss, G., and Hutchinson, D., 1974, Sources and disposition of pituitary prolactin in maternal circulation, amniotic fluid, fetus and placenta in the pregnant rhesus monkey, *Endocrinology* **98**:1364.

Kann, G., and Denamur, R., 1974, Possible role of prolactin during the oestrous cycle and gestation in the ewe, *J. Reprod. Fertil.* **39**:473.

Karg, H., and Schams, D., 1974, Prolactin release in cattle, *J. Reprod. Fertil.* **39**:463.

Knight, J. W., Bazer, F. W., and Wallace, H. D., 1974, Effect of progesterone induced increase in uterine secretory activity on development of the porcine conceptus, *J. Anim. Sci.* **39**:743.

Knight, J. W., Bazer, F. W., Thatcher, W. W., Franke, D. E., and Wallace, H. D., 1977, Conceptus development in intact and unilaterally hysterectomized–ovariectomized gilts: Interrelations among hormonal status, placental development, fetal fluids and fetal growth, *J. Anim. Sci.* **44**:620.

Kraeling, R. R., Rampacek, G. B., Cox, N. M., and Kiser, T. E., 1979, Suppression of prolactin secretion in lactating sows with bromocryptine (CB-154), *Proc. Am. Soc. Anim. Sci. Tucson*, p. 311.

Lehmeyer, J. E., and MacLeod, R. M., 1972, Suppression of pituitary tumor function by alkaloids, *Proc. Am. Assoc. Cancer Res.* **13**:90.

Lloyd, H. M., Meares, J. D., and Jacobi, J., 1975, Effects of estrogen and bromocryptine on *in vivo* secretion and mitosis in prolactin cells, *Nature (London)* **225**:497.

Lockett, M. F., and Nail, B., 1965, A comparison of the renal actions of growth and lactogenic hormones in rats, *J. Physiol.* **181**:192.

McCance, R. A., and Dickerson, J. W. T., 1957, The composition and origin of the fetal fluids of the pig, *J. Embryol. Exp. Morphol.* **5**:43.

McCance, R. A., and Widdowson, E. M., 1953, Renal function before birth, *Proc. R. Soc. London Ser. B* **141**:488.

McCarthy, E. F., 1946, The osmotic pressure of human fetal and maternal sera, *J. Physiol.* **104**:433.

McGovern, P. T., 1976, Dose of progesterone and allantoic fluid volume in conceptuses in ovariectomized goats, *Am. J. Physiol.* **181**:1.

Mainoya, J. R., 1972, Effects of prolactin on absorption of water and ions by the rat intestine, *Am. Zool.* **12**:112 (abstract).

Mainoya, J. R., 1975, Further studies on the action of prolactin on fluid and ion absorption by the rat jejunum, *Endocrinology* **96**:1190.

Mainoya, J. R., Bern, H. A., and Regan, J. W., 1974, Influence of ovine prolactin on transport of fluid and sodium chloride by the mammalian intestine and gall-bladder, *J. Endocrinol.* **63**:311.

Manku, M. S., Mtabaji, J. P., and Horrobin, D. F., 1975, Effect of cortisol, prolactin and ADH on the amniotic membrane, *Nature (London)* **258**:78.

Meites, J., Lu, K. H., Wuttke, W., Welsch, C. W., Nagasaw, H., and Quadri, S. K., 1972, Recent studies on functions and control of prolactin secretion in rats, *Recent Prog. Horm. Res.* **28**:471.

Mellor, D. J., 1970, Distribution of ions and electrical potential difference between mother and fetus at different gestational ages in goats and sheep, *J. Physiol.* **207**:133.

Meschia, G., 1955, Colloidal osmotic pressures of fetal and maternal plasmas of sheep and goats, *Am. J. Physiol.* **181**:1.

Meschia, G., Battaglia, F. C., and Barron, D. H., 1957, A comparison of the freezing points of fetal and maternal plasmas of sheep and goats, *Q. J. Exp. Physiol.* **42**:163.

Meshia, G., Wolkoff, A. S., and Barron, D. H., 1958, Difference in electric potential across the placenta of goats, *Proc. Natl. Acad. Sci. USA* **44**:483.

Miller, R. K., and Berndt, W. D., 1974, Characterization of neutral amino acid accumulation by human term placental slices, *Am. J. Physiol.* **227**:1236.

Moriarity, C. M., and Hogben, A. M., 1970, Active Na^+ and Cl^- transport by the chick chorioallantoic membrane, *Biochim. Biophys. Acta* **219**:463.

Niall, H. D., Hogan, M. L., Saver, R , Rosenblum, I. Y., and Greenwood, F. C., 1971, Pituitary and placental lactogenic and growth hormones: Evolution from a primordial gene reduplication, *Proc. Natl. Acad. Sci. USA* **68**:866.

Nicoll, C. S., Yaron Z., Nutt, N., and Daniels, E., 1970, Effects of ergotamine tartrate on prolactin and growth hormone secretion by rat adenohypophysis *in vitro*, *Biol. Reprod.* **5**:59.

Prystowsky, H., 1958, Fetal blood studies. VIII. Some observations on the transient fetal bradycardia accompanying uterine contractions in the human, *Bull. Johns Hopkins Hosp.* **102**:1.

Ramsey, D. H., and Bern, H. A., 1972, Stimulation by ovine prolactin of fluid transfer in everted sacs of rat small intestine, *J. Endocrinol.* **53**:453.

Ramsey, E. M., Corner, G. W., Jr., Long, W. N., Jr., and Stran, H. M., 1959, Studies of amniotic fluid and intervillous space pressures in the rhesus monkey, *Am. J. Obstet. Gynecol.* **77**:1016.

Reiser, S., and Christiansen, P. A., 1972, Relative effectiveness of extracellular sodium in supporting leucine uptake by isolated intestinal epithelial cells, *Proc. Soc. Exp. Biol. Med.* **140**:362.

Reynolds, S. R. M., 1960, Regulation of the fetal circulation, *Clin. Obstet. Gynecol.* **3**:834.

Riddle, O., 1963, Prolactin in vertebrate function and organization, *J. Natl. Cancer Inst.* **31**:1039.

Robertson, H. A., and King, G. J., 1974, Plasma concentrations of progesterone, oestrone, oestradiol 17-β and of oestrone sulphate in the pig at implantation during pregnancy and at parturition, *J. Reprod. Fertil.* **40**:133.

Schultz, S. F., and Curran, P. F., 1970, Coupled transport of sodium and organic solutes, *Annu. Rev. Physiol.* **36**:51.

Schultz, S. F., and Zalusky, R., 1964, Ion transport in isolated rabbit ileum. I. Short-circuit current and Na fluxes, *J. Gen. Physiol.* **47**:567.

Skou, J. C., 1965, Enzymatic basis for active transport of Na^+ and K^+ across cell membranes, *Physiol. Rev.* **45**:596.

Soloff, M. S., 1975. Uterine receptor for oxytocin: Effects of estrogen, *Biochem. Biophys. Res. Commun.* **65**:205.

Stanley, J. E., and Fleming, W. R., 1967, Effect of prolactin and ACTH on the serum and urine sodium levels of *Fundulus kansac*, *Comp. Biochem. Physiol.* **20**:199.

Stewart, M. E., and Terepka, A. R., 1969, Transport functions of the chick chorioallantoic membrane, *Exp. Cell Res.* **58**:93.

Tuft, P. H., and Boving, B. G., 1970, The forces involved in water uptake by the rabbit blastocyst, *J. Exp. Zool.* **174**:165.

Ussing, H. H., and Zerahn, K., 1951, Active transport of sodium as the source of electric current in the short-circuited isolated frog skin, *Acta Physiol. Scand.* **23**:110

Utida, S., Hirano, T., Oide, H., Ando, M., Johnson, D. W., and Bern, H. A., 1972, Hormonal control of the intestine and urinary bladder in teleost osmoregulation, *Gen. Comp. Endocrinol. Suppl.* **3**:317.

Watlingtin, C. O., Smith, T. C., and Huf, E. G., 1970, Direct electrical currents in metabolizing epithelial membranes, *J. Physiol. Biochem.* **3**:49.

Wheeler, K. P., Inui, Y., Hollenberg, P. E., Eavenson, E., and Christensen, H. N., 1965, Relation of amino acid transport to sodium ion concentration, *Biochim. Biophys. Acta* **109**:620.

Wislocki, G. B., 1935, On the volume of fetal fluids in sow and cat, *Anat. Rec.* **63**:183.

Wuttke, W., Cassell, E., and Meites, J., 1971, Effects of ergocornine on serum prolactin and LH, and on hypothalamic content of PIR and LRF, *Endocrinology* **88**:737.

13

CRITICAL REVIEW OF EMBRYO TRANSFER PROCEDURES WITH CATTLE

G. E. SEIDEL, Jr.

More offspring have resulted from transferring bovine embryos than from embryos of all other species combined. Recent survey data from North America indicate that at least 17,000 bovine pregnancies were produced commercially in 1979 at a cost of about $20,000,000 (Seidel, 1981). It is estimated that more than 50,000 bovine embryos were transferred worldwide in 1980, and probably 25,000 calves will result. Although the first successful bovine embryo transfer was reported in 1951 (Willett *et al.*, 1951), there was no commercial application until the early 1970s.

The application of embryo transfer technology is facilitated by a very active professional organization, the International Embryo Transfer Society. Currently, there are nearly 500 members from more than 20 countries. While the species of major interest to this group is cattle, there is also active interest in about a dozen other species, including primates. Currently the second most important commercial species is the horse, but swine, goats, sheep, and rabbits are also being propagated by commercial embryo transfer.

The motives of people who purchase bovine embryo transfer services are generally profit oriented. Few people realize that the propagation of most cattle by embryo transfer is only superficially related to genetic progress in terms of increased meat or milk production. This is because high genetic potential for these traits, although necessary, is not sufficient for commanding high prices. A number of other factors, some of them subtle like color or popular blood lines, affect prices when dealing with elite cattle. The

G. E. Seidel, Jr. • Animal Reproduction Laboratory, Colorado State University, Fort Collins, Colorado 80523.

economics of the industry are discussed in more detail elsewhere (Seidel, 1981; Seidel and Seidel, 1981).

The technology for bovine embryo transfer was initially developed at universities and research institutes, to a great extent by extrapolation from other species, particularly rabbits and sheep. However, by the mid-1970s, the flow of information was as much from industry to universities and research institutes as in the other direction. In the past decade, a number of technological advances occurred, including the use of prostaglandin $F_{2\alpha}$ in superovulation regimens, development of nonsurgical methods of embryo recovery and transfer, and the preservation of embryos by freezing to liquid nitrogen temperature. Determination of the sex of embryos, producing identical twins, and *in vitro* fertilization will probably have commercial application within 5 years.

Recent research support for embryo transfer has come primarily from the industry, frequently through work done with cattle owned by the companies themselves. Governmental agencies and universities have also been involved in the development of embryo transfer technology, but on a more limited scale. At this time, it appears that the private sector will have the dominant role in the development of *in vitro* fertilization and embryo transfer technology for most, if not all, nonlaboratory species.

Tremendous amounts of research have been done concerning bovine embryo transfer, and large files of data have been accumulated. There appear to be three broad reasons for reviewing experimental work in this area: (1) the information may be useful for improving bovine embryo transfer procedures; (2) it may be helpful for reproduction of cattle outside of the context of embryo transfer; and (3) some information might profitably be extrapolated to other species, particularly in designing relevant experiments.

The rationale for choosing the particular areas of bovine embryo transfer for review includes personal preference, availability of appropriate experimental data, and potential usefulness of the analyses. Some excellent reviews already exist, e.g., Foote and Onuma (1970), Gordon (1975), and Betteridge (1977a).

Normalcy of Superovulated Ova

All but a few percent of the tens of thousands of calves produced from embryo transfer have been from donors treated with gonadotropins in order to induce superovulation; approximately 10 times as many pregnancies can be obtained per donor per attempted embryo collection with superovulation than with single ovum recoveries (Seidel, 1981). To date there is no information from any appropriately controlled study to determine if calves from superovulation are different from those from untreated donors. From anecdotal information, the calves produced do not appear to have more problems or abnormalities than normal. However, as we shall see, there are some problems along the way.

Before proceeding further, superovulation must be placed in context, as must any procedure modifying the biology of an organism. A few words about artificial insemination (AI) in cattle will illustrate this point. Most of the dairy cows in North America and practically all of them in a number of other countries are inseminated artificially. The procedure is obviously successful and has numerous advantages, but many differences from natural mating must be imposed for success. These include: (1) site of semen deposition (vaginal for the bull, uterine for AI); (2) number of sperm (billions for the bull, tens of millions for AI); (3) timing (various times during estrus for the bull, late in estrus or early metestrus for AI); and (4) additives to semen (none for the bull, many for AI such as milk, egg yolk, buffers, antibiotics, cryoprotectants if frozen, etc.) (Foote, 1980). In the same way, successful superovulation entails many differences from normal reproduction. Ovulation frequently is deliberately induced at a different time in the reproductive cycle from normal; animals sometimes are prepuberal; and ovulation may occur over a longer period of time than normal and insemination may, therefore, be timed differently. While superovulation is often successful, there can be problems. A clear example of this is inducing ovulation at the wrong stage of follicular development in pigs (Hunter *et al.*, 1976); if ovulation occurred too early, oocytes remained in the germinal vesicle stage and frequently were polyspermic. Another example is superovulating prepuberal calves without first preparing the oviduct and uterus with appropriate steroids (Seidel *et al.*, 1971). Embryos degenerated within a few days in that environment.

One factor that is clearly different in superovulated animals is elevated steroid concentrations in blood: estradiol-17β during follicular growth and progesterone later (Saumande, 1978; Spilman *et al.*, 1973). This probably alters sperm transport and causes ova to move from the oviduct to the uterus earlier or later than normal, depending on the particular circumstances. Possibly altered ratios of steroid hormones are more critical than the absolute levels, and this is further complicated by superovulation regimens. For example, gonadotropins with long half lives may have effects that linger for many days (Schams *et al.*, 1979).

Although a few superovulation methods lead to some abnormal embryos, there does not appear to be a single study showing an increased incidence of abnormalities in the offspring produced under reasonable circumstances, although one must deal with the problems of multiple births if one induces this condition in monotocous species.

Probably the most thorough study of offspring from superovulated vs. unsuperovulated embryos is that of Maurer *et al.* (1968) with rabbits. They found a 60% ($N = 243$) survival rate to term from transferring embryos resulting from superovulation with FSH, 45% ($N = 143$) with embryos from

PMSG, and 55% ($N = 152$) from unsuperovulated ones; none of these were significantly different from each other. They recovered embryos from the oviducts at the two- and four-cell stages. Had they waited to recover the embryos from the uterus some days later, the superovulated ones might have suffered due to crowding or other adverse effects.

There are a number of studies concerning the normality of superovulated ova in rodents, with results ranging from completely normal offspring to considerable abnormalities in embryos. There seem to be no reasonably controlled studies showing increased abnormalities in the young actually born. References and discussion may be found in Fleming and Yanagimachi (1980) and Maudlin and Fraser (1977).

Studies comparing superovulated to unsuperovulated bovine ova are limited. Elsden et al. (1978) found a pregnancy rate of 71% ($N = 69$) for unsuperovulated ova vs. 59% ($N = 358$) ($p < 0.05$) for superovulated ova. Pregnancy rates for morphologically abnormal embryos were slightly higher in the superovulated group: 22% ($N = 76$) vs. 12% ($N = 8$). Although all embryos for this study were collected from the same population of donors, it was not a controlled study. On the average, superovulated embryos were held in culture longer between recovery and transfer than unsuperovulated ones and were transferred to slightly less desirable recipients in terms of estrous cycle synchrony with the donors. These biases were probably small, however. In any case, the data show that superovulated embryos were not very different, if at all, from unsuperovulated ones. A few more superovulated embryos were classified as retarded (18% vs. 10%), but numbers per group were small (76/434 vs. 8/77).

Probably the clearest difference between superovulated and unsuperovulated bovine ova at the time of recovery is fertilization rate. Elsden et al. (1976) found a fertilization rate of 70% ($N = 179$) for superovulated ova and 89% ($N = 36$) ($p < 0.05$) for unsuperovulated ova from the same population. Although there are no other studies comparing this directly, nearly all studies on superovulation show fertilization rates between 50 and 80% (Betteridge, 1977b), and those studies concerning unsuperovulated bovine ova show fertilization rates of 80–100% (Ayalon, 1978; Callaghan and King, 1980). The reasons for this difference are unknown, but problems with sperm transport and ovulation over a period of time are likely possibilities. If superovulated ova were transferred to the reproductive tract of a properly inseminated, untreated animal at the time of ovulation, fertilization rates might be normal; this hypothesis, however, remains to be tested.

A Note on Experimental Design

Many studies with bovine embryo transfer are retrospective analyses, as much of the data accumulated have been from commercial or semicommercial situations involving clinical like material. Even with strictly experimental work, one has a multicomponent system that includes superovulation, insemination, embryo recovery, embryo culture for at least several hours, frequently some method of synchronizing the estrous cycles of recipient and donor, transfer of the embryos per se, and criteria for evaluation of success. In doing an experiment concerning one or two of these components, one automatically accumulates data on the others, such as the length of time embryos were kept *in vitro* between collection and transfer. Frequently, these accumulated data, which are incidental to the main purpose of the experiment, are analyzed. Such analyses are not always ideal, because the experiments were not designed with them in mind. Although retrospective studies frequently provide valuable information, they are especially subject to changes over time, such as improving skills, which can confound results when new techniques are introduced. A more serious problem lies in developing hypotheses from retrospective examination of data; many of the differences observed are due to chance and/or confounding of various factors. When interesting hypotheses arise from such procedures, experiments should be designed to test them properly.

Another important point to keep in mind when evaluating bovine embryo transfer experiments is whether embryos or recipients are the limiting factor. In most commercial situations, the objective is to obtain as many pregnancies as possible; therefore, all but the worst appearing embryos are transferred. In many experimental situations, recipients instead of embryos are limited, and only the very best appearing embryos are transferred, which leads to high pregnancy rates and disappointing results when the treatments are applied commercially.

Morphological Evaluation of Embryos

It is possible for experienced personnel to classify bovine embryos into categories that accurately reflect probabilities of pregnancy after transfer. The data of Table I illustrate this well. In some cases data from two subclasses from the original references have been combined for brevity. The work of Shea *et al.* (1976) actually represents eight classifications; the second row of Table I concerns 8- to 12-cell embryos that by and large were somewhat retarded relative to the morulae collected at the same time (row 3). Thus, the pregnancy rates range from 18 to 60%. Shea *et al.* had two even poorer classifications: 1- to 3-cell embryos with a pregnancy rate of 4% ($N = 55$) and 4- to 7-cell embryos with a pregnancy rate of 14% ($N = 122$). There would have been larger differences among groups in some of the studies if subgroups had not been combined for publication and if very poor embryos had been transferred instead of discarded.

Table I

Pregnancy Rates and Morphological Evaluation of Embryos

| | Highest rating → | | | | | | IV → Lowest rating | |
| | I | | II | | III | | IV | |
Authors	N	% Pregnant	N	% Pregnant	N	% Pregnant	N	% Pregnant
Drost et al. (1975)	27	67	7	14				
Shea et al. (1976)[a]	33	42	338	42	294	36	45	18
Shea et al. (1976)[b]	506	60	1831	56	401	45	18	33
Elsden et al. (1978)	275	63	152	58	42	31	42	12
Elsden et al. (1979)	227	63	41	32				
Nelson et al. (1979)	1098	61	284	52	86	34		
Markette (1980)	673	59	138	55	99	26		
Markette (1980)	193	67	20	25				
Schneider et al. (1980)	1809	70	694	55				
Tervit et al. (1980)	22	59	18	17				
Shea (1981)	679	56	130	44				
Wright (1981)	1748	64	438	45	100	33		

[a] Eight- to twelve-cell embryos.
[b] Morulae.

The morphological evaluations are clearly not perfect (Shea *et al*., 1976), and frequently one is surprised by the development of poor embryos. One such embryo transferred in our laboratory developed into a calf that sold at public auction for $131,000. Under some circumstances morphological evaluations can be supplemented to good effect with biochemical measurements such as glucose uptake (Renard *et al*., 1980b) or measures of enzyme activity (Schilling *et al*., 1979). Such information might be especially useful in evaluating embryos that have been frozen and thawed and/or cultured for long periods of time. Morphological evaluations of embryos stressed by these treatments appear to be less reliable than those of freshly collected embryos (Tervit and Elsden, 1981).

Morphological Normalcy of Superovulated Ova with Time

The percentage of morphologically abnormal embryos recovered from superovulated cattle increases with time (Table II). These data are in agreement with Seidel *et al*. (1978), who, however, only looked at two time periods. This is circumstantial evidence that the environment in the reproductive tract of the superovulated donor is harmful to embryos. There are several problems with this conclusion. First, although morphological evaluations are very useful (Table I), they are imperfect; some embryos that appear degenerate are capable of developing into calves, and many normal-appearing embryos are not. Second, there are no similar large accumulations of morphological information concerning unsuperovualted embryos; a very similar pattern might occur. Third, pregnancy rates are much lower with morphologically normal early embryos relative to later stage embryos (Table VII); this may be partially related to the inability to evaluate early embryos accurately.

On the other hand, there is some evidence that placing superovulated cleavage-stage bovine embryos into the rabbit oviduct leads to a higher proportion of normal embryos when they are recovered from the rabbit several days later compared to those that remained in the superovulated cow for a comparable period of time (Boland *et al*., 1976, 1978; Trounson *et al*., 1976). A possible caveat with these results is that not all bovine ova are recovered from the rabbit, and the missing ones may be the degenerate ones. Another consideration in analyzing the data in Table II is that none of the studies concerns superovulation with FSH (Elsden *et al*., 1978), which may not perturb steroid concentrations as much as PMSG (Schams *et al*., 1979).

A special case, the superovulated prepuberal calf, appears to show a similar trend to that in Table II (Seidel *et al*., 1971), which would not be unexpected for the immature reproductive tract. One further point is that the apparent decrease in abnormalities on Days 11 and 12 (Table II) may be an

Table II

Degenerate and Retarded Embryos after Different Lengths of Time in the Superovulated Cow

Authors	Days embryos recovered postestrus										
	2	3	4	5	6	7	8	9	10	11	12
Newcomb et al. (1976)											
% Abnormal		2		18	24	27	52				
N		133		313	268	274	151				
Boland et al. (1978)											
% Abnormal	0	4	14	45	37						
N	169	589	314	393	131						
Renard and Heyman (1979)											
% Abnormal					30	49	48	48	43	34	36
N					149	185	151	132	197	76	104

artifact because of the much lower recovery rate on these days (data not presented). Possibly some of the abnormal embryos were destroyed or expelled from the reproductive tract by this time.

The practical consequences of data like those in Table II are complicated by other considerations such as the impracticality of recovering embryos nonsurgically prior to Day 6, and the need to use certain stages of optimal success with freezing, sexing, and other manipulations. Additional work is needed to clarify the effects of superovulation on the oviduct, uterus, and the embryos developing there.

In Vitro Culture of Bovine Embryos

Embryos must be kept *in vitro* between collection and transfer. This immediately raises practical questions such as what medium to use, the temperature for culture, the nature of the container, how long embryos can be kept without decreasing viability, etc. The standard practice for routine embryo transfer is to recover embryos in the morning, and transfer them by the end of the day. For storing embryos during this interval, phosphate-buffered saline (PBS) with various slight modifications and enriched with fetal calf serum is used almost universally, either at ambient temperature or at 37° C.

No attempt will be made to review methods of freezing embryos or cooling them to 5–10° C for long-term storage. Rather, I will concentrate on the problem of keeping embryos viable for about a day. Earlier work was reviewed by Seidel (1977). Data to be discussed (Table III) are limited to studies in which two or more treatments were compared, and embryos were transferred to determine pregnancy rates.

Clearly, embryos can be cultured for up to 24 hr without great declines in pregnancy rates. The early studies by Rowson *et al.*, (1969, 1972) were the first to indicate that pregnancy rates did not decline after some hours *in vitro*. However, many of the studies in Table III show decreased pregnancy rates with increased time under *in vitro* conditions. Furthermore, some studies show marked differences among culture media. Extreme caution must be exercised, however, in interpreting these data. Many of the media are bicarbonate buffered and require 5% CO_2 atmosphere for maintenance of pH, although this is complicated by the exact formulations (e.g., Hanks' vs. Earle's salts) and additions of serum and Hepes buffer. A 5% CO_2 atmosphere was not used for some of the studies in which it would have been appropriate, and even when used, it was sometimes not maintained uniformly because of constantly moving embryos in and out of the incubator or gassed container. The problem of maintaining a 5% CO_2 atmosphere under extensive experimental or commercial conditions is the reason why PBS is used so extensively despite

Table III

Embryonic Survival *in Vivo* after Culture *in Vitro* at 30–38°C

Authors	Treatments	N	% Fetal development	Comments
Seidel (1974)	TCM 199 + Hepes + 5% serum	88	53	1–10 hr *in vitro*, 8-cell to morulae
	Modified Ham's F10 + BSA	102	43	
Boland et al. (1975)	TCM 199	12	17	0–3 hr *in vitro* at 30°C, nonsurgical transfer
	PBS + 15% FCS	12	33	
Drost et al. (1975)	4–7 hr *in vitro*	12	50	TMC 199 + HEPES + 10% FCS 8-cell to morulae
	7–11 hr *in vitro*	15	80	
Sreenan et al. (1975)	0–2 hr *in vitro*	62	73	TCM 199, no additives, 8-cell to blastocysts
	2–8 hr *in vitro*	48	42	
Hahn and Hahn (1976b)	TCM 199 + HEPES + 10% FCS	7	0	Blastocysts, 4–8 hr *in vitro*
	Modified PBS + 10% FCS	13	69	
Shea et al. (1976)	0–3 hr *in vitro*	967	60	TCM 199 + Hepes + 10% FCS, morulae
	3–6+ hr *in vitro*	161	57	
Hahn et al. (1978)	1–4 hr *in vitro*	27	63	Morulae and blastocysts, modified PBS
	20–24 hr *in vitro*	11	45	
	32–36 hr *in vitro*	30	3	
Peters et al. (1978)	Immediate transfer	70	56	Morulae, twinned, Ham's F10 + 10% FCS
	24 hr *in vitro*	48	40	
Renard et al., (1978)	Immediate transfer	34	59	Blastocysts, twinned, nonsurgical transfer, Menezo's B-2 medium
	24 hr *in vitro*	26	27	
Renard et al. (1980a)	Immediate transfer	83	49	Day 10–12 blastocysts, nonsurgical transfer, Menezo's B-2 medium
	24 hr *in vitro*	45	33	
Schneider et al. (1980)	Immediate transfer	50	60	Morulae and blastocysts, BMOC-3 + 10% FCS
	24 hr *in vitro*	47	62	
Tervit and Elsden (1981)	Immediate transfer	20	25	Blastocysts after freezing and thawing
	24 hr in Ham's F10 + 10% FCS	10	20	
	24 hr in PBS + 10% FCS	10	0	

the fact that CO_2 is required for certain synthetic reactions (Kane, 1978) and is, therefore, indispensible for the long-term well-being of embryos. Work of Hahn *et al.*, (1978) also hints at this (data not presented here).

Bedirian *et al.* (1979) reported a 44% pregnancy rate when embryos were exported from Canada to Europe in PBS enriched with bovine serum. The time between collection and transfer ranged from 18 to 33 hr, and an attempt was made to keep the embryos at 37° C throughout the process. Schneider *et al.* (1980) had excellent success with culturing embryos (Table III); they used recipients in estrus 12–36 hr after the donors and obtained best results with those in estrus 12 hr after the donor, suggesting that in their system embryos developed at approximately normal rates. Nevertheless, under most conditions bovine embryos probably develop considerably more slowly *in vitro* than *in vivo*, which makes selection of synchronized recipients perplexing.

The study by Renard *et al.* (1980a; Table III) showed that initial pregnancy rates after transfer of embryos cultured for 24 hr were similar to the embryos transferred immediately (70% vs. 62%), but that subsequent embryonic mortality was much higher for the cultured group. This requires further study and suggests that pregnancy rates at less than 60 days of gestation may be misleading.

When bovine embryos are of questionable morphology, it is frequently useful to culture them for several hours or even overnight; sometimes their appearance improves remarkably. The data in Table III suggest that it might be best to culture less than 24 hr under such circumstances. Renard *et al* (1980b) have recently shown that glucose uptake over a 20-hr period *in vitro* might be an excellent criterion for evaluating Day 11–12 bovine embryos. Possibly, times shorter than 20 hr should also be evaluated.

The central problem with *in vitro* culture of bovine embryos is the lack of basic information on what bovine embryos require. Essentially nothing is known about metabolic pathways or preferred substrates for bovine embryos. Clearly, the bovine embryo is not too particular, as most survive fairly well for short times *in vitro* and very well in the ligated rabbit oviduct (Boland *et al.*, 1978; Trounson *et al.*, 1976). It is almost a certainty that preimplantation bovine embryos eventually will be cultured *in vitro* for some days with essentially normal rates of development.

Stage of the Estrous Cycle to Initiate Superovulation

The efficacy with which prostaglandin $F_{2\alpha}$ or suitable analogues lyse the bovine corpus luteum has provided great flexibility in superovulating cattle. The current universal procedure is to give the prostaglandin 1 to 3 days after initiating gonadotropin treatment. As prostaglandin $F_{2\alpha}$ is effective on Days 5–16+ of the bovine estrous cycle, gonadotropin treatment can be started on

Table IV

Initiation of Superovulation at Various Stages of the Estrous Cycle[a]

Authors	Days	N	Success	Days	N	Success	Days	N	Success	Criteria of success
Phillippo and Rowson (1975)	4–7	32	6	8–12	58	34	—	—	—	% > 6 Fertilized ova
Hahn et al. (1976)	5–10	13	3.7	11–14	15	2.1	15–16	16	2.1	No. of normal embryos
Betteridge (1977b)	3–8	16	38	8–12	58	78	13–16	9	56	% > 2 Ovulations
Sreenan and Gosling (1977)	3	10	3.6	10	16	4.7	—	—	—	No. of fertilized ova
Sreenan et al. (1978)	7–8	15	5.1	9–11	84	14.5	12–14	10	11.1	No. of ovulations
Greve et al. (1979)	9	17	3.1	10–11	46	3.3	12–13	20	4.1	No. of normal embryos
Hasler et al. (1979)	9–10	—[b]	8.8	11–12	—[b]	10.2	13–14	—[b]	9.3	No. of ova recovered
Schilling et al. (1980)	8–9	25	2.4	10–11	65	1.9	12–13	17	3.1	No. of normal embryos

[a] Considers only studies where luteolysis was induced by prostaglandin $F_{2\alpha}$ or its analogues.
[b] 160 superovulations for all groups combined.

Days 3–16 of the cycle. A number of early studies indicated that Days 8–12 were optimum for initiating treatment with gonadotropins (Betteridge, 1977b). A summary of studies concerning this matter is shown in Table IV. There is no consistent pattern in these data except perhaps that it is best to stay away from Days 3–7. A prudent policy might be to initiate treatment between Days 9 and 14 whenever possible. A possibility that remains to be studied is that different superovulation regimens may have different optimal starting times. Until more is known about normal follicular growth in cattle, it will be necessary to rely on the kinds of studies in Table IV.

Regimens for Inseminating Superovulated Cows

Currently the standard practice for superovulated cattle is to inseminate on two or three occasions with two to six times the total normal amount of semen. In commercial practice, frozen semen is almost always used. There are only a few studies that have examined this problem critically (Table V). In four of the five studies concerning fresh vs. frozen semen, fresh semen was best. However, slightly more sperm were inseminated with fresh rather than frozen semen in two of the four studies, and one of the studies concerned prepuberal calves. There does appear to be some small advantage to using fresh semen. Semen of mediocre quality can lead to disastrous results with superovulated cows, particularly if frozen (Newcomb et al., 1980; Callaghan and King, 1980).

From Table V, there appears to be some advantage to insemination on two or three occasions. There are a number of anecdotal accounts of good fertilization rates when superovulated cows were inseminated once with one dose of high-quality frozen semen. However, from the experimental data available, it is probably worth the investment of using multiple doses of semen on multiple occasions if the semen is not too expensive, particularly in the absence of information about the bull's fertility.

The best evidence that sperm may not reach superovulated ova in the same numbers as with untreated cattle comes from the work of Bellows et al. (1969). They found considerably fewer sperm in the zona pellucida after natural mating of superovulated heifers relative to untreated controls (about 10 sperm vs. more than 50; $p < 0.01$). Additional work of this sort would be highly desirable with artificial insemination of frozen semen.

Side of Transfer

The embryo of the untreated cow remains in the uterine horn ipsilateral to the ovary with the ovulation site and developing corpus luteum; the bovine fetus also develops in that uterine horn with very rare exceptions (Scanlon,

Table V

Seminal Treatments for Superovulated Cattle

Authors	Fresh semen	Frozen semen	Criteria	Comments
Onuma et al. (1970)	72 (68)	33 (33)	% Cleavage (No. of ova)	Donors were calves
McKenzie and Kenney (1973)	67 (49)	29 (75)	% Cleavage (No. of ova)	More sperm in fresh than frozen treatment
Sreenan and Beehan (1976)	71 (23)	61 (20)	% Cleavage (No. of donors)	More sperm in fresh than frozen treatment
Seidel et al. (1978), Expt. I	4.2 (15)	5.2 (13)	No. of normal embryos (No. of donors)	
Seidel et al. (1978), Expt. II	7.1 (40)	4.0 (36)	No. of normal embryos (No. of donors)	

	Frequency of insemination (8- to 24-hour intervals)				
	1X	2X	3X	4X	Criteria
Onuma et al. (1970)		44 (38)	58 (63)		% Cleavage (no. of ova)
Seidel et al. (1978)		5.2 (15)		4.4 (13)	No. of normal embryos (No. of donors)
Critser et al. (1980)	2.8 (24)[a]		4.5 (26)		No. of normal embryos (No. of donors)
Newcomb (1980)	70	88	88		% Fertilized[b]

[a] A triple dose of semen with one insemination yielded 3.7 cleaved ova ($N = 26$).
[b] Approximately 50 donors total; data pooled from various insemination regimens.

Table VI

Effect of Side of Transfer on Pregnancy Rate

Authors	Ipsilateral transfers		Contralateral transfers	
	N	% Pregnant	N	% Pregnant
Newcomb and Rowson (1976)	13	46	13	0
Sreenan (1976a)	31	61	22	18
Tervit et al. (1977)	28	50	28	36
Newcomb et al. (1978)[a]	20	85	20	30
Del Campo et al. (1979)	15	67	15	13
Holzer et al. (1979)[b]	576	39	55	18

[a] Embryos were also transferred to the opposite sides nonsurgically.
[b] Least-squares means.

1972). It is of interest to note that the first successful bovine embryo transfer resulted from transfer contralateral to the corpus luteum (Willett et al., 1951) However, experiments have shown a considerable advantage to ipsilateral transfer (Table VI). In most studies, pregnancy rates were very low with contralateral transfers, but in the study by Tervit et al. (1977) they were not significantly different from ipsilateral transfers. Their work is among the best in terms of documenting that the pregnancies actually were on the side indicated because they slaughtered most of the recipients to examine uteri directly. Apparently, much remains to be learned about contralateral embryo transfer involving only one embryo. Almost certainly the lowered pregnancy rate is due to failure to maintain the corpus luetum (Christie et al., 1979) because of the failure of the local luteotropic or antiluteolytic mechanism, not because of some environmental difference between ipsilateral and contralateral uteri. Various experiments with twinning support this idea, although these experiments can be very difficult to interpret in the context of ipsilateral vs. contralateral transfer (Sreenan, 1978; Newcomb and Rowson, 1980).

Stage of Embryonic Development and Surgical Transfer

Bovine embryos are routinely transferred to the uterus; surprisingly, transfer of bovine embryos to the oviduct remains essentially unstudied. Most but by no means all superovulated bovine embryos pass from the oviducts to the uterus between 3 and 5 days after the onset of estrus (Newcomb et al., 1976; Betteridge et al., 1980); it is commonly held that embryos in unsuperovulated cows move to the uterus 4 days after the beginning of estrus, but extensive data are not available (Crisman et al., 1980). A number of studies were summarized by Betteridge (1977a) in which embryos were transferred between 3 and 16 days after estrus. Few of the studies had as a major goal determining which day of pregnancy was best for recovery and transfer of embryos; rather, most were of

Table VII

Pregnancy Rates from Transferring Embryos Surgically at Different
Stages of Gestation

Day of gestation	Nelson et al. (1975)		Newcomb and Rowson (1975)		Hasler et al. (1980)	
	N	% Pregnant	N	% Pregnant	N	% Pregnant
3	54	30	67	10	28	18
4	194	54	51	55	135	49
5	141	63	40	72	232	53
6	43	63	23	87	109	58
7			10	70	10	50

a survey nature. Three such studies are summarized in Table VII. There is
some overlap in the animals used in the studies by Nelson et al. (1975) and
Hasler et al. (1980). The studies are in good agreement with each other that
pregnancy rates are very low when embryos are transferred to the uterus on
Day 3, increase substantially on Day 4, and plateau after Day 5 (also see Shea,
1981). Pregnancy rates may decline slightly after Day 7 with surgical transfer
(Elsden et al., 1978), but this requires additional study. Newcomb and
Rowson (1975) even transferred some Day 2 embryos to the uterus, but no
pregnancies resulted. The numbers per group in Table VII are fairly low in
some cases so that confidence intervals would be wide. The actual days of
gestation for the study of Hasler et al. (1980) are 2.5–3, 3.5–4, etc., whereas
those of Nelson et al. (1975) are grouped on the basis of 3–3.5, 4–4.5, etc. The
low pregnancy rates on Day 3 are probably due to an inappropriate
environment. It is interesting that the pregnancy rate for Day 4 embryos
placed in Day 3 uteri was 47% compared to 12% for Day 3 embryos in Day 3
uteri (Newcomb and Rowson, 1975).

Although these studies appear fairly conclusive, some early work,
admittedly with small numbers, indicated that pregnancy rates were greater
than 90% when Day 3 and Day 4 embryos were transferred to the uterus
(Sreenan and Beehan, 1974; Sreenan et al., 1975; Rowson et al., 1972). The
reason for these very high pregnancy rates with early embryos in earlier
studies is unclear. Possibilities include (1) more intense selection of embryos,
with embryos being discarded when they showed the slightest defect; (2)
different methods of transferring embryos, e.g., to the very tip of the uterine
horn in contrast to less precise localization of embryo deposition in the studies
with larger numbers; (3) an embryo was placed in each uterine horn in the
studies reporting high pregnancy rates, in contrast to placement of a single
embryo in the horn ipsilateral to the corpus luteum in the larger studies; and
(4) none of the studies, large or small, were expressly designed to study this

phenomenon as evidenced by the uneven subclass numbers. The data were simply studied in retrospect. Which of these reasons (or others) explain the differences in pregnancy rates when younger embryos are transferred to the uterus remains to be determined. Although the studies summarized in Table VII are convincing, it must be admitted that pregnancy rates can be fairly high with Day 3 and Day 4 embryos under some circumstances.

Considering only studies with reasonable numbers of observations, it appears that the highest pregnancy rate after transfer of normal embryos singly to the ipsilateral horn of the uterus of perfectly synchronized recipients was 83% (38/46 embryos, Days 5–7 of gestation) (Newcomb and Rowson, 1975). More sophisticated methods of selecting embryos such as determining glucose uptake (Renard *et al.*, 1980b) may lead to even higher pregnancy rates. Pregnancy rates with embryo transfer are sometimes higher than those normally achieved with conventional reproduction in well-managed herds (Seidel, 1981).

Donor-Recipient Estrous Cycle Synchrony

Probably the most venerable principle of embryo transfer biology is that the donor and recipient must be at similar stages of their reproductive cycles for high rates of success. Because of profound cyclical changes in the reproductive tract, this principle is intuitively sensible; it is also supported by empirical evidence (Table VIII).

The interactions between the reproductive tract and the embryo may be divided into two components: (1) nutritive, regulative, and other environmental influences of the reproductive tract on the embryo, and (2) influences of the embryo on the reproductive system, especially the luteotropic or antiluteolytic effects that change the cyclic corpus luteum to a corpus luteum of pregnancy. Asynchronous embryo transfer is worthy of study for many reasons. For example, how do synchrony requirements relate to different reproductive cycle lengths among and within females? There is also the very practical question of how much asynchrony in either direction can be tolerated without substantial changes in pregnancy rates.

Table VIII summarizes studies with bovine embryo transfer in which synchrony was analyzed. It is obvious that only a few, if any, of the investigations concerned synchrony as the primary objective. Rather, the usual practice was to use the most synchronous animals available (sufficient perfectly synchronous recipients were frequently unavailable) and analyze synchrony in retrospect.

Rowson *et al.* (1969) conducted the first study of bovine embryo transfer with sufficient numbers of pregnancies available for analyzing synchrony. Based primarily on anecdotal evidence, they concluded that a deviation of 2

Table VIII

Effect of Recipient-Donor Estrous Cycle Synchrony on Pregnancy Rates

	Recipient after donor										Recipient before donor									
	−2		−1.5		−1		−0.5		0		+0.5		+1		+1.5		+2		
Authors	N	%	N	%	N	%	N	%	N	%	N	%	N	%	N	%	N	%	Comments
Rowson et al. (1972)	10	30			23	52			23	91			23	57			10	40	Some twinned
Sreenan and Beehan (1974)					7	71			24	92									Some twinned
Newcomb and Rowson (1975)					26	58			63	73			35	60					Day 3 ova excluded
Seidel et al. (1975b)							91	52	266	57	75	49							
Sreenan et al. (1975)					13	62			50	82			9	67					All twinned
Hansen (1976)					23	65	127	55	73	51	11	55							
Shea et al. (1976)					556[a]	49			1126	62			334[b]	59					
Kunkel and Stricklin (1978)			239[c]	59					353	59					346[d]	47			
Trounson et al (1978b)	12	50	31	52	112	57	311	61	32	44	277	57	10	30					Frozen embryos
Nelson et al. (1979)									586	58			100	54	26	38	13	54	
Newcomb (1979)					26	38			16	62			28	50					Nonsurgical
Schneider et al. (1980)							593	61	1488	67	475	66							
Wright (1981)			115	41	301	58	620	61	747	59	374	68	98	61	27	59			Nonsurgical

[a] −0.5 to −1.5 days.
[b] +0.5 to +1.5 days.
[c] −1 to −3.5 days.
[d] +1 to +3.5 days.

days in either direction from exact synchrony between estrous cycles of donors and recipients could be tolerated. However, a more detailed analysis of greater accumulations of their data (first row of Table VIII) showed that pregnancy rates were drastically reduced with asynchrony of only 1 day, even further reduced with 2 days, and only 10% (1/10, data not presented in Table VIII) with asynchrony of 3 days. Many of the studies that followed gave similar results, i.e., pregnancy rates decline as asynchrony increases. However, the more recent studies with hundreds of transfers per subgroup indicate that synchronization requirements are not as strict as previous studies indicated, and that there may even be some advantage when the recipient is in estrus $\frac{1}{2}$–1 day before the donor. Halley *et al.* (1979) also point out that pregnancy rates in their large study were highest when the recipient was in estrus prior to the donor, although they did not present these data. This situation is especially fortuitous for commercial embryo transfer companies because they can obtain high pregnancy rates by using recipients in estrus prior to donors before dipping into the pool of recipients in estrus after the donors, which in turn can be used for donors on subsequent days. The data currently available indicate that asynchrony of 1–1.5 days in either direction does not drastically lower pregnancy rates and that a difference of 2 days will frequently lead to pregnancy, which is what Rowson *et al.* (1969) concluded originally.

The data from many of the studies from 1972 to 1975 were confounded by additional treatments and may for that reason show large declines in pregnancy rates with slight asynchrony. Many of the recipients were twinned, and some studies have relatively more twinned recipients in the more synchronous groups. Although pregnancy rates in twinned recipients were not significantly higher than nontwinned ones, the potential for failure to detect true differences is enormous with studies of that kind and size. It is also possible that synchrony requirements are different for twinning than for single transfers, especially when pregnancy rates with synchronous twinning are in the 90% range.

Probably the most important difference between the earlier and the later studies with respect to synchrony requirements is age of embryos. It is quite probable that older embryos have less stringent requirements for synchrony, possibly because there is less change in the reproductive tract throughout the luteal phase than during the transition between follicular and luteal phases. Some of the studies in Table VIII allude to this possibility.

The data in Table VIII have some potential artifacts. Because of the knowledge that synchrony is important, the best embryos tend to be transferred to the most synchronous recipients and, at least in many commercial contexts, the worst embryos tend to be kept until the end of the day, which makes this situation even worse because poor embryos are held *in vitro* longer. This problem probably also arises in some experiments not involving commercial work. It is therefore probable that requirements for synchrony are even less stringent than suggested in Table VIII. Another artifact concerns the detection of estrus, which tends to be more intense and accurate with the few valuable donors than with the many less valuable recipients. As synchrony is generally timed from the onset of estrus, such practices would lead to some recipients having actually begun estrus perhaps half a day earlier than what was recorded. This factor, plus the likelihood that slightly older embryos (relative to the reproductive tract) should be more efficacious in rescuing the corpus luteum from luteolysis, suggest that a recipient in estrus shortly after the donor might be the ideal choice. There is such evidence for small laboratory mammals (Marsk, 1977; Beier, 1974). However, for cattle, the data surprisingly suggest that it may be slightly preferable for recipients to be in estrus before the donor. Therefore, there is some factor overriding those suggested above. One possibility is that erring on the side of a younger uterus is more damaging than erring in the opposite direction due to the composition of uterine secretions. A second, attractive hypothesis is that the superovulated embryo is somehow slightly different from the unsuperovulated one in one of the following senses: (1) ovulation (and fertilization) may occur earlier or at least over a longer period of time in superovulated than unsuperovulated cows, making the superovulated embryos older relative to the onset of estrus; (2) superovulated embryos may be at a different site from normal (Newcomb et al., 1976); or (3) embryos in superovulated reproductive tracts may sometimes be slightly speeded up in development relative to normal because of higher levels of progesterone (Spilman et al., 1973; Schams et al., 1979) and/or related endocrine effects. Lawson (1977) cites data that sheep embryos elongate more rapidly when

Table IX

Effect of Site of Surgical Transfer on Embryo Survival Rate

Authors	Mid to base of uterine horn		2–4 cm From uterotubal junction		Comments
	N	% Survival	N	% Survival	
Boland et al. (1976)	19	21	21	57	Contralateral transfers to mated recipients
Sreenan (1976a)	20	60	20	65	One embryo transferred to each uterine horn
Christie et al. (1980)	29	45	30	73	
Newcomb et al. (1980)	80	61	80	69	One embryo transferred to each uterine horn
Rowe et al. (1980)	20	45	20	60	

transferred to uteri at more advanced stages of the luteal phase than if left in synchronous uteri. This work has been extended by Wilmut and Sales (1981) and provides credence for the possibility that superovulated bovine embryos are speeded up developmentally. Apparently no one has studied differences in synchrony requirements for superovulated vs. unsuperovulated embryos. A final comment is that different methods of superovulation may result in different synchrony requirements.

From the evidence discussed, the possibility that recipients can be made even more receptive than normal should not be discounted. There are several studies in progress concerning hCG injections that appear promising. Another possibility is modifying reproductive events other than onset of estrus, such as the onset of blastokinin production, to add additional flexibility to current procedures of estrous cycle synchronization (Beier, 1974).

Factors Affecting Pregnancy Rates after Nonsurgical Transfer

Pregnancy rates after nonsurgical embryo transfer are lower than with surgical methods, but the reasons are not clear. Some factors have been ruled out. Sham-transfer studies to previously inseminated recipients (Seidel *et al.*, 1975a) and embryo transfers to the contralateral horn of previously inseminated recipients (e.g., Sreenan and McDonagh, 1979) did not lower pregnancy rates. Therefore, potential deleterious effects of entry into the uterus through the cervix, such as ejection of embryos, trauma to the endometrium, or introduction of microorganisms, appear to be minor problems. One factor that may be a problem is placement of the embryo. Several studies in which embryos were deposited surgically in different areas of the uterine horns are summarized in Table IX. Three of the studies concerned twinning, which confuses interpretation. However, there is some advantage in transferring to the uterine tip in each study. In the study by Christie *et al.* (1980), which did not involve twinning, the pregnancy rate at the tip was definitely higher than that from transfers lower in the horn. The study by Boland *et al.* (1976), which concerns contralateral (to the corpus luteum) transfers only, strongly suggests an effect independent of a luteotropic mechanism. However, the study by Newcomb *et al.* (1980) fails to bear this out. There may also be interactions with age of embryo and whether cows or heifers are used as recipients, as cows have considerably longer uteri.

A factor that seems to have profound effects on success rates of nonsurgical transfer is differences among technicians (Table X). This may be related to different sites of embryo deposition or other factors; the causes of the technician differences are unknown, although experience appears to be very important. Similar differences, although of a smaller magnitude, are

Table X
Technician Effects with Nonsurgical Transfer

Authors	Technician A		Technician B		Technician C	
	N	% Pregnant	N	% Pregnant	N	% Pregnant
Bowen et al. (1978)	22	27	17	18	52	13
Halley et al. (1979)	161	46	481	24	—	—
Elsden et al. (1980)	48	33	35	26	—	—
Rowe et al. (1980)	40	58	40	35	—	—
Schneider et al. (1980)	145	53	153	48	125	28
Curtis et al. (1981)	60	35	60	13	—	—
de los Santos-Valadez et al. (1981)	29	41	40	30	—	—

common among artificial insemination technicians. It has been shown that these differences are usually related to site of semen deposition, and further, that most technicians with low success rates can be retrained successfully (Graham, 1966).

The skill of the technician in quickly and atraumatically passing the inovulation device through the cervix and up the uterine horn to the site of deposition of the embryo may be as important as proper site of deposition. Boland et al. (1976), when transferring embryos nonsurgically to the contralateral uterine horn of inseminated heifers, obtained 32% (8/25) pregnancies with easy transfers but only 17% (4/23) when transfers were difficult. Bowen et al (1978) obtained 20% pregnancies (18/88) with normal transfers but none (0/6) when difficulties were encountered. Similarly, Wright (1981) obtained a pregnancy rate of 59% ($N = 2218$) with easy transfers and 50% ($N = 46$) with difficult ones. Furthermore, two recent papers (Rowe et al., 1980; Tervit et al., 1980) provide evidence that the faster (and therefore probably easier) transfers result in higher pregnancy rates, although data from Curtis et al. (1981) are less clear on this point. In the next decade considerable effort must be invested in finding the reasons for technician differences in nonsurgical embryo transfer success rates so that this problem can be solved or circumvented.

The stage of development of the embryos at the time of nonsurgical transfer may also affect success rates (Table XI). Half of the studies cited show marked advantages in transferring more advanced embryos, at least up to 10–11 days after estrus, while the other half show no such advantage. The more extensive data concerning surgical transfers presented in Table VII are in agreement with data in Table XI that embryos should be transferred at least 5–6 days after the beginning of estrus. However, it is likely that artifact is responsible for some of the differences found in Table XI. For example, it is easier to evaluate older embryos, and some of the results are probably due to

Table XI

Pregnancy Rates from Transferring Embryos Nonsurgically at Different Stages of Gestation

Authors	Days	N	% Pregnant	Days	N	% Pregnant	Days	N	% Pregnant
Lawson et al (1975)	3–5	20	10	6–9	40	38	—	—	—
Hahn and Hahn (1976a)	5	14	7	6	24	29	7	17	65
Renard et al (1977)[a]	6–7	23	30	9–10	36	50	—	—	—
Brand et al. (1978)	6–8	32	37	11–12	29	34	—	—	—
Heyman et al (1978)[a]	7–9	34	35	10–11	30	57	12–13	26	38
Jillella and Baker (1978)	6–7	6	67	8–9	15	47	—	—	—
Trounson et al. (1978a)	6–7	24	33	8–9	24	58	—	—	—
Halley et al. (1979)	6	170	24	7	274	26	8	142	42
Newcomb (1979)	7	27	48	8	27	52	10	21	48
Elsden et al (1980)	6–7	48	31	9–10	35	29	—	—	—
Shea (1981)	7	366	58	8	234	56	9	62	53
Wright (1981)	6.5	260	60	7	1612	59	8	210	65

[a] Most transfers were bilateral (twins) and fetal survival rates are given.

stricter culling of older embryos. Another problem is the nature of the experimental design. From the unequal subclass numbers, one would surmise that these experiments were not designed specifically to study age of embryos at transfer, and it appears possible that the older embryos were transferred later in some experiments than the younger embryos, hence after the technicians had more experience. In the absence of details about how experiments were conducted, one must be aware that these kinds of biases may be present.

One perplexing problem with nonsurgical embryo transfer is that fetal losses seem high between 35 and 60 days of gestation (Table XII). Kummerfeld et al. (1978) found a 7% loss between Days 25 and 75 with artificially inseminated dairy cows. A similar study by Bulman and Lamming (1979) showed 12% pregnancy loss in this time period. The only major study of embryonic and fetal mortality in recipients receiving embryos surgically showed a 9% loss of pregnancies (13/147) between Days 25 and 60 (Markette et al., 1980). From Table XII, it appears that fetal losses after Day 25 with nonsurgical transfer are approximately double those with surgical transfer or artificial insemination. Sreenan (1976b) also mentions a 20% rate of resorption with nonsurgical transfer. These losses are even higher when embryos are cultured. As discussed earlier, Renard et al. (1980a) found a 46% loss of pregnancies between Days 21 and 60 for embryos cultured for 24 hr vs. a 29% loss (Table XII) for those cultured less than 8 hr. Possibly, insults such as freezing will also lead to large embryonic and fetal wastage when followed by nonsurgical transfer. Information on pregnancy losses from earlier

Table XII
Fetal Loss between Various Intervals after
Nonsurgical Transfer

Authors	N	% Fetal loss	Interval
Hahn and Hahn (1976a)	14	29	Days 42–90
Brand et al. (1978)	27	11	Days 60–90
Jillella and Baker (1978)	16	31	Days 45–90
Christie et al. (1980)	14, 15[a]	12	Days 16–25
	15, 20[a]	17	Days 25–42
Renard et al. (1980a)	58	10	Days 21–28
		7	Days 28–35
		12	Days 35–60
Tervit et al. (1980)	31	13	Days 42–slaughter[b]
Curtis et al. (1981)	40	28	Days 35–60
de los Santos-Valadez et al. (1981)	27	11	Days 35–60

[a] Separate groups of animals slaughtered sequentially.
[b] Recipients slaughtered 4–168 days later.

nonsurgical transfer studies concerns only small numbers of pregnancies; however, a cursory examination of published data reviewed by Foote and Onuma (1970) and Brand and Drost (1977) indicates very high losses of pregnancy.

The cause of this high level of wastage is unknown, but clearly deserves study. It further indicates that it would be wise to use at least 60 days of gestation as an endpoint of pregnancy for nonsurgical transfer studies; some studies have used 6 weeks of gestation as an endpoint.

Embryonic survival rates with twinning have not been discussed because of difficulties in interpretation. There is some evidence that two embryos are more luteotropic than one, and thus embryo survival rates may be higher than with single transfers. This, however, may depend on where the embryos are placed, the preferred sites being one embryo in the tip of each uterine horn (Newcomb et al., 1980).

Conclusions

Superovulation and embryo transfer have apparently become a permanent component of the armamentarium used by North American cattle breeders. A fringe benefit of this work is increased knowledge of bovine reproduction outside of the context of embryo transfer. It is possible that this information will be of greater net economic benefit over the next decade than the actual use of embryo transfer, which, although extensive, is still used for only a small fraction of 1% of all cattle.

As with most things, our ignorance exceeds our knowledge for most aspects of superovulation, in vitro storage of embryos, and embryo transfer methodology. Basic information on bovine reproduction, although scant, has been indispensible for developing efficacious technology. In recent years more research has been done in this field by private industry than by universities or governmental research laboratories, although frequently it has been a joint enterprise.

Although there have been some very well-designed experiments, much of the experimental material with bovine embryo transfer is of clinical nature, and therefore great care must be taken in its interpretation. Even so, much has already been learned from the large volumes of data and more can be gleaned by further analyses.

The procedures used are successful: the reproductive capacity of valuable donor cows can be amplified more than 10-fold on the average (Seidel, 1981). It would seem wise for researchers who work with mammalian reproduction to be cognizant of the work with bovine embryo transfer, so they can learn from mistakes made and take advantage of knowledge available.

ACKNOWLEDGMENTS

The help of my colleagues at the Colorado State University Embryo Transfer Unit in preparing this review is greatly appreciated. Our research has been supported in part by the Colorado State University Experiment Station through Regional Project W-112, Reproductive Performance in Beef Cattle and Sheep.

References

Ayalon, N., 1978, A review of embryonic mortality in cattle, *J. Reprod. Fertil.* **54**:483–493.

Bedirian, K. N., Mills, M. S., Bligh, P. J., Geroldi, R., and Kilmer, B. A., 1979, Commercial export of bovine embryos from Canada to Europe, *Theriogenology* **11**:3–4.

Beier, H. M., 1974, Oviductal and uterine fluids, *J. Reprod. Fertil.* **37**:221–237.

Bellows, R. A., Anderson, D. C., and Short, R. E., 1969, Dose–response relationships in synchronized beef heifers treated with follicle stimulating hormone, *J. Anim. Sci.* **28**:638–644.

Betteridge, K. J., 1977a, *Embryo Transfer in Farm Animals*, Canada Department of Agriculture, Ottawa.

Betteridge, K. J., 1977b, Techniques and results in cattle: Superovulation, in: *Embryo Transfer in Farm Animals* (K. J. Betteridge, ed.), Canada Department of Agriculture, Ottawa, pp. 1–9.

Betteridge, K. J., Eaglesome, M. D., Randall, G. C. B., and Mitchell, D., 1980, Collection, description, and transfer of embryos from cattle 10–16 days after oestrus, *J. Reprod. Fertil.* **59**:205–216.

Boland, M. P., Crosby, T. F., and Gordon, I., 1975, Twin pregnancy in cattle established by nonsurgical egg transfer, *Br. Vet. J.* **131**:738–740.

Boland, M. P., Crosby, T. F., and Gordon, I., 1976, Induction of twin pregnancy in heifers using a simple nonsurgical technique, *Proc. 8th Int. Congr. Anim. Reprod. A.I.* **III**:241–244.

Boland, M. P., Crosby, T. F., and Gordon, I., 1978, Morphological normality of cattle embryos following superovulation using PMSG, *Theriogenology* **10**:175–180.

Bowen, J. M., Elsden, R. P., and Seidel, G. E., Jr., 1978, Nonsurgical embryo transfer in the cow, *Theriogenology* **10**:89–95.

Brand, A., and Drost, M., 1977, Embryo transfer by nonsurgical methods, in: *Embryo Transfer in Farm Animals* (K. J. Betteridge, ed.), Canada Department of Agriculture, Ottawa, pp. 31–34.

Brand, A., Aarts, M. H., Zaayer, D., and Oxender, W. D., 1978, Recovery and transfer of embryos by nonsurgical procedures in lactating dairy cattle, in: *Control of Reproduction in the Cow* (J. M. Sreenan, ed.), Nijhoff, The Hague, pp. 281–291.

Bulman, D. C., and Lamming, G. E., 1979, The use of milk progesterone analysis in the study of oestrous detection, herd fertility and embryonic mortality in dairy cows, *Br. Vet. J.* **135**:559–567.

Callaghan, B. D., and King, G. J., 1980, Determination of the fertilization rate of A.I. sires, *Theriogenology* **14**:403–410.

Christie, W. B., Newcomb, R., and Rowson, L. E. A., 1979, Embryo survival in heifers after transfer of an egg to the uterine horn contralateral to the corpus luteum and the effect of treatments with progesterone or hCG on pregnancy rates, *J. Reprod. Fertil.* **56**:701–706.

Christie, W. B., Newcomb, R., and Rowson, L. E. A., 1980, Nonsurgical transfer of bovine eggs: Investigation of some factors affecting embryo survival, *Vet. Rec.* **106**:190–193.

Crisman, R. O., McDonald, L. E., and Wallace, C. E., 1980, Oviduct (uterine tube) transport of ova in the cow, *Am. J. Vet. Res.* **41**:645–647.

Critser, J. K., Rowe, R. F., Del Campo, M. R., and Ginther, O. J., 1980, Embryo transfer in cattle: Factors affecting superovulatory response, number of transferable embryos, and length of post-treatment estrous cycles, *Theriogenology* **13**:397–406.

Curtis, J. L., Elsden, R. P., and Seidel, G. E., Jr., 1981, Nonsurgical transfer of bovine embryos, *Theriogenology* **15**:124 (abstract).

Del Campo, M. R., Rowe, R. F., and Ginther, O. J., 1979, Relationship between side of embryo and transfer and pregnancy rate in cattle, *Proc. 71st Annu. Meet. Am. Soc. Anim. Sci.* p. 290 (abstract).

de los Santos-Valadez, S., Elsden, R. P, and Seidel, G. E., Jr., 1981, unpublished.

Drost, M., Anderson, G. B., Cupps, P. T., Horton, M. B., Warner, P. V., and Wright, R. W., Jr., 1975, A field study on embryo transfer in cattle, *J. Am. Vet. Med. Assoc.* **166**:1176–1179.

Elsden, R. P., Hasler, J. F., and Seidel, G. E., Jr., 1976, Nonsurgical recovery of bovine eggs, *Theriogenology* **6**:523–532.

Elsden, R. P., Nelson, L. D., and Seidel, G. E., Jr., 1978, Superovulating cows with follicle stimulating hormone and pregnant mare's serum gonadotrophin, *Theriogenology* **9**:17–26.

Elsden, R. P., Nelson, L. D., and Seidel, G. E., Jr., 1979, Embryo transfer in fertile and infertile cows, *Theriogenology* **11**:17–26.

Elsden, R. P., Nelson, L. D., and Seidel, G. E., Jr., 1980, unpublished.

Fleming, A. D., and Yanagimachi, R., 1980, Superovulation and superpregnancy in the golden hamster, *Dev. Growth Differ.* **22**:103–112.

Foote, R. H., 1980, Artificial insemination, in: *Reproduction in Farm Animals* (E. S. E. Hafez, ed.), Lea & Febiger, Philadelphia, pp. 521–545.

Foote, R. H., and Onuma, H., 1970, Superovulation, ovum collection, culture and transfer: A review, *J. Dairy Sci.* **53**:1681–1692.

Gordon, I., 1975, Problems and prospects in cattle egg transfer, *Irish Vet. J.* **29**:21–30, 39–62.

Graham, E. F., 1966, The use of a dye indicator for testing, training and evaluating technicians in artificial insemination, *Proc. 1st Natl. Assoc. Anim. Breeders Tech. Conf. A.I. Bovine Reprod.*, pp. 57–60.

Greve, T., Lehn-Jensen, J., and Rasbech, N. O., 1979, Morphological evaluation of bovine embryos recovered nonsurgically from superovulated dairy cows on days 6½ to 7½: A field study, *Ann. Biol. Anim. Biochim. Biophys.* **19**:1599–1611.

Hahn, J., and Hahn, R., 1976a, Experiences with nonsurgical techniques, in: *Egg Transfer in Cattle* (L. E. A. Rowson, ed.), EEC Publication EUR 5491, Luxembourg, pp. 199–204.

Hahn, J., and Hahn, R., 1976b, Experiences with ova transfer in cattle, *World Rev. Anim. Prod.* **12**:51–58.

Hahn, J., Hahn, R., Luhmann, F., Baumgartner, G., Lorrmann, W., and Zoder, H. F., 1976, Ergebnisse der Superovulation bei farsen nach kombinierter PMSG/PGF$_{2\alpha}$-Behandlung, *Berl. Muench. Tieraerztl. Wochenschr.* **89**:89–93.

Hahn, J., Moustafa, L. A., Schneider, U., Hahn, R., Romanowski, W., and Roselius, R., 1978, Survival of cultured and transported bovine embryos following surgical and nonsurgical transfers, in: *Control of Reproduction in the Cow* (J. M. Sreenan, ed.), Nijhoff, The Hague, pp. 356–362.

Halley, S. M., Rhodes, R. C., III, McKellar, L. D., and Randel, R. D., 1979, Successful superovulation, nonsurgical collection and transfer of embryos from Brahman cows, *Theriogenology* **12**:97–108.

Hansen, H. B., 1976, Pregnancy rate in cattle in relation to oestrus synchronization and cell stages, in: *Egg Transfer in Cattle* (L. E. A. Rowson, ed.), EEC publication EUR 5491, Luxembourg, pp. 223–227.

Hasler, J. F., Bartlett, C., and McCauley, A., 1979, Effect of dose of FSH and day of treatment on superovulation of lactating Holsteins, *Proc. 71st Annu. Meet. Am. Soc. Anim. Sci.* p. 302 (abstract).

Hasler, J. F., Bowen, R. A., Nelson, L. D., and Seidel, G. E., Jr., 1980, Serum progesterone concentrations in cows receiving embryo transfers, *J. Reprod. Fertil.* **58**:71–77.

Heyman, Y., Renard, J. P., Ozil, J. P., and du Mesnil du Buisson, F., 1978, Cervical embryo transfer at different stages in cattle, in: *Control of Reproduction in the Cow* (J. M. Sreenan, ed.), Nijhoff, The Hague, pp. 330–335.

Holzer, G., Nelson, L. D., and Seidel, G. E., Jr., 1979, unpublished.

Hunter, R. H. F., Cook, B., and Baker, T. G., 1976, Dissociation of response to injected gonadotropin between the Graafian follicle and oocyte in pigs, *Nature (London)* **260**: 156–158.

Jillella, D., and Baker, A. A., 1978, Transcervical transfer of bovine embryos, *Vet. Rec.* **103**:574–576.

Kane, M. T., 1978, Culture of mammalian ova, in: *Control of Reproduction in the Cow* (J. M. Sreenan, ed.), Nijhoff, The Hague, pp. 383–397.

Kummerfeld, H. L., Oltenacu, E. A. B., and Foote, R. H., 1978, Embryonic mortality in dairy cows estimated by nonreturns to service, estrus, and cyclic milk progesterone patterns, *J. Dairy Sci.* **51**:1773–1777.

Kunkel, R. M., and Stricklin, W. R., 1978, Donor–recipient asynchrony, stage of embryo development, and the post-transfer survival of bovine embryos, *Theriogenology* **9**:96 (abstract).

Lawson, R. A. S., 1977, Research applications of embryo transfer in sheep and goats, in: *Embryo Transfer in Farm Animals* (K. J. Betteridge, ed.), Canada Department of Agriculture, Ottawa, pp. 72–78.

Lawson, R. A. S., Rowson, L. E. A., Moor, R. M., and Tervit, H. R., 1975, Experiments on egg transfer in the cow and ewe: Dependence of conception rate on the transfer procedure and stage of the oestrous cycle, *J. Reprod. Fertil.* **45**:101–107.

McKenzie, B. E., and Kenney, R. M., 1973, *In vitro* culture of bovine embryos, *Am. J. Vet. Res.* **34**:1271–1275.

Markette, K. L., 1980, Bovine embryonic mortality estimated by serum progesterone patterns and observed estrus, M.S. thesis, Colorado State University.

Markette, K. L., Seidel, G. E., Jr., and Elsden, R. P., 1980, Embryonic loss after bovine embryo transfer, *Theriogenology* **13**:105 (abstract).

Marsk, L., 1977, Developmental precosity after asynchronous egg transfer in mice, *J. Embryol. Exp. Morphol.* **39**:129–137.

Maudlin, I., and Fraser, L. R., 1977, The effect of PMSG dose on the incidence of chromosomal anomalies in mouse embryos fertilized *in vitro*, *J. Reprod. Fertil.* **50**:275–280.

Maurer, R. R., Hunt, W. L., Van Vleck, L. D., and Foote, R. H., 1968, Developmental potential of superovulated rabbit ova, *J. Reprod. Fertil.* **15**:171–175.

Nelson, L. D., Bowen, R. A., and Seidel, G. E., Jr., 1975, Factors affecting bovine embryo transfer, *J. Anim. Sci.* **41**:371–372 (abstract).

Nelson, L. D., Elsden, R. P., and Seidel, G. E., Jr., 1979, unpublished.

Newcomb, R., 1979, Surgical and nonsurgical transfer of bovine embryos, *Vet. Rec.* **105**: 432–434.

Newcomb, R., 1980, Investigation of factors affecting superovulation and nonsurgical embryo recovery from lactating British Friesian cows, *Vet. Rec.* **106**:48–52.

Newcomb, R., and Rowson, L. E. A., 1975, Conception rate after uterine transfer of cow eggs in relation to synchronization of oestrus and age of eggs, *J. Reprod. Fertil.* **43**:539–541.

Newcomb, R., and Rowson, L. E. A., 1976, Aspects of nonsurgical transfer of bovine eggs, *Proc. 8th Int. Congr. Anim. Reprod. A.I.* **III**:262–265.

Newcomb, R., and Rowson, L. E. A., 1980, Investigation of physiological factors affecting nonsurgical transfer, *Theriogenology* **13**:41–49.

Newcomb, R., Rowson, L. E. A., and Trounson, A. O., 1976, The entry of superovulated eggs into the uterus, in: *Egg Transfer in Cattle* (L. E. A. Rowson, ed.), EEC Publication EUR 5491, Luxembourg, pp. 1–15.

Newcomb, R., Christie, W. B., and Rowson, L. E. A., 1978, Comparison of the fetal survival rate in heifers after the transfer of an embryo surgically to one uterine horn and nonsurgically to the other, *J. Reprod. Fertil.* **52:**395–397.

Newcomb, R., Christie, W. B., and Rowson, L. E. A., 1980, Fetal survival rate after the surgical transfer of two bovine embryos, *J. Reprod. Fertil.* **59:**31–36.

Onuma, H., Hahn, J., and Foote, R. H., 1970, Factors affecting superovulation, fertilization, and recovery of superovulated ova in prepuberal cattle, *J. Reprod. Fertil.* **21:**119–126.

Peters, D. F., Anderson, G. B., BonDurant, R., Cupps, P. T., and Drost, M., 1978, Transfer of cultured bovine embryos, *Theriogenology* **10:**337–342.

Phillippo, M., and Rowson, L. E. A., 1975, Prostaglandins and superovulation in the bovine, *Ann. Biol. Anim. Biochim. Biophys.* **15:**233–240.

Renard, J. P., and Heyman, Y., 1979, Variable development of superovulated bovine embryos between day 6 and day 12, *Ann. Biol. Anim. Biochim. Biophys.* **19:**1589–1598.

Renard, J. P., Heyman, Y., and du Mesnil du Buisson, F., 1977, Unilateral and bilateral cervical transfer of bovine embryos at the blastocyst stage, *Theriogenology* **7:**189–194.

Renard, J. P., Menezo, Y., Saumande, J., and Heyman, Y., 1978, Attempts to predict the viability of cattle embryos produced by superovulation, in: *Control of Reproduction in the Cow* (J. M. Sreenan, ed.), Nijhoff, The Hague, pp. 398–417.

Renard, J. P., Heyman, Y., and Ozil, J. P., 1980a, Importance of gestation losses after nonsurgical transfer of cultured and noncultured bovine blastocysts, *Vet. Rec.* **107:**152–153.

Renard, J. P., Philippon, A., and Menezo, Y., 1980b, *In vitro* uptake of glucose by bovine blastocysts, *J. Reprod. Fertil.* **58:**161–164.

Rowe, R. F., Del Campo, M. R., Critser, J. K., and Ginther, O. J., 1980, Embryo transfer in cattle: Nonsurgical transfer, *Am. J. Vet. Res.* **41:**1024–1028.

Rowson, L. E. A., Moor, R. M., and Lawson, R. A. S., 1969, Fertility following egg transfer in the cow: Effect of method, medium, and synchronization of oestrus, *J. Reprod. Fertil.* **18:**517–523.

Rowson, L. E. A., Lawson, R. A. S., Moor, R. M., and Baker, A. A., 1972, Egg transfer in the cow: Synchronization requirements, *J. Reprod. Fertil.* **28:**427–431.

Saumande, J., 1978, Relationships between ovarian stimulation by PMSG and steroid secretion, in: *Control of Reproduction in the Cow* (J. M. Sreenan, ed.), Nijhoff, The Hague, pp. 169–194.

Scanlon, P. F., 1972, Frequency of transuterine migration of embryos in ewes and cows, *J. Anim. Sci.* **34:**791–794.

Schams, D., Menzer, C., Schallenberger, E., Hoffmann, B., Prokopp, A., Hahn, J., and Hahn, R., 1979, Superovulation beim Rind: Hormonprofile bei Stimulation mit Serum-gonadotropin (PMSG) bzw. hypophysarem FSH, *Zuchthygiene* **14:**11–25.

Schilling, E., Smidt, D., Sacher, B., Petac, D., and El Kaschab, S., 1979, Diagnosis of the viability of early bovine embryos by fluorescence microscopy, *Ann. Biol. Anim. Biochim. Biophys.* **19:**1625–1629.

Schilling, E., Sacher, B., and Smidt, D., 1980, Qualitat von Eiern und Embryonen superovulierter Kuhe, *Zuchthygiene* **15:**30–34.

Schneider, H. J., Jr., Castleberry, R. S., and Griffin, J. L., 1980, Commercial aspects of bovine embryo transfer, *Theriogenology* **13:**73–85.

Seidel, G. E., Jr., 1974, Maintaining the viability of bovine embryos outside the cow, *Proc. Soc. Study Breed. Soundness*, 9 pp.

Seidel, G. E., Jr., 1977, Short-term maintenance and culture of bovine embryos, in: *Embryo*

Transfer in Farm Animals (K. J. Betteridge, ed.), Canada Department of Agriculture, Ottawa, pp. 20–24.

Seidel, G. E., Jr., 1981, Superovulation and embryo transfer in cattle, *Science* **211**:351–358.

Seidel, G. E., Jr., and Seidel, S. M., 1981, The embryo transfer industry, in: *New Technologies in Animal Breeding* (B. G. Brackett, G. E. Seidel, Jr., and S. M. Seidel, eds.), Academic Press, New York, in press.

Seidel, G. E., Jr., Larson, L. L., and Foote, R. H., 1971, Effects of age and gonadotropin treatment on superovulation in the calf, *J. Anim. Sci.* **33**:617–622.

Seidel, G. E., Jr., Bowen, J. M., Homan, N. R., and Okun, N. E., 1975a, Fertility of heifers with sham embryo transfer through the cervix, *Vet. Rec.* **97**:307–308.

Seidel, G. E., Jr., Bowen, R. A., and Nelson, L. D., 1975b, unpublished.

Seidel, G. E., Jr., Elsden, R. P., Nelson, L. D., and Hasler, J. F., 1978, Methods of ovum recovery and factors affecting fertilization of superovulated bovine ova, in: *Control of Reproduction in the Cow* (J. M. Sreenan, ed.), Nijhoff, The Hague, pp. 268–280.

Shea, B. F., 1981, Evaluating the bovine embryo, *Theriogenology* **15**:31–42.

Shea, B. F., Hines, D. J., Lightfoot, D. E., Ollis, G. W., and Olson, S. M., 1976, The transfer of bovine embryos, in: *Egg Transfer in Cattle* (L. E. A. Rowson, ed.), EEC Publication EUR 5491, Luxembourg, pp. 145–152.

Spilman, C. H., Seidel, G. E., Jr., Larson, L. L., Vukman, G. R., and Foote, R. H., 1973, Progesterone, 20β-hydroxypregn-4-en-3-one, and luteinizing hormone levels in superovulated prepuberal and postpuberal cattle, *Biol. Reprod.* **9**:116–124.

Sreenan, J. M., 1976a, Egg transfer in the cow: Effect of site of transfer, *Proc. 8th Int. Congr. Anim. Reprod. A.I.* **III**:269–272.

Sreenan, J. M., 1976b, General discussion, in: *Egg Transfer in Cattle* (L. E. A. Rowson, ed.), EEC Publication EUR 5491, Luxembourg, p. 390.

Sreenan, J. M., 1978, Nonsurgical embryo transfer in the cow, *Theriogenology* **9**:69–83.

Sreenan, J. M., and Beehan, D., 1974, Egg transfer in the cow: Pregnancy rate and egg survival, *J. Reprod. Fertil.* **41**:497–499.

Sreenan, J. M., and Beehan, D., 1976, Methods of induction of superovulation in the cow and transfer results, in: *Egg Transfer in Cattle* (L. E. A. Rowson, ed.), EEC Publication EUR 5491, Luxembourg, pp. 19–34.

Sreenan, J. M., and Gosling, J. P., 1977, The effect of cycle stage and plasma progesterone level on the induction of multiple ovulations in heifers, *J. Reprod. Fertil.* **50**:367–369.

Sreenan, J. M., and McDonagh, T., 1979, Comparison of the embryo survival rate in heifers following artifical insemination, nonsurgical blastocyst transfer or both, *J. Reprod. Fertil.* **56**:281–284.

Sreenan, J. M., Beehan, D., and Mulvehill, P., 1975, Egg transfer in the cow: Factors affecting pregnancy and twinning rates following bilateral transfers, *J. Reprod. Fertil.* **44**:77–85

Sreenan, J. M., Beehan, D., and Gosling, J. P., 1978, Ovarian responses in relation to endocrine status following PMSG stimulation in the cow, in: *Control of Reproduction in the Cow* (J. M. Sreenan, ed.), Nijhoff, The Hague, pp. 144–158.

Tervit, H. R., Elsden, R. P., 1981, Development and viability of frozen-thawed cattle embryos, *Theriogenology* **15**:395–403.

Tervit, H. R., Havik, P. G., and Smith, J. F., 1977, Egg transfer in cattle: Pregnancy rate following transfer to the uterine horn ipsilateral or contralateral to the functional corpus luteum, *Theriogenology* **7**:3–10.

Tervit, H. R., Cooper, M. W., Goold, P. G., and Haszard, G. M., 1980, Nonsurgical embryo transfer in cattle, *Theriogenology* **13**:63–71.

Trounson, A. O., Willadsen, S. M., Rowson, L. E. A., and Newcomb, R., 1976, The storage of cow eggs at room temperature and at low temperatures, *J. Reprod. Fertil.* **46**:173–178.

Trounson, A. O., Rowson, L. E. A., and Willadsen, S. M., 1978a, Nonsurgical transfer of bovine embryos, *Vet. Rec.* **102**:74–75.

Trounson, A. O., Shea, B. F., and Ollis, G. W., and Jacobson, M. E., 1978b, Frozen storage and transfer of bovine embryos, *J. Anim. Sci.* **47**:677–681.

Willett, E. L., Black, W. G., Casida, L. E., Stone, W. H., and Buckner, P. J., 1951, Successful transplantation of a bovine ovum, *Science* **113**:247.

Wilmut, I., and Sales, D. I., 1981, Effect of an asynchronous environment on embryonic development in sheep, *J. Reprod. Fertil.* **61**:179–184.

Wright, J. M., 1981, Nonsurgical embryo transfer in cattle: Embryo–recipient interactions, *Theriogenology* **15**:43–56.

EPILOGUE

LUIGI MASTROIANNI, Jr.

Mammalian fertilization, confined as it is to the nurturing lumen of the oviduct, is inaccessible to sequential scrutiny. Through *in vitro* fertilization, observations can now be carried out at the laboratory bench. The contributions to this volume have provided a comprehensive review of the physiological and biochemical events associated with fertilization, as observed *in vitro*. Techniques developed for *in vitro* fertilization and embryo culture have also received concentrated attention. Developed largely through trial and error over years, these are now established as practical laboratory tools for the evaluation of the events that occur early in reproduction.

A review of mammalian fertilization is an exercise in comparative biology. Techniques have been developed for *in vitro* fertilization in a number of species. Although there are distinct species differences, the process presents many characteristics in common. Observations in marine forms have also proved useful, and a wealth of information has accumulated from the study of nonmammalian species in which extracorporeal fertilization is the rule.

Attention was first focused on the methods used for collection of gametes in laboratory animals. Standard techniques vary significantly among species, particularly in terms of the source of gametes. Ova are recovered from the ovarian follicle, from the surface of the ovary following ovulation, or from the oviduct. Depending on the method of recovery, the oocyte is affected by different conditions in the female reproductive tract prior to collection that may influence the overall process *in vitro*. Spermatozoa are harvested from the epididymis, or ejaculated spermatozoa are used. There are substantial

LUIGI MASTROIANNI, Jr. • Department of Obstetrics and Gynecology, University of Pennsylvania, School of Medicine, Philadelphia, Pennsylvania 19104.

differences between epididymal and ejaculated spermatozoa, the latter having been exposed to the seminal plasma.

Capacitation of the spermatozoa, defined as acquisition of fertilizing ability through exposure to the female reproductive tract, displays marked species variation. Capacitation is associated with changes in both metabolism and sperm surface components. Although changes in sperm metabolism and in the biophysical characteristics of the sperm membrane can be considered separately, both are part of the sperm maturation process that occurs prior to fertilization.

Alterations in the sperm membrane have been extensively investigated. Components that appear on or disappear from the sperm surface have been evaluated, and changes in the sperm membrane prior to fertilization have been explored with immunochemical techniques. There is marked species variation in the time required for capacitation, hamster, human, and mouse spermatozoa completing the process in a much shorter time than rabbit spermatozoa. The likely sequence of events, as summarized by Oliphant and Eng, begins with initial dissociation of acrosomal-stabilizing factor (ASF) from the sperm membrane. ASF is a high-molecular-weight glycoprotein acquired from the seminal plasma. The membrane-altered spermatozoon, under the continued influence of female reproductive tract fluids, then exhibits increased metabolism. This is associated with influx of calcium. The acrosome reaction occurs as the outer acrosomal membrane is dissociated, resulting finally in acquisition of the ability to penetrate the oocyte. The acrosome reaction may be a separate event, and although it may justifiably be considered apart from capacitation, it represents a continuum of ther processes that culminate in fertilizing ability.

The importance of species differences was highlighted further by review of the systems utilized for ovum recovery and transfer in the rhesus monkey. In this spontaneously ovulating mammal, follicular ova have been employed. Their fertilizability is materially affected by the timing of recovery in relation to the anticipated time of ovulation. Development of the follicle has been monitored by determinations of peripheral levels of gonadotropins and estrogens. In the monkey, as in the rabbit and human, recovery of the follicular oocyte from the dominant follicle must be delayed until reinitiation of the meiotic process is well under way and the oocyte is "mature" as suggested by release of the first polar body. The presence of a mature ovulatory follicle is implied when serum estradiol levels exceed 150 pg/ml preceded by an LH surge 12–20 hr earlier. The methods utilized for timing of follicular ovum recovery are still imprecise, and in experiments carried out by Kreitmann, Nixon, and Hodgen, only 39% of recovered ooctyes exhibited evidence of full maturation, in spite of meticulous hormonal monitoring. The fertilizability of some of these ova was established by transferring them to the previously ligated oviduct for *in vivo* fertilization.

Of particular importance are the reported observations on the function of the monkey corpus luteum following ovum extraction. Although the length of the luteal phase is not altered, initial progesterone levels are significantly lower than normal. Aspiration of the follicle may be associated with removal of substantial numbers of progesterone-producing luteinized granulosa cells from the follicle wall. These experiments emphasize the technical difficulties associated with ovum recovery in the primate species.

Numerous culture media have been proposed for the support of *in vitro* fertilization and embryo culture. Media that have been used successfully have been characterized with regard to their ability to provide satisfactory conditions for both fertilization and embryonic development. The culture media employed have certain ingredients in common, but by and large they represent only slight modifications of a basic Krebs–Ringer bicarbonate solution or Tyrode's solution. In general their ionic concentrations mimic those of mammalian blood but differ significantly from those observed in oviductal fluid.

The energy sources commonly employed in tissue culture have been utilized for both *in vitro* fertilization and embryonic development. The osmotic pressures of the numerous media that have been used vary. Protein content appears to be important, as it has been shown that protein not only sustains the viability of spermatozoa in culture but is also important for the acrosome reaction. For regulation of pH, the bicarbonate–CO_2 buffer system yields the best overall results. In experiments in the hamster, a chemically defined sperm motility factor, isolated from follicular fluid, enhances *in vitro* fertilization. Although satisfactory culture media that support mammalian *in vitro* fertilization are provided by simple balanced salt solutions, supplemented with appropriate energy sources and protein, it is likely that the "ideal" environmental conditions have not as yet been defined.

The criteria for successful *in vitro* fertilization must be stringently defined. Inasmuch as parthenogenetic cleavage occurs without benefit of spermatozoa, we must look to evidence other than cleavage to be sure that fertilization has in fact occurred. Disintegration of nonfertilized ova into structures that superficially resemble cells occurs with some frequency. The presence of a slit in the zona does not necessarily indicate sperm penetration, as it can be artifactual. The morphological criteria that support the conclusion that fertilization has occurred prior to cleavage include the presence of components of the fertilizing sperm in the vitellus, two well-developed pronuclei with characteristic nuclei, and two polar bodies, observed in the same specimen. The ultimate criterion for *in vitro* fertilization lies in the successful transfer of the embryo into a recipient with subsequent establishment of pregnancy, followed by delivery of young exhibiting normal karyotypes. Short of this, the effectiveness of *in vitro* fertilization procedures can be assessed only by rigid application of the morphological criteria cited above.

Conditions appropriate for postfertilization culture of the embryo have been reviewed in detail. The criteria utilized for assessing normal *in vitro* development include cleavage that coincides temporally with that observed within the oviduct, viability of the blastomeres after cleavage as determined by fluorescent staining, successful completion of maturation to the blastocyst stage, and most cogently, of course, continued normal development following transfer. Only in two species, mouse and man, have normal offspring been produced without prior exposure to the oviductal environment. This suggests that presently available culture systems do not always adequately duplicate the environment provided *in vivo*.

The stage of development at which the embryo is normally transferred from the oviduct to the uterus varies among species. Development to the morula or early blastocyst stage within the oviduct occurs in the rabbit, while in the rhesus monkey and man the embryo reaches the uterus prior to morula formation. Thus, in the latter species it is not necessary to culture beyond the early stages prior to transfer. Observations on further embryonic development *in vitro* do, however, provide an opportunity to address the basic issues surrounding mammalian differentiation and on that basis there is clear justification for the development of culture systems that will support later development.

The developing embryo constitutes a dynamic structure that demands changing *in vitro* conditions. Apart from the medium itself, a number of variables must be considered in the experimental design, and efforts have been made to duplicate the environment provided by the female reproductive tract. These experiments provide some insight into the conditions that allow development to proceed efficiently *in vitro*. For embryo culture, as for *in vitro* fertilization, a bicarbonate buffer system appears pivotal for the regulation of pH. Temperature control is also critical, and the efficiency with which the zygote and embryo are handled *in vitro* materially influences the end result. The oxygen concentration provided is also critical, and there appear to be some species differences in this regard. Development proceeds most efficiently when the embryo is transferred to another culture medium following fertilization, removing it from the initial sperm-containing medium. It has been suggested that slightly lowered pH and a slightly decreased oxygen concentration favor utilization of nutrients by the zygote and through the early stages.

The conditions for successful *in vitro* embryonic development vary among species. In general, levels of potassium, calcium, magnesium, and phosphate employed are similar to those observed in serum. It would appear that calcium is essential to ensure membrane stability and permeability, especially as development proceeds to the morula stage. A gradual change in requirements for energy substrates has been observed, pyruvate, oxaloacetate, lactate, or phosphoenolpyruvate supporting optimal development. Subsequent to the eight-cell stage, the mouse embryo is capable of developing normally in glucose only. In other species, however, the combination of substrates that support normal development varies substantially. In general, the addition of serum albumin to the culture medium provides stability as development progresses. There are marked species differences in the requirement for either protein or amino acids. In addition to its role in maintaining pH, bicarbonate is important in sustaining *in vitro* blastocyst formation and blastocyst expansion.

Recently, media have been developed that support the *in vitro* development of cow embryos. Success followed the efforts to duplicate the known composition of sheep oviductal fluid. Comparative studies suggest that additional experimental effort is required if we are to establish appropriate conditions for uniformly successful *in vitro* development and to single out the variations in compositions that enhance or retard such development.

After the techniques used in the recovery and conditioning of gametes and the *in vitro* requirements for fertilization and development were examined, consideration was given to issues of sperm–egg interaction. The acrosome reaction occurs prior to penetration. This is associated with loss of the outer acrosomal membrane and release of its enzyme-rich contents. At least 11 acrosomal enzymes have been identified, hyaluronidase and the trypsinlike enzyme, acrosin, receiving concentrated attention. The role of these enzymes is still not completely clear, but the suggestion has been advanced that acrosin is associated with penetration through the zona pellucida. It is established that the acrosome reaction affects sperm–egg fusion, which occurs at the postacrosomal region or equatorial segment. Sperm motility also influences fusion as does calcium, pH, and temperature. Sperm–egg fusion is a necessary step in the penetration process.

Much information on the basic process of fertilization has been derived from studies in nonmammalian systems. Events in common include the acrosome reaction, release of proteinase, and the presence of an extracellular egg coating, the zona pellucida in mammals or the vitelline layer in the sea urchin. There is also sperm–egg specificity. The sea urchin offers the advantage of providing massive numbers of eggs for biochemical study in contrast to the limited numbers available even in such a prolific egg provider as the mouse. That not withstanding, sperm-specific receptor glycoproteins have been isolated from both the mammalian zona pellucida and the marine vitelline layer. A protein, referred to as "bindin," thought to be important in mediating species-specific sperm–egg adhesion, has been isolated from sperm acrosomal granules. A bindin receptor glycoprotein has been identified in the egg vitelline layer.

After the oocyte is penetrated a reaction occurs that blocks entry of additional spermatozoa. Depending on the species, the "block to polyspermy" may occur at the level of the zona pellucida, at the level of the plasma membrane, or both. The changes in the zona associated with this phenomenon have two components. One involves the ability of the zona to react to sperm, and the other is associated with a change in the biophysical characteristics of the zona, referred to as "hardening," defined as increased resistance to dissolution. These are separate events.

The oocyte contains membrane-surrounded cytoplasmic structures, the cortical granules, which are located in greatest number at the periphery of the cell. They produce a serine proteinase that alters the zona receptors to sperm. Cortical granules also produce an ovoperoxidase that may be responsible for zona hardening. Although cortical granules have been implicated in the block to polyspermy, their premature release from eggs in the zona-free state does not inhibit fertilization. The mechanism behind the plasma membrane block is unknown. Recent extensions of earlier observations in marine forms to the mouse have suggested the possibility that there is an electrically mediated block at the level of the plasma membrane.

Sperm binding is associated with the presence of sperm receptors, whose activity is affected adversely by proteolytic enzymes and antizona antibodies. Efforts to isolate zona receptors suggest that they are glycoproteins, and a component with a molecular weight of 83 kd has been implicated. It has been clearly demonstrated that sperm binding to the zona requires calcium.

Supernumerary sperm that may have penetrated the vitellus can be seen in the form of cytoplasmic droplets in the process of being extruded from the vitellus after penetration. This suggests that under some circumstances the oocyte itself is capable of removing extra spermatozoa that have entered. This mechanism, although interesting, is certainly not the principal controller of polyspermy in mammalian systems.

The cortical reaction and its association with the block to polyspermy has been studied extensively in the sea urchin. This system involves both a rapid and a delayed block to polyspermy. Activation of the egg is associated with changes in the fertilization membrane. This is equivalent to the zona hardening observed in mammalian forms. However, clearly identifiable physiological differences between sea urchins and mammals have been observed. In the sea urchin a sperm filament, a product of the acrosome, is extruded prior to penetration.

On contact with the sperm, the sea urchin egg membrane instantaneously exhibits changes in potential from negative to positive. This immediately blocks further sperm fusion and is referred to as the "rapid block to polyspermy." There follows extrusion of the cortical granules, a secretory event that brings about alterations in the vitelline layer. Proteinases are released from the cortical granules that produce a delayed but permanent block to polyspermy at the level of the vitelline layer. These proteolytic enzymes elevate the vitelline layer and remove sperm receptors. Fertilization is also associated with synthesis of hydrogen peroxide, which brings about an ovoperoxidase-induced hardening of the vitelline layer. These events are associated with the so-called "slow block to polyspermy." Peroxidase inhibitors have been used successfully to isolate the fertilization membranes for biochemical analysis. Activation of the egg involves membrane depolarization, a transient increase in levels of intracellular free calcium, triggering of cortical granule release, and finally a sodium-dependent elevation in intracellular pH that turns on protein and DNA synthesis.

Consideration has been given to the chromosomal abnormalities that occur with some frequency in gametes and early embryos. The causal relationship between such genetic defects and deficiencies in the fertilization process or early development can be efficiently explored in mammalian models with extracorporeal techniques. Aneuploidy, abnormality in chromosome number, has been observed with great frequency in human specimens following spontaneous abortion. The defect may have been produced during meiosis, at the time of fertilization, or by nondisjunction during the first mitotic division. Evidence has accumulated, largely in the mouse model, that the incidence of oocyte or embryonic chromosomal abnormalities can be influenced variably by maternal age, radiation, the method used for oocyte maturation, and temperature. In the rabbit but not in the mouse, an increased incidence of aneuploidy is observed following hormonally induced superovulation. Fortunately, chromosomally abnormal human embryos are disposed of by nature with great efficiency, and spontaneous abortion or embryonic resorption are the rule, estimated to occur in over 90% of affected pregnancies.

Techniques have been developed to create mouse embryos that are monosomic or trisomic for any of the 19 different autosomes. Nullisomic spermatozoa, those lacking an autosome, are capable of fertilization, producing monosomic embryos that develop through the blastocyst stage. This experimental model has been most useful in sorting out the influence of specific chromosomes on early development. Mouse systems have also been devised to produce completely identical twins by separating the blastomeres at the two-cell stage. It is then possible to karyotype one of the resulting blastocysts and to carry out metabolic and biochemical studies on the other. These studies open the way for a systematic investigation of both the functional and the molecular consequences of aneuploidy.

In vitro culture systems have been used to explore transfer of fluid and ions during early development. Prior to implantation the blastocyst displays a dramatic increase in volume. This occurs as a result of active transport across the trophectoderm membrane. It is associated with the development of Na^+/K^+ ATPase in the membranes of the blastocyst as well as other developmental changes.

The pig embryo has been used as a model to study alterations in the embryo *in vitro*. There is active transport into the allantoic sac, which is formed from the hindgut, and rapid expansion occurs between Days 18 and 30. Within the embryo there is a series of fluid exchanges. As the embryo matures, exchange across the placental membrane is modulated by hormones. They exert their influence on the external or chorionic layer of the embryo. Ratios of steroid hormones affect transport, and a positive exchange is influenced by a high progesterone/estrogen ratio. Permeability and transport are also affected by prolactin and human placental lactogen. The latter is thought to enhance amino acid availability to the fetus through its effect on placental active-transport processes.

Experimental manipulation of gametes and embryos in cattle has special significance in societal terms. As reviewed by Dr. Seidel, whose final chapter in this volume has brought us full circle, techniques of fertilization and embryo transfer have been used successfully to produce genetically more efficient animals. Ability to understand and control reproduction through *in vitro* techniques has already had a substantial impact on food production.

In this comprehensive consideration of *in vitro* fertilization and embryo culture, initial attention was focused on the technical aspects of gamete recovery and culture. Subsequently, the detailed biochemical and biophysical events associated with fertilization and early development were considered. The use of *in vitro* systems has done much to ferret out the complex sequence of events that occur during early development. The impact of these techniques in the large-animal field is readily appreciated. Their implications, in terms of our ability to develop new and acceptable contraceptive techniques and to provide systems useful in the diagnosis and treatment of human infertility, are equally cogent. There is little doubt that information that has accumulated thus far from *in vitro* fertilization studies and embryo culture in both laboratory and domestic animals has contributed greatly to our understanding of early reproductive processes. In spite of herculean efforts, there are still significant gaps in our knowledge. These clearly justify ongoing emphasis on laboratory experimentation if we are to continue to define systems that will lead to successful clinical applications in the management of human reproduction problems.

INDEX